Young Bok Jung • Sang Hak Lee
Seong Hwan Kim • Jeong-Ku Ha

Treatment of the Cruciate Ligaments Injuries

Using Rectangular or Oval Shape Tunnel

Springer

Young Bok Jung
Hyundae General Hospital
Namyangju-Si, Kyonggi-do, Korea (Republic of)

Sang Hak Lee
School of Medicine
Kyung Hee University
Seoul, Korea (Republic of)

Seong Hwan Kim
Chung-Ang University Hospital
Seoul, Korea (Republic of)

Jeong-Ku Ha
Seoul Jump Orthopedic Clinic
Seoul, Korea (Republic of)

ISBN 978-981-95-9038-4 ISBN 978-981-95-9039-1 (eBook)
https://doi.org/10.1007/978-981-95-9039-1

This Springer imprint is published by the registered company Springer Nature Singapore Pte Ltd.
The registered company address is: 152 Beach Road, #21-01/04 Gateway East, Singapore 189721, Singapore

Foreword

Knee ligament injuries are relatively common and related to sports or daily activities. So, it is imperative that general orthopedic surgeons (not even knee specialists), physiotherapists, and other allied health professionals remain up-to-date on the most current concepts in treatment and management of these injuries. Although there are a lot of evolving concepts for novel methods for treatment of ligament injury in the past decade, and too much information is provided to select it properly, this book will provide an up-to-date and comprehensive approach for managing knee ligament injuries. Young-Bok Jung is an orthopedic surgeon internationally recognized for his expertise in knee surgery and, specifically, PCL and posterolateral corner injury, as the author of more than 100 related scientific articles. He is a Past-President of the Korean Orthopedic Association, the Korean Knee Society, the Korean Arthroscopy Society and the Korean Orhtopaedic Society for Sports Medicine. I hope you really share the author's sound experience and reasonable concept for knee injury management.

Icheon Elijah Hospital
Icheon, Republic of Korea

Ho-Joong Jung

Editor's Preface

The motivation for writing this book is to share with others the knowledge I have gained from my experience and the patients I have operated on, and hopefully to help in the treatment of patients.

Recently, when the anatomy of the cruciate ligament was rediscovered, i.e., the cruciate ligament is not round but flat, in the past, arthroscopic round tunnel was made in cruciate ligament reconstruction, but since the rounded rectangular tunnel technique has been used since last for 7–8 years, I have seen more cases, in side to side difference test using the KT 1000 arthrometer test same as the normal side in and also easier to do in revision ACL, PCL reconstruction, so I decided to write this book to publicize the advantages of using the rounded rectangular dilator and the oval-shaped dilator. We made videos to useful to take over each one's skill to see the arthroscopic surgery of the ligament and meniscus repair technique which will be helpful to the surgeons. Chapter 1. Introduced anatomy of the ACL PCL which is not round but flat. Chapter 2 ACL active conservative Treatment. Chapter 3. Surgical treatment of the ACL injury with ramp lesion , meniscal injuries, round tunnel and using rounded rectangular or oval shape dilator. Chapters 4, 5, and 6 ACL with combined ligament injury Chap. 7 ACL revision surgery, Chap. 8 Rehabilitation after ACL reconstruction Chap. 9 Conservative treatment of the PCL injury Chap. 10 PCL reconstruction Chap. 11 Management PLC injury, Chap. 12 PCL revision reconstruction, Chap. 13 Multiligament injuries, ACL, PCL with combine injuries. I would like to thank Drs. Sang Hak Lee, Sung Hwan Kim, Jeuk Lee, Du-Bin Yang, and Jung-Ku Ha, and I would like to thank Springer, Stephanie Sibin, for accepting my suggestions without question. I would like to thank my teacher, Professor Myung Sang Moon, who recommended me to write the book in English. I would like to thank my wife for her support in writing this book, and I would like to appreciate God's blessings upon me.

Seoul, South Korea Young Bok Jung

Associate Editor's Preface

In the realm of orthopedic surgery, the significance of the knee joint—a complex and critical junction of bones, cartilage, and ligaments—cannot be overstated. Serving as the fulcrum for human mobility, the knee is exposed to a spectrum of injuries and degenerative conditions that challenge both diagnosis and treatment. It is with this focus that we introduce this book, dedicated solely to the intricate world of ligament and meniscus surgery of the knee.

Ligament injuries in the knee are incredibly common, affecting athletes, laborers, and individuals from all walks of life. Whether it's an acute tear of the anterior cruciate ligament (ACL) or chronic laxity of the posterior cruciate ligament (PCL), the implications are significant, affecting not just mobility but also quality of life. Thus, this book aims to serve as an authoritative text covering all aspects of knee ligament surgery—from basic anatomy and biomechanics to cutting-edge surgical techniques and rehabilitation protocols.

The contents of this book are carefully curated to cater to various audiences. For the orthopedic resident, it offers a step-by-step guide to surgical procedures, complete with nuanced tips and pitfalls to avoid. For the seasoned orthopedic surgeon, it provides a comprehensive overview of the latest research and advances in imaging, graft selection, anatomical theories, biomechanical studies, recent surgical techniques, and minimally invasive techniques.

The surgical realm is notably collaborative. Therefore, this book also aims to bridge the gaps between knee specialists, residents, general orthopedic surgeons, physiotherapists, and other healthcare professionals involved in the care of patients with knee ligament injuries. The chapters on surgical technique, postoperative care, and rehabilitation are structured to serve as a guide for a multidisciplinary approach to patient recovery.

Each chapter of this book is penned by experts in the field, ensuring that the information is both current and reliable. Wherever possible, we have supplemented the text with high-quality images, illustrative figures, and video demonstrations to facilitate a deeper understanding of the subject matter.

In closing, this book is not just an academic exercise; it is a commitment to advancing the quality of care for patients plagued by knee sports medicine issues. We owe a debt of gratitude to the surgeons, clinicians, researchers, and medical writers who have contributed to this book, each of whom has enriched the text in their own unique way.

We hope that this work will serve as a cornerstone for anyone looking to expand their knowledge and skills in the ever-specialized field of knee ligament surgery. Thank you for engaging with this text, and we look forward to the contributions that you will make to this vital area of orthopedic medicine.

Your journey through the landscape of knee sports medicine and ligament surgeries of the knee begins here.

We hope that this preface serves its purpose effectively and sets the tone for the in-depth exploration of knee ligament surgery that follows. Thank you for choosing this book as your guide.

Seoul, South Korea Seong Hwan Kim

Acknowledgments

First and foremost, I would like to thank Ms Stephanie Sibin for her efforts and careful corrections and for accepting my application. I also thank Ms Lauren Kim; Drs. NAM, Hyun-Cheul, Lee, Sang-Hak, Kim sung-hwan, Ha, Jeong-Ku; and Dr. Lee, Jeuk, and Yang Du Bin, for help in writing this book.

Contents

Part I

Anatomy of Cruciate Ligaments

Basic Anatomy of the Anterior and Posterior Cruciate Ligaments

1

Abstract

The reconstruction procedure of ACL and PCL is increasing nowadays. The ultimate goal of ligament reconstruction procedure, such as ACL reconstruction or PCL reconstruction, is to restore the normal anatomy and, furthermore, perform satisfying outcome of the patient. Therefore, the knowledge about basic anatomy of ACL and PCL is essential. This chapter will provide you a brief but essential anatomy, which is necessary for performing ACL or PCL reconstruction.

Keywords

ACL · PCL anatomy

1.1 Anatomy of ACL

ACL is a band of connective tissue that originates at the medial side of the lateral femoral condyle and runs an oblique course to the insertion at the medial tibial eminence. It is an intra-articular, extra-synovial ligament because it is enveloped in the synovial membrane, which protects the ligament from the synovial fluid. The width of the ACL ranges from 7 ~ 12 mm, fans out toward its insertion at the tibia, with the narrowest in the mid-substance area of the ACL. Its primary role is a restraint to anterior tibial translation and plays a secondary role, which is a restraint to internal rotation of the knee.

There was a debate about the size and location of the femoral attachment of the ACL until the early 2000s. Several cadaveric studies were performed to find out the accurate anatomy of the ACL. Mochizuki et al. described the ACL femoral attachment, differentiating the main attachment of the mid-substance ACL fibers and the attachment of the thin fibrous tissue, which is termed "fan-like extension fibers". The study revealed static and dynamic observation of the fan-like extension fibers. The fan-like extension fibers, which extends from the mid-substance fibers, came into contact with the margin of articular cartilage of the posterior condyle, showing no change of its attachment location during the range of motion of the knee, compared to those of the mid-substance ACL fibers, which curved anteriorly when the knee was flexed.

The cutline along the valley of attachment of the fold was also evaluated, showing significantly smaller area of attachment of the mid-substance fiber compared to that of attachment of the fan-like extension fiber.

The resected area (Mochizuki et al 2014).

Smigielski et al. also found out that the ACL formed a flat ribbon-like ligament from its femoral insertion to mid-substance from his cadaveric study, showing continuity with the posterior femoral cortex (Fig. 1.1).

Y. B. Jung et al., *Treatment of the Cruciate Ligaments Injuries*,
https://doi.org/10.1007/978-981-95-9039-1_1

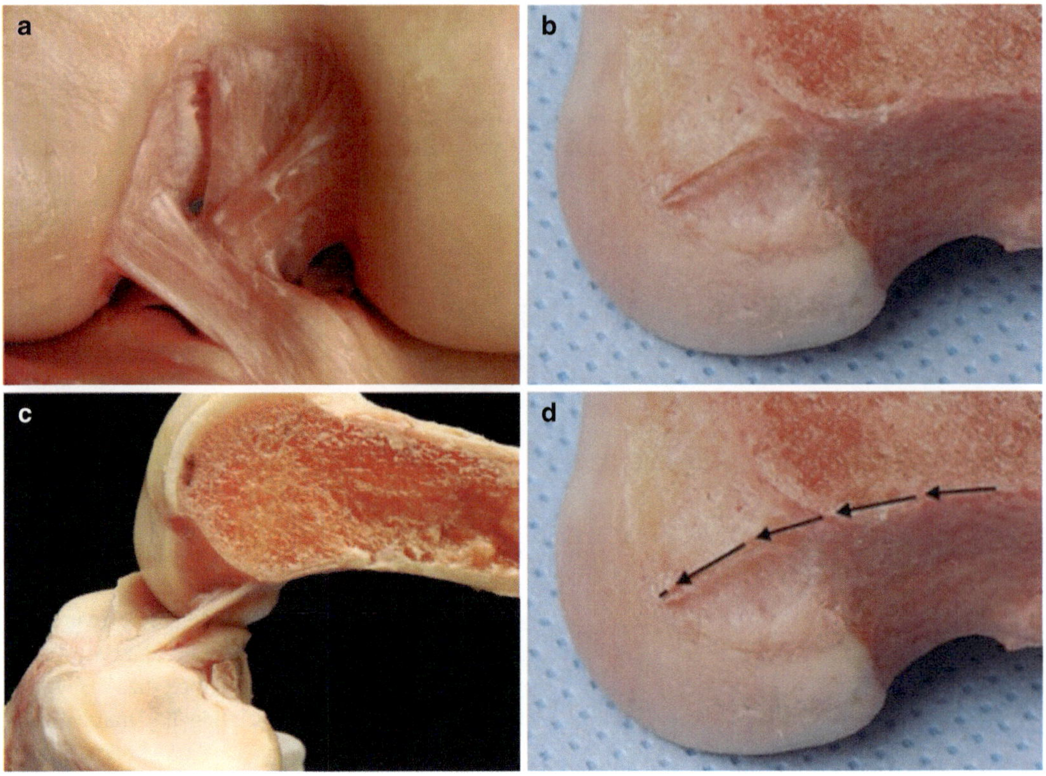

Fig. 1.1 (**a**) ACL shape is flat, not round. (**b–d**) Ribbon shape (flat) ACL fiber showing continuity with the posterior femoral cortex (Smigielski et al. 2015)

A study aimed to investigate the tibial insertion site of the ACL was also performed. Siebold et al. revealed that the "direct" "C"-shaped tibial insertion runs from along the medial tibial spine to the anterior aspect of the lateral meniscus, forming a "raindrop-like" ring structure with outer fibers of the anterior and posterior horn of the lateral meniscus. The indirect fibers extended from the direct fibers fan out anteriorly, forming a "duckfoot"-like footprint with the direct fiber footprint.

1.2 Anatomy of PCL

PCL is a band of connective tissue, which originates at the lateral side of the medial femoral condyle and runs an oblique course to the insertion at the depression just inferior to the joint line, between the two tibial plateaus, posterior to the tibial spine. It is an intra-articular, extra-synovial ligament because it is enveloped in the synovial membrane, which protects the ligament from the synovial fluid. The width of PCL ranges from 10 ~ 15 mm. It consists of two functional bundles, which are the anterolateral (AL) and posteromedial (PM) bundles.

It's primary role is a restraint to posterior tibial translation at all flexion angles. It also has a role in restraining tibial rotation. In the past, the anterolateral bundle and posteromedial bundle were believed to have independent functions, but recent studies revealed that both bundles play a role in restraining posterior tibial translation at all flexion of the knees.

The femoral attachment of PCL has a wide variation in shape and size. Several landmarks are used to identify the anterolateral bundle and the posteromedial bundle. The medial intercondylar ridge defines the proximal end of the insertion of the PCL, while the medial bifurcate ridge separates the footprints of two bundles, and while

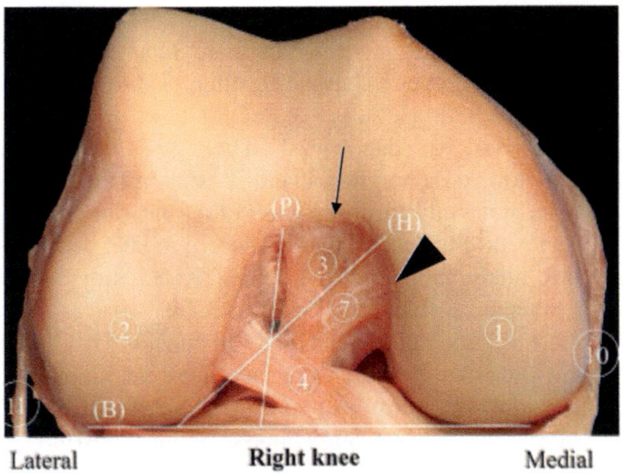

Fig. 1.2 The anterior view of the knee joint showing PCL (arrow) and the ligament of Humphrey (arrowhead). (Tomohiro et al. 2017)

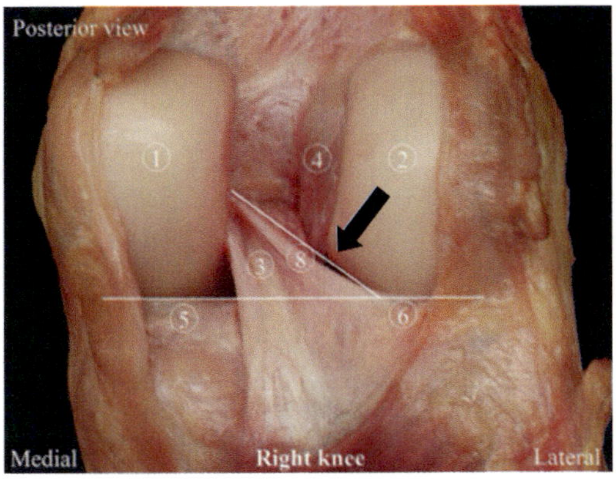

Fig. 1.3 (a) Posterior view of the right knee showing the ligament of Wrisberg (black arrow). (Tomohiro et al. 2017)

knee is flexed, the slope of each bundle changes, differentiating the plane of each bundle.

The area of the femoral footprint of the anterolateral bundle is slightly larger than the posteromedial bundle (55% vs 45%), while the cross-sectional area of the anterolateral bundle itself was significantly larger than that of the posteromedial bundle, and this explains why the anterolateral bundle is a major contributor to PCL strength. The distance between the center of each bundle's footprint is approximately 12 mm, and the distance between the distal margin of each footprint and the notch articular cartilage was 1 ~ 2 mm and 5 ~ 6 mm.

The tibial attachment of PCL is rather consistent in shape and size compared to the femoral attachment. The tibial insertion of PCL, which is the PCL fossa, has a trapezoidal shape and becomes wider inferiorly. The anterolateral bundle attaches at the superolateral aspect of the footprint, while the posteromedial bundle attaches at the inferomedial portion.

Johannsen et al. performed a cadaveric study, analyzing the relationship between PCL and several landmarks of the knee joint. He found out that the lateral meniscus posterior root center was about 12.7 mm medial to the most anterior edge of the PCL tibial footprint, while the medial meniscus posterior root attachment center was about 8.2 mm anteromedial from the PCL tibial footprint.

As our goal is to achieve good outcomes after PCL reconstruction, understanding not only the anatomy of the PCL but also the anatomy of the ligaments of Humphrey and Wrisberg is also critical. These meniscofemoral ligaments are named based on their location in relation to the PCL, which is the anterior meniscofemoral ligament, which is the ligament of Humphrey, and the posterior meniscofemoral ligament, which is the ligament of Wrisberg.

The ligament of Humphrey runs obliquely to the medial intercondylar notch, showing approximately 8.9 mm in width and 2.2 mm thick at the area of femoral insertion. Due to its relatively wide and robust appearance, there is a possibility of misidentification as a posteromedial bundle of the PCL (Fig. 1.2).

The ligament of Wrisberg is thinner than the ligament of Humphrey and has an anatomical variability, which makes the anatomy of the PCL more ambiguous. In some cases, a thin oblique superficial ligament covering the posterior site of the PCL was observed attached to the tibia more laterally than the PCL. It was found in the knees that had no ligament of Wrisberg and was named the "tibiofemoral" ligament. It is obviously different from Wrisberg's ligament but can be considered a subtype of Wrisberg's ligament functionally (Fig. 1.3).

Although a wide variation exists, a typical relationship exists among ligaments' bony attachment sites.

Further Reading

1. Zantop T, Petersen W, Freddie HF. Anatomy of the anterior cruciate ligament. Oper Tech Orthop. 2005;15:20–8.
2. Forsythe B, Harner C, Martins CAQ, Shen W, Lopes OV Jr, Freddie HF. Topography of the femoral attachment of the posterior cruciate ligament. JBJS. 2009;90–A:249–55.
3. Mochizuki T, Fujishiro H, Nimura A, Kanukrauh PM, Yasuda K, Muneta T, Akita K. Anatomic and histologic analysis of the mid-substance and fan-like extension fibers of the anterior cruciate ligament during knee motion, with special reference to the femoral attachment. Knee Surg Sports Traumatol Arthrosc. 2014;22(2):336–44.
4. Shearn JT, Grood ES, Noyes FR, Levy MS. One- and two-strand posterior cruciate ligament reconstructions: cyclic fatigue testing. J Orthop Res. 2015;23:958–63.
5. Smigielski R, Zdanowicz U, Drwiega M, Ciszek B, Ciszkowska-Lyson B, Siebold R. Ribbon like appearance of the midsubstance fibers of the anterior cruciate ligament close to its femoral insertion site: a cadaveric study including 111 knees. Knee Surg Sports Traumatol Arthrosc. 2015;23:3143–50.
6. Kato T, Smigielski R, Ge Y, Zdanowicz U, Ciszek B, Ochi M. Posterior cruciate ligament is twisted and flat structure: new prospective on anatomical morphology. Knee Surg Sports Traumatol Arthrosc. 2018;26(1):31–9.

Part II

Treatment of Anterior Cruciate Ligament (ACL) Injury

2 Active Conservative (Nonsurgical) Treatment of Acute ACL Injury

Abstract

The treatment of an anterior cruciate ligament injury requires either conservative or surgical treatment, depending on the extent of the injury, the degree of damage to the cruciate ligament, and the stage of injury. Active conservative treatment involves immobilizing the knee in a long-leg or cylindrical cast at 10–20° of flexion for 2–3 weeks, followed by wearing an ACL brace for 4–6 weeks. This approach is suitable for young, active patients who are highly cooperative. If the ACL is not severely damaged and anterior instability is isolated, the injury is acute with Lachman grade 1 instability (a 2–5 mm difference side-to-side). During cast immobilization, swelling subsides. Then, inside the cast, the patient's tiny leg movements will happen, and the cast will need to be changed, usually weekly. The doctor should also recommend that the patient do QSE and SLR exercises to reduce thigh muscle atrophy.

Another method is muscle-strengthening exercises and rehabilitation treatment to help the patient return to their pre-injury state quickly, improving knee joint function and building up functional activity after an ACL injury.

Keywords

Acute · ACL · Active conservative treatment Long-leg cast

2.1 Principles of Treatment of Anterior Cruciate Ligament

As the number of sports populations increases, especially soccer, basketball, etc., the frequency of anterior cruciate ligament (ACL) injury is increasing due to the increase in other accidents. The number of ACL reconstructions is increasing every year. According to US statistics, more than 200,000 cases of ACL injury occur each year, and more than 100,000 cases of ACL reconstruction have been performed recently. However, there is still a reported failure rate of more than 10–20%. Anterior cruciate ligament reconstruction is one of the most frequently performed surgical procedures in orthopedics. In other recent reports, failure rates for primary reconstructions range from 0.7% to 8%.

Treatment of the ACL injuries includes

1. Conservative treatment:
   A. Active conservative treatment, i.e., immobilization with a long-leg cast or cylinder cast immobilization to improve the natural

Y. B. Jung et al., *Treatment of the Cruciate Ligaments Injuries*,
https://doi.org/10.1007/978-981-95-9039-1_2

healing force of the injured ACL and then to reduce anterior instability.

B. The other method, muscle-strengthening exercise and rehabilitation treatment for rapid return to the pre-injury state to improve knee joint function and build up functional activity, after ACL injury.

There are two different ways of nonsurgical treatment of ACL injury. In other words, if the anterior cruciate ligament is not severely damaged, and the anterior instability is isolated acute ACL injury with Lachman grade 1 instability (2–5 mm). And the synovium covering the ACL is relatively well preserved, even if the synovial fluid does not interfere with the healing of the injured ACL. In the MRI, the indication for active conservative treatment is almost completely torn; the shape of the entire ACL is maintained in a straight line, not completely distorted, and the sheath of the ACL is also relatively well preserved. In this case, we can do the active conservative treatment. The active conservative treatment induces natural healing of the ACL rupture by a long-leg cast immobilization (or cylinder cast) at 10–20 degree flexion of the knee for 3–6 weeks, and then take an ACL brace for 6 weeks while continuing thigh muscle-strengthening exercises from the beginning, partial weight-bearing with crutches for 6 weeks, in well cooperative, young active patients. The other conservative treatment method, muscle-strengthening exercise and rehabilitation treatment for rapid return to the pre-injury state, for improving knee joint function and building up functional activity, after anterior cruciate ligament injury. In our clinical experiences, in about ten cases treated with an active conservative method, such as long-leg plaster immobilization for 3–6 weeks and then an ACL brace for 6 weeks, their knee stability was improved, as shown by a negative Lachman test and a negative pivot shift test in most of them. In two of the active conservative-treated cases (ten cases), we had done ACL reconstruction with the remnant-preserve technique, which was to get excellent results. According to Ahn et al., 48 patients were observed for 21 months after conservative treatment; 41 cases (87%) were negative for the Lachman test, and in 36 cases (76%), the pivot shift test was negative, and the IKDC score was 91 and KT 2000 arthrometer side-to-side difference was 2.85 mm.

2.2 Cases of ACL Conservative Treatments

Case 1: ACL Conservative Treatment for Your Athlete

A 14-year-old male patient with no history of knee problems presented to the outpatient department complaining of pain in his left knee. He injured his left knee 2 weeks ago while playing football at school. There were no specific findings on the plain radiograph taken immediately after the injury, and the Lachman test grade 1 was checked on physical examination (Fig. 2.1).

He underwent conservative treatment with an ACL brace. Six weeks after the injury, the Lachmann test was negative, and he achieved a range of motion of 0–90° (Fig. 2.2).

Based on the KT-2000 arthrometer maximum manual test (MMT), 8.5 mm right and 8.5 mm left were checked (Fig. 2.3).

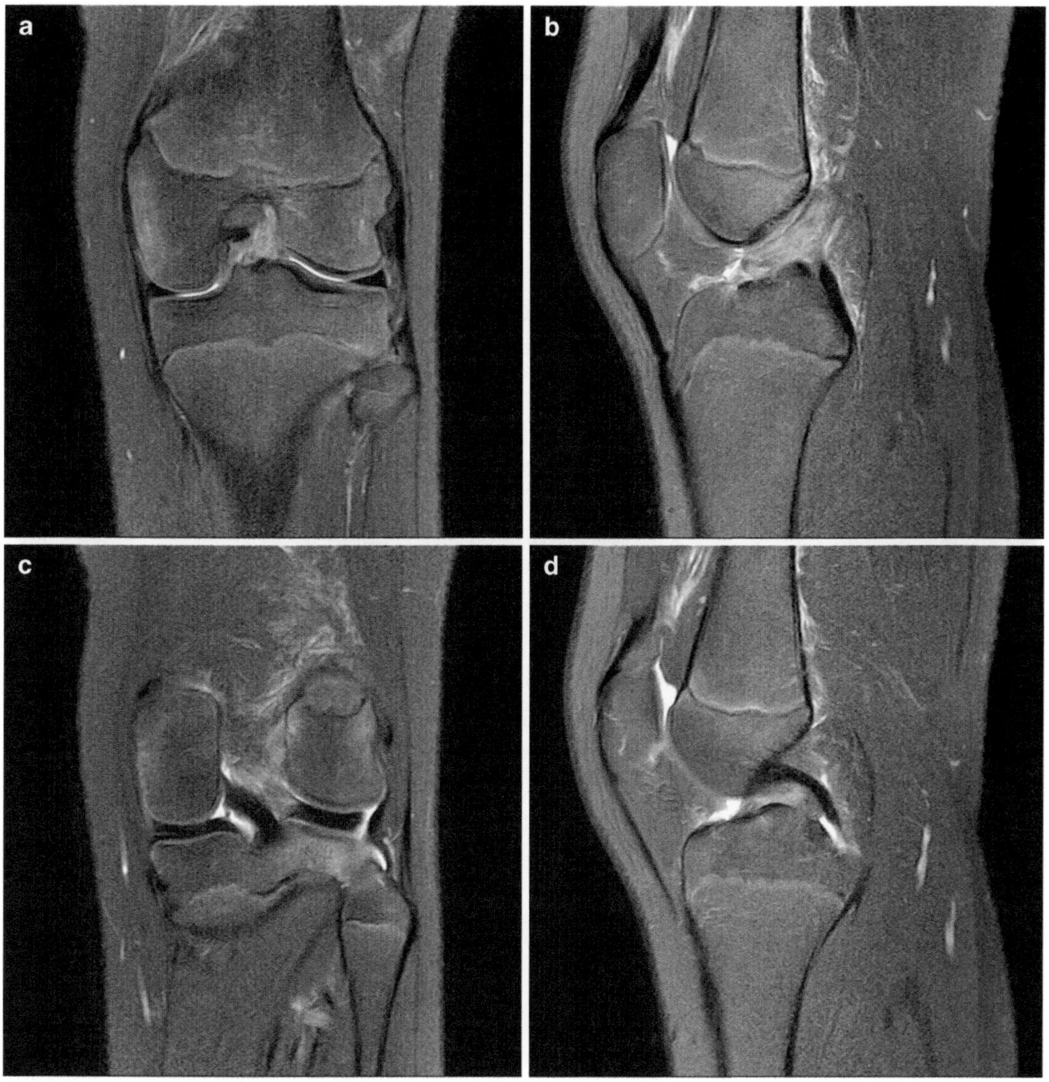

Fig. 2.1 The ACL is injured at mid-substance (**a, b**), but its continuity and shape are relatively well preserved. (**a–d**) The other ligament injury is not visible on the MRI

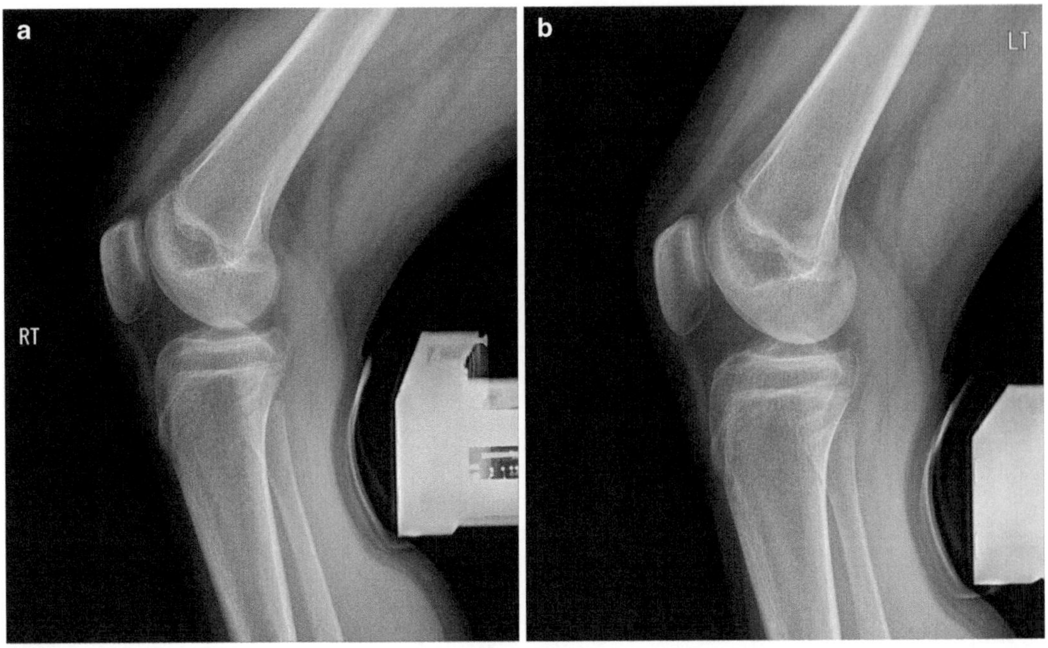

Fig. 2.2 (**a, b**) Seven months after active conservative treatment. In a stress view, there is no definite instability

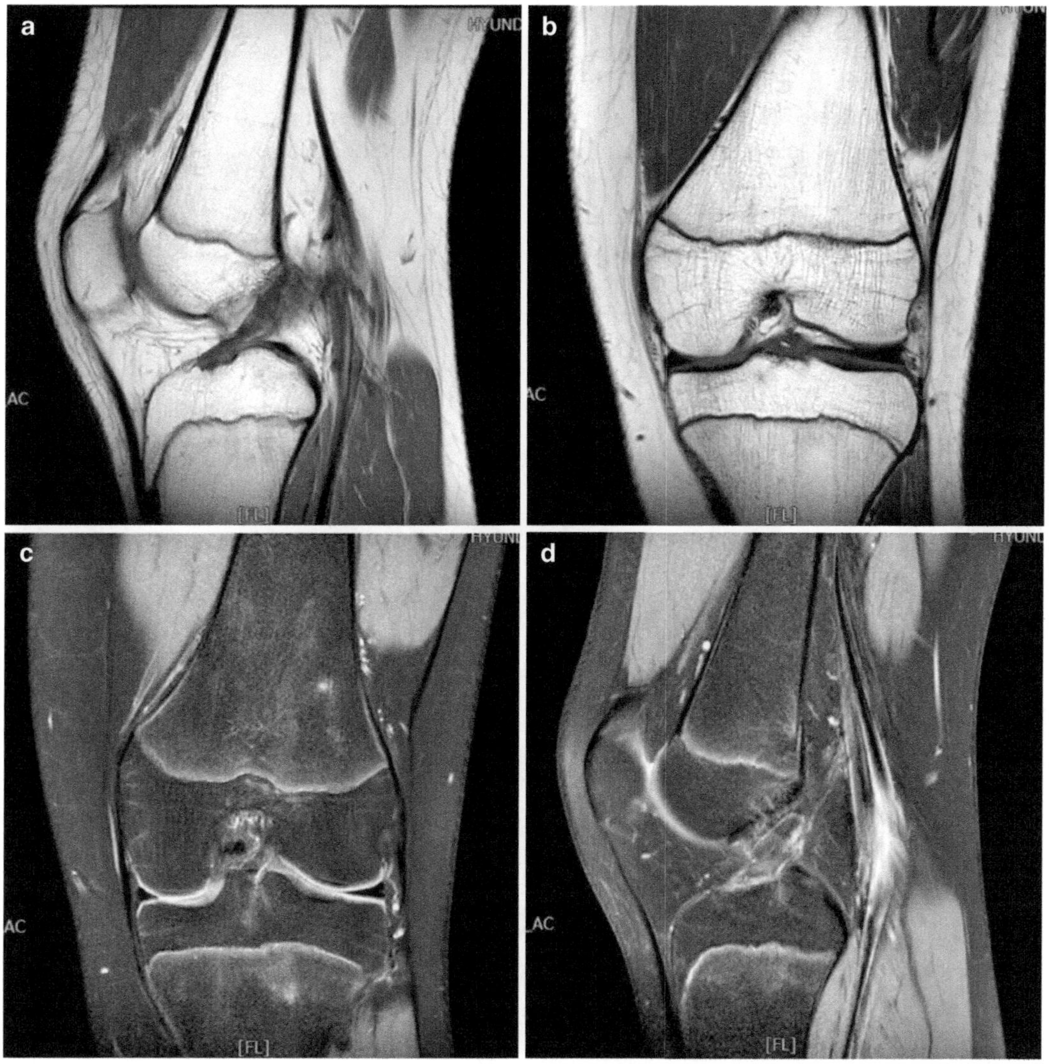

Fig. 2.3 (**a**, **b**) 7 months after active conservative treatment. ACL shows good continuity at T1. (**c, d**) 7 months after active conservative treatment. ACL shows good continuity at the T2 MRI film

Case 2: ACL Conservative Treatment for Middle-Aged Patient

A 48-year-old male patient with no history of knee problems presented to the outpatient clinic complaining of pain in his right knee. He injured his right knee after a fall. There were no specific findings on the plain radiograph taken immediately after the injury, and effusion grade 2, Lachman test grade 2, and KT-2000 arthrometer maximum manual test (MMT) of 10 mm right and 8 mm left were checked (Figs. 2.4 and 2.5).

He was then treated conservatively with a long-leg cast for 2 weeks and then changed to an ACL brace with a 90° block for 4 weeks. Final outpatient follow-up (10 weeks after injury) showed that the Lachman test was negative, with no effusion, and no pain. After 5 years, we followed up with him by telephone and found no specific symptoms, indicating a good outcome.

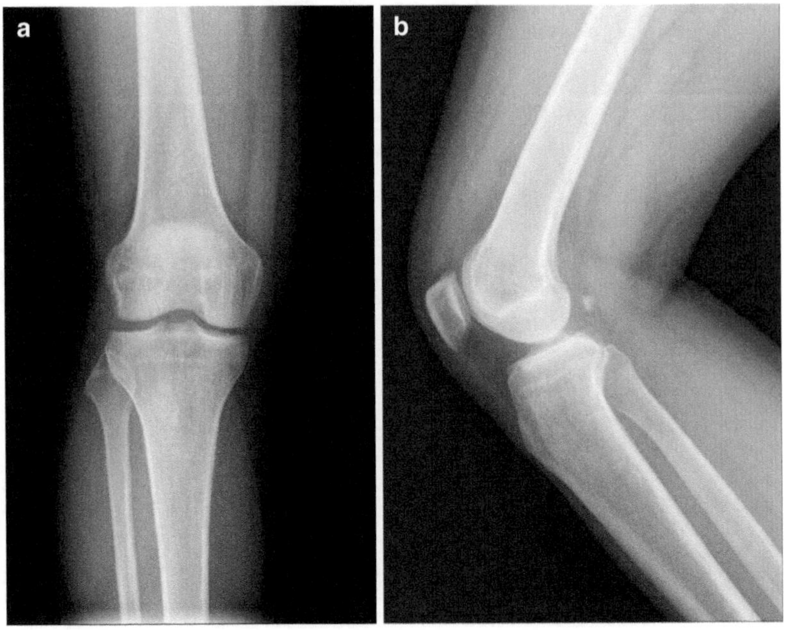

Fig. 2.4 (**a, b**) There is no specific abnormal finding on the plain radiograph

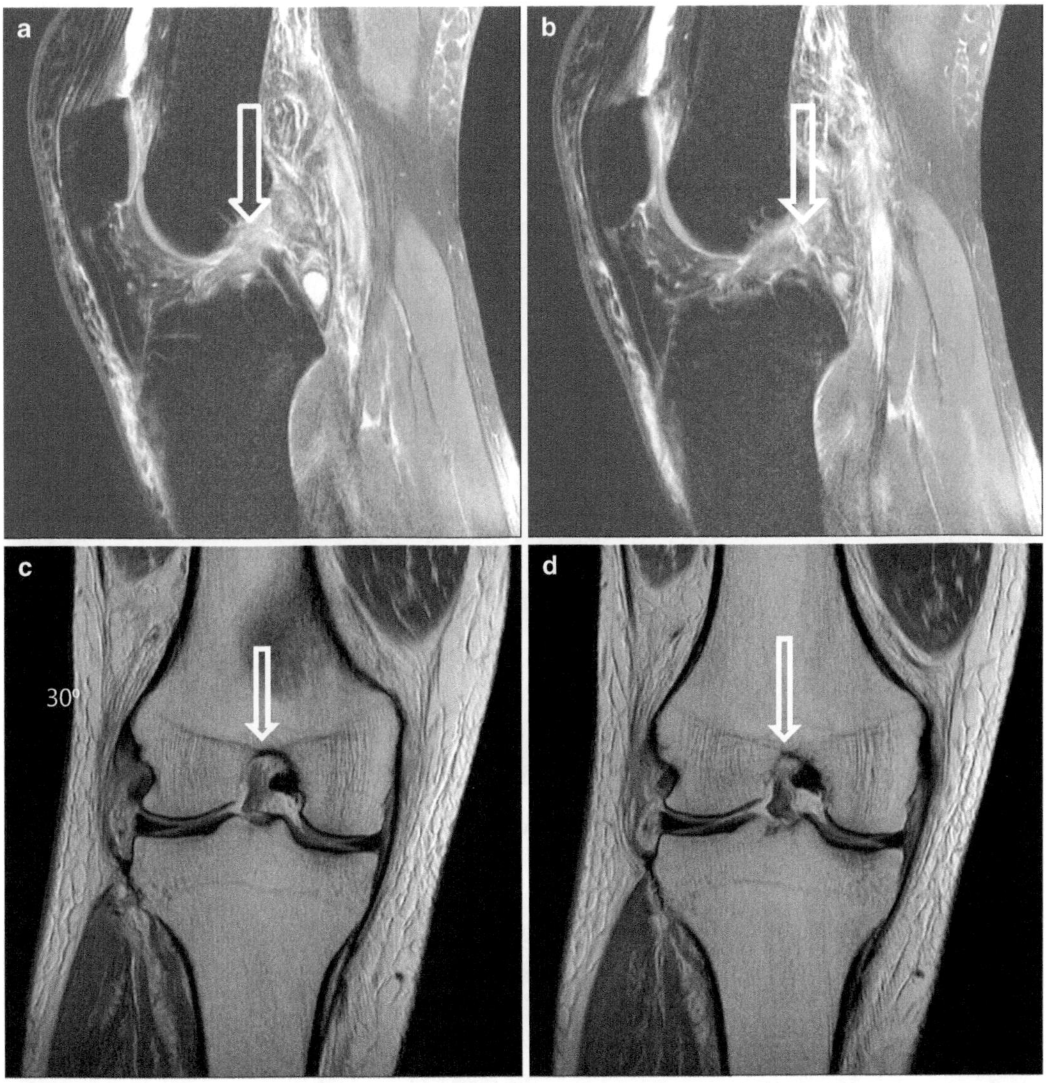

Fig. 2.5 (**a, b**) ACL discontinuity at proximal substance rupture, but ACL shape is straight and well preserved, and synovial tissue is covered and not completely disrupted (**a–d**)

Case 3: ACL Conservative Treatment

A 23-year-old male patient complained of right knee pain. He was injured while playing basketball 4 days ago. His right knee was hit directly on the anteromedial side. There were no specific findings on the X-ray taken immediately after the injury, and Lachman test grade 1, varus and valgus stress test negative, and posterior drawer test negative were confirmed on physical examination (Figs. 2.6, 2.7, 2.8, and 2.9).

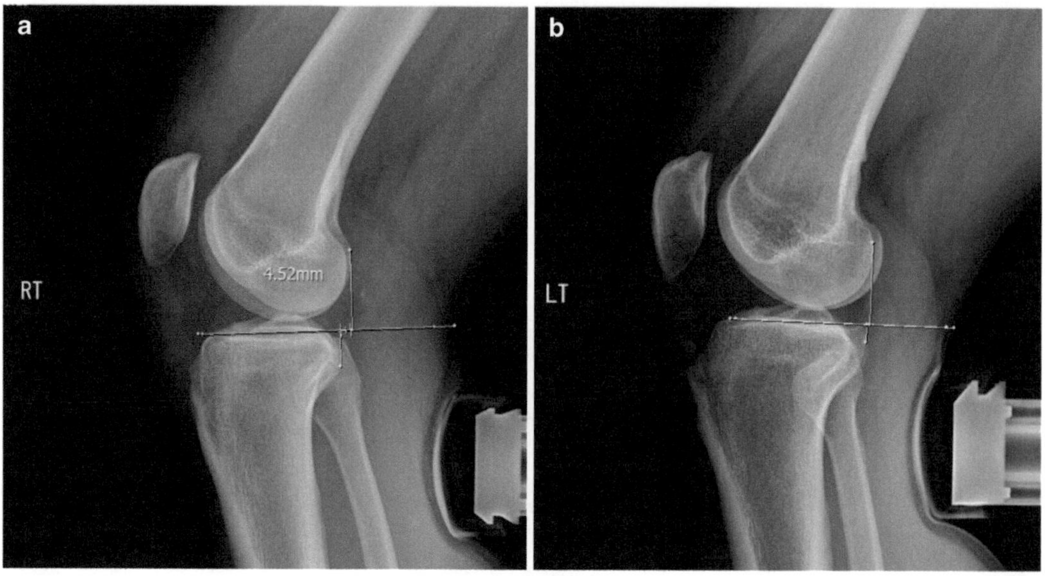

Fig. 2.6 (**a**, **b**) A 4.5 mm side-to-side difference was checked compared to the unaffected side in the pull stress test imaging

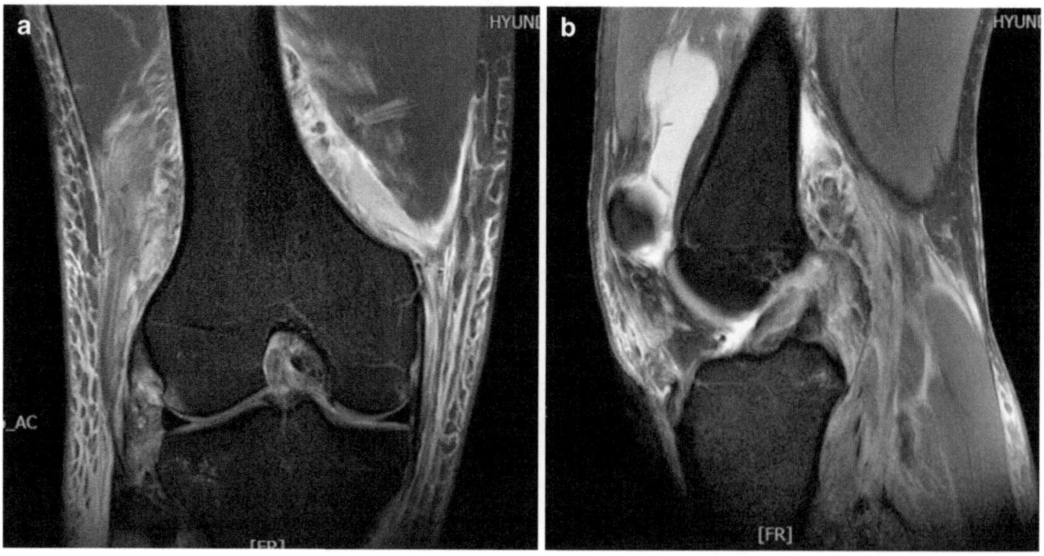

Fig. 2.7 (**a**, **b**) Four days after injury. MRI shows a proximal ACL tear; the shape of the ACL is relatively straight and well-preserved in the MRI image

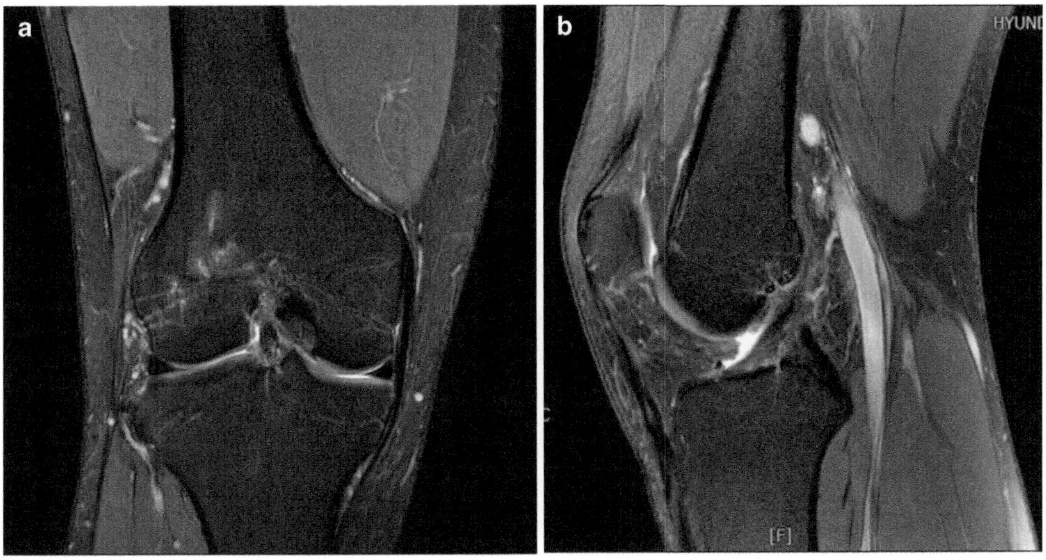

Fig. 2.8 (**a, b**) 17 months after active conservative treatment. MRI: ACL continuity looks good compared to MRI 4 days after trauma. Lachman test is negative, and pivot shift test is negative on physical examination

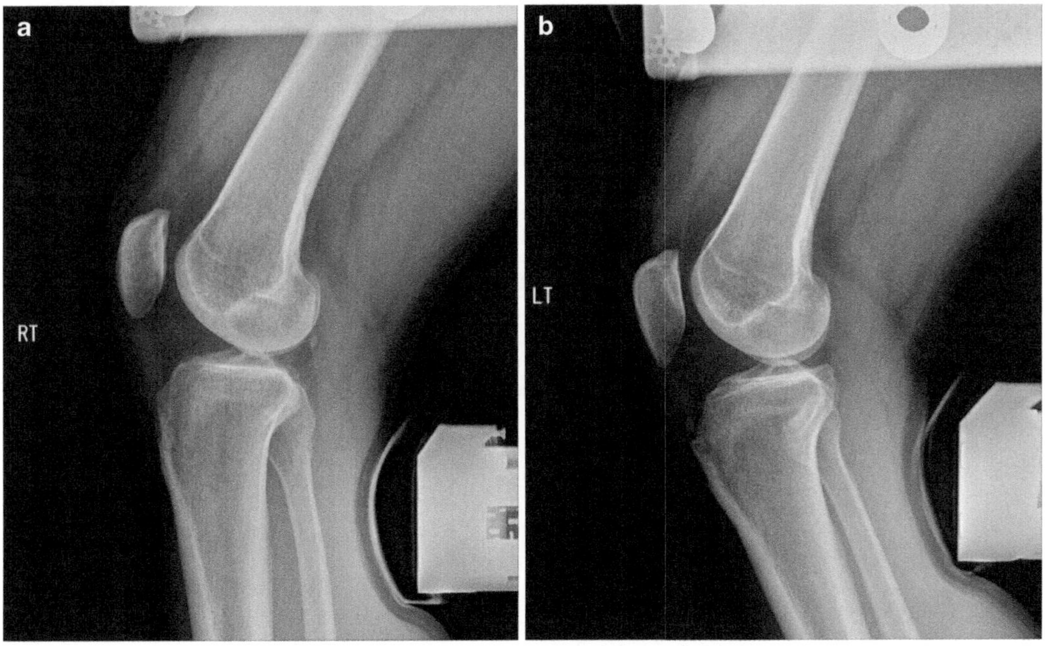

Fig. 2.9 (**a, b**) 52 months after active ACL conservative treatment. KT1000 arthrometer maximum manual test (MMT); 10 mm right, 8–9 mm left and Lachman test is negative, and pivot shift test is negative on physical examination. He is able to perform normal activities

References

1. Jung YB, Tae SK, Yum JK, JS KIM. Conservative (active) treatment for injured anterior cruciate ligament- two cases report-the Korean. J Arthroscopy. 1997;1(1):112–5.
2. Harris KP, Driban JB, Sitler MR, Cattano NM, Balasubramanian E, Hootman JM. Tibiofemoral osteoarthritis after surgical or nonsurgical treatment of anterior cruciate ligament rupture: a systematic review. J Athl Train. 2017;52:507–17.
3. Monk AP, Davies LJ, Hopewell S, Harris K, Beard DJ, Price AJ. Surgical versus conservative interventions for treating anterior cruciate ligament injuries. Cochrane Database Syst Rev. 2016;4:CD011166.
4. Tsoukas D, Fotopoulos V, Basdekis G, Makridis KG. No difference in osteoarthritis after surgical and non-surgical treatment of ACL-injured knees after 10 years. Knee Surg Sports Traumatol Arthrosc. 2016;24:2953–9.
5. Ardern CL, Sonesson S, Forssblad M, Kvist J. Comparison of patient-reported outcomes among those who chose ACL reconstruction or non-surgical treatment. Scand J Med Sci Sports. 2017;27:535–44.
6. Ahan JW, Lee SH. Conservative treatment of anterior cruciate ligament injury. Adv. Knee Arthroscopy. 2009;179

Surgical Treatment of the ACL Injury

3

Abstract

It is difficult to diagnose an acute anterior cruciate ligament (ACL) injury through physical examination because patients cannot relax their muscles due to pain. Patients with an acute ACL injury are examined by comparing the affected side with the uninjured side. The Lachman and pivot shift tests are positive with full muscle relaxation. Stress film using a KT 1000 or 2000 arthrometer shows a difference of more than 3–5 mm between the knees of patients with an acute ACL injury (the knee ROM is nearly within the normal range, and the swelling has subsided). It usually takes 2–3 weeks for the swelling to subside and for a nearly full range of motion (ROM) to be achieved. If ACL surgery is performed too early, arthrofibrosis will occur, and the knee joint will become stiff. However, if there is a locked meniscus bucket handle tear or knee dislocation or subluxation, surgery should be performed as early as possible for reduction. When we perform ACL remnant preservation and wrap over the graft, healing of the reconstructed ACL graft, especially synovialisation, will be much better (Figs 3.36 and 3.37).

According to Nakase et al., the rounded rectangular femoral tunnel ACL reconstruction (RFTR) group had a larger femoral tunnel area than the anatomic single-bundle ACL reconstruction (ASBR) group (average area: 53.1 ± 4.0 mm² vs. 46.1 ± 7.0 mm², $P < 0.01$). The RFTR group had better anteroposterior stability and higher Lysholm scores than the ASBR group (average side-to-side difference for anterior tibial translation, 0.6 ± 0.8 mm vs. 1.6 ± 1.4 mm; $P < 0.01$; average Lysholm score, 98.5 ± 2.1 vs. 97.5 ± 3.5; $P < 0.01$). There were significant differences in rotational laxity between the groups (negative pivot shift, 94.3% vs. 92.3%; $P < 0.01$). No significant difference was noted in the IKDC subjective score between the two groups. The surgeon should carefully check for combined injuries, such as posteromedial or posterolateral instability (PLRI) and meniscal injury. Neglecting PLRI and other combined injuries will result in failure of the ACL reconstruction.

Keywords

ACL · Arthrofibrosis · Rounded rectangular tunnel · PLRI. Posteromedial

3.1 Treatment of the Acute ACL Injury

In the case of acute ACL, it is difficult to diagnose by physical examination because the patient cannot relax his or her muscles due to pain.

Supplementary Information The online version contains supplementary material available at https://doi.org/10.1007/978-981-95-9039-1_3.

Y. B. Jung et al., *Treatment of the Cruciate Ligaments Injuries*,
https://doi.org/10.1007/978-981-95-9039-1_3

3.2 Surgical Indication of ACL Injury

1. A patient with an acute ACL injury is examined by comparing both sides; Lachman test and pivot shift test are positive, with full muscle relaxation. In the KT 1000 or 2000 arthrometer, stress film shows more than 3–5 mm differences between both knees (Figs. 3.29a, b and 3.32a, b). The knee ROM is nearly within the normal range and has subsided swelling. The time of surgery, usually 2–3 weeks, takes to subside swelling to get nearly full ROM. If ACL surgery is done too early, arthrofibrosis will occur, and knee joint stiffness will result. Exceptionally, if the meniscus bucket handle tear is in a locking state (Fig 3.41a), knee dislocation or subluxation status should be addressed as early as possible for the reduction.
2. Chronic ACL Injury

   Young patients, even old patients, who have no severe cartilage degenerative change (under KL grade 1–2) and whose knee joint alignment is good. Activity is good for the patient.

   Lachman test, definite positive and Pivot shift test; definite positive, giving way history.

   ACL reconstruction should be done; otherwise, OA change will occur earlier.
3. ACL with a combined injury, such as posteromedial (Fig. 3.31) or posterolateral instability (Figs. 3.29 and 3.30)

3.3 Surgical Technique: Using a Rounded Rectangular Dilator

The four-stranded autogenous hamstring tendons, including semitendinosus and gracilis tendons, are harvested with an autogenous hamstring tendon diameter of less than 8 mm; the tibialis allograft is used as a hybrid graft technique to increase the diameter of the graft to 9–11 mm. Whenever possible, the remnant preservation or pullout suture techniques during ACL reconstruction are performed according to the remnant tissue morphologies (Video 3.1). When we do ACL remnant preservation and pullout suture over the graft, the reconstructed ACL graft healing, especially synovialization, will be much better (Figs. 3.36 and 3.37). The ACL graft was healing beautifully; it looked like ligamentum mucosa-like tissue was seen (Fig. 3.37). Following systematic arthroscopic examination, single-bundle anatomic ACL reconstruction is performed through the low anteromedial (AM) portal. The establishment of the femoral tunnel starts at 90* of knee flexion to ensure close proximity to the anatomical position. The guide pin is first located, then finalized at nearly 120* flexion knee position through the low AM portal, with gradual flexion from the 90* knee position under arthroscopic visualization. At first marking point (guide pin starting point with awl or electrocautery) and then arthroscope (sheath and scope) change through lower AM portal to confirm correct position or not, to see intercondylar ridge and posterior femoral cortical line, which is as such, a linear ACL femoral origin arising in continuity with the posterior femoral cortex (Smigielsky et al. 2015. KSSTA) (Figs. 3.1a, b and 3.6a, b). The ACL femoral attachment is centered on and spreads posterior to the extended line of the posterior femoral cortex (Fig. 3.34a) (Amis and Jacob, KSSTA 1998).

The guide pin is placed at the 9- and 10-o'clock position for the right knee and the 2- and 3-o'clock position for the left knee. During the establishment of the rectangular femoral tunnel, the direction of the long axis of the rectangular dilator is aligned parallel to the femoral footprint of the ACL (Fig. 3.2). Because it is sometimes difficult to visualize the entire femoral footprint of the ACL in a nearly full-flexion knee position(120°), especially with the remnant preservation technique, the cartilage upper margin of the posterior femoral condyle could be used as a good alternative anatomical landmark for the rectangular femoral tunnel (Fig. 3.3). Using a 6 mm(small women) or 7 mm offset guide is put on the just above posterior femoral condylar articular upper margin, which is a good landmark to get ACL femoral tunnel starting point. With

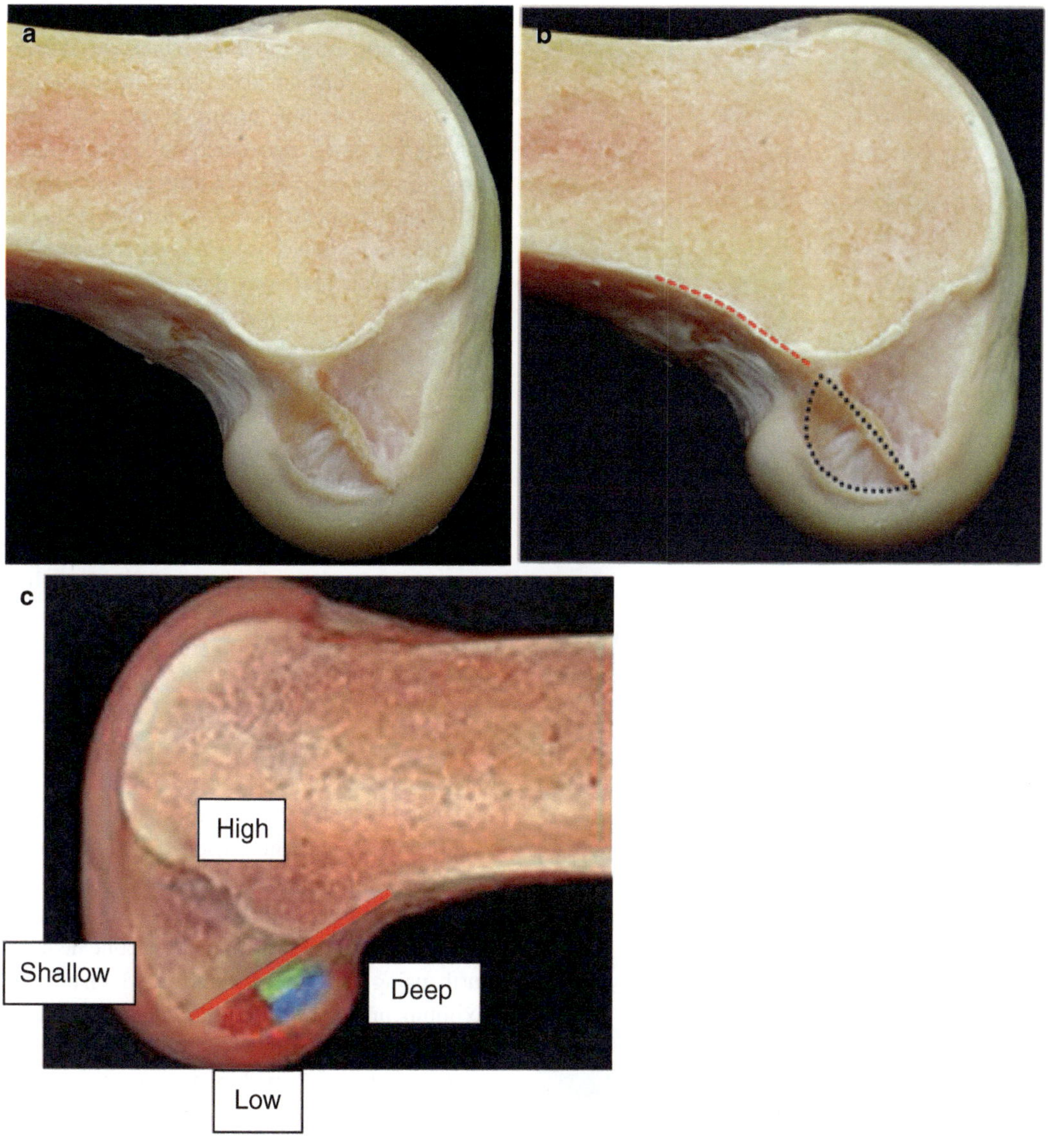

Fig. 3.1 Ribbon-like structure was shown. (Smigielski et al., Bone Joint J 2016). Cadaver specimens showing (**a**) the left knee joint, lateral femoral condyle viewed from the medial side. Femoral anterior cruciate ligament (ACL) attachment is visualized; (**b**) black dots—crescent shape of ACL femoral attachment extended from the intercondylar ridge (resident's ridge) to the posterior articular margin of the lateral femoral condyle; red dashed line—posterior femoral cortex; (**c**) continuous line from the posterior femoral cortex could be a reference of ACL footprint

the knee in nearly full flexion (more than 120° of flexion), an Ultrabutton drill pin (Smith and Nephew Co.) is inserted through the accessory low anteromedial portal, penetrating the lateral side of the thigh, to create a femoral tunnel of 4.5 mm diameter, to create a round femoral tunnel to pass the Ultrabutton. Subsequently, we used the original, rounded rectangular dilators, which are available in various sizes. In all cases, dilate entire 25–30 mm of the femoral tunnel (Fig. 3.34a). A tibial tunnel is established slightly anterior to the center of the ACL tibial footprint

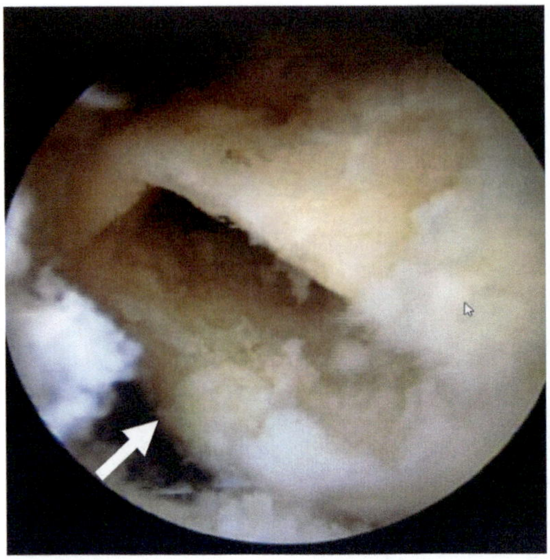

Fig. 3.2 Femoral rectangular tunnel

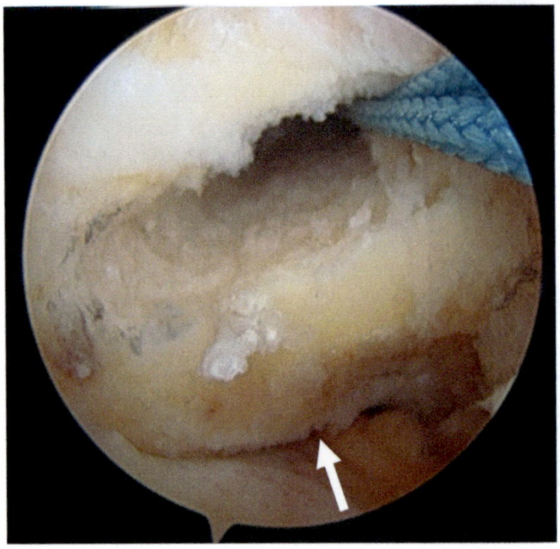

Fig. 3.3 The cartilage upper margin of the posterior femoral condyle, white arrow

(3–5 mm anterior to the inner margin of the anterior horn of the lateral meniscus) with a 45–50 tibial guide angle and a guide pin insert, and check the point is correct or not. During the establishment of the rectangular tibial tunnel, the direction of the long axis of the rectangular dilator is aligned parallel to the tibial footprint of the ACL to avoid damage to the anterior horn of the menisci. Additionally, the anterior margin of the proximal tibial plateau could be used as a supplemental reference for the long axis of the rectangular dilator, which is also aligned parallel. To avoid cortical fracture during tunnel establishment, the 5 or 6 mm cannulated drill and a smaller dilator, usually size 5× 10 mm (same size as 8 mm round reamer), should be used at first, and the dilator size should be increased sequentially. The quadrupled graft was then passed consecutively through the tibial and femoral tunnels and fixed with cyclic loading using the cortical suspension device (Ultrabutton, Smith and Nephew, London, UK) at the femoral side and Intrafix—nonabsorbable interference screw fixation between four bundles of tendon (Depuy Co.)—at the tibial side with the knee at 0–10° flexion. Back-up fixation with a post-tie screw fixation or bone staple (Arthrex Inc.) on tibia is applied depending on the graft length (Video 3.2).

Wen et al. reported four theories to explain the advantage of the oval femoral tunnel technique. First, an oval femoral tunnel provides a larger surface area for better blood supply from the adjacent cancellous bone surrounding the femoral tunnel. Second, an oval femoral tunnel closely resembles ACL anatomic insertions and restores natural ACL morphology. Third, the grafts used in an oval femoral tunnel should not easily rotate, and this is advantageous for tendon-bone healing. Fourth, using the dilator technique, which ensures maximum preservation of the cancellous bone, leads to better mechanical stability. Zhao et al. reported that a flattened bone sacrifice of the medial tibial plateau tunnel accelerated tendon-bone healing in the early period after ACL reconstruction in a rabbit model.

According to Nakase et al., the rounded rectangular femoral tunnel ACL reconstruction (RFTR) group had a larger femoral tunnel area than the anatomic single-bundle ACL reconstruction (ASBR) group (average area, 53.1 ± 4.0 mm^2 vs. 46.1 ± 7.0 mm^2; $P < 0.01$). RFTR group had better anteroposterior stability and higher Lysholm scores than the ASBR group (average side-to-side difference for anterior tibial translation, 0.6 ± 0.8 mm vs. 1.6 ± 1.4 mm; $P < 0.01$;

average Lysholm score, 98.5 ± 2.1 vs. 97.5 ± 3.5; $P < 0.01$). Differences in rotational laxity between the groups were significant (negative pivot shift, 94.3% vs. 92.3%; $P < 0.01$). No significant difference was noted in the IKDC subjective score between the two groups. The RFTR group had significantly larger femoral bone tunnels immediately after surgery; however, no significant differences were observed in bone tunnel area on the 3-month postoperative CT (106.2 ± 23.8 mm^2 vs. 102.1 ± 24.8 mm^2; $P = 0.264$). The bone tunnel enlargement ratio was significantly lower in the RFTR group (73 ± 38% vs. 107±41%; $P < 0.01$). The graft length change was 1.0 ± 0.7 mm with the isometric reconstruction technique and 3.4 ± 0.9 mm with the anatomic rectangular tunnel technique (ART).

The native ACL exhibits an intrinsic length change of 3–6 mm; therefore, the ART technique may more closely replicate the biomechanical function of the native ACL. (Excursion of bone-patella tendon-bone grafts during the flexion-extension movement in anterior cruciate ligament reconstruction.

According to Jiayi Shao et al. [39], in the rounded rectangular tunnel group, the average percentage of ACL tibial footprint covered by the tunnel is 70.8% ± 2.5%, which is significantly higher than that in the round tunnel group (48.2% ± 6.4%) ($P = 0.012$). As for the anterior root of the lateral meniscus (ARLM) attachment area (Figs. 3.4a, b and 3.5a–c) in the round tunnel group, there was a significant decrease (22.5% ± 5.9%) in the anterior root of the lateral meniscus attachment area after tibial tunnel reaming compared with the intact state ($P < 0.001$). Conversely, in the rounded rectangular tunnel group, the ARLM attachment area is not significantly affected by tibial tunnel reaming. Rounded-rectangular tibial tunnel was able to better cover the native ACL tibial footprint and significantly lower the risk of iatrogenic injury to the ARLM attachment than the round tibial tunnel during ACL reconstruction in a cadaver study (Orthopedic J. of Sports med V10 (3) 2022 Mar) (Fig. 3.4a, b).

The advantage of the rounded rectangular tunnel compared to the round tunnel:

1. RFTR group had a larger femoral tunnel area than the anatomic single-bundle ACL reconstruction (ASBR) group (average area, 53.1 ± 4.0 mm^2 vs. 46.1 ± 7.0 mm^2; $P < 0.01$).
2. RFTR group had better anteroposterior stability and higher Lysholm scores than the ASBR

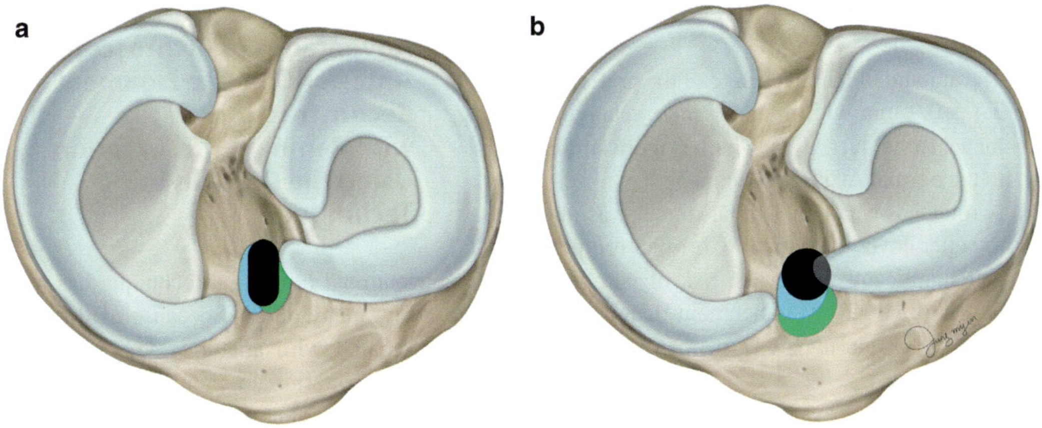

Fig. 3.4 (**a**, **b**) Diagram of footprint coverage in (**a**) the RRT and (**b**) the RT group. The ACL tibial tunnel is shown in black, the ACL tibial footprint in blue, the ARLM attachment in green, and the tibial plateau in yellow. *ACL* anterior cruciate ligament, *ARLM* anterior root of lateral meniscus, *RRT* rounded-rectangular tunnel, *RT* round tunnel. (Shao Jiayi et al. [39])

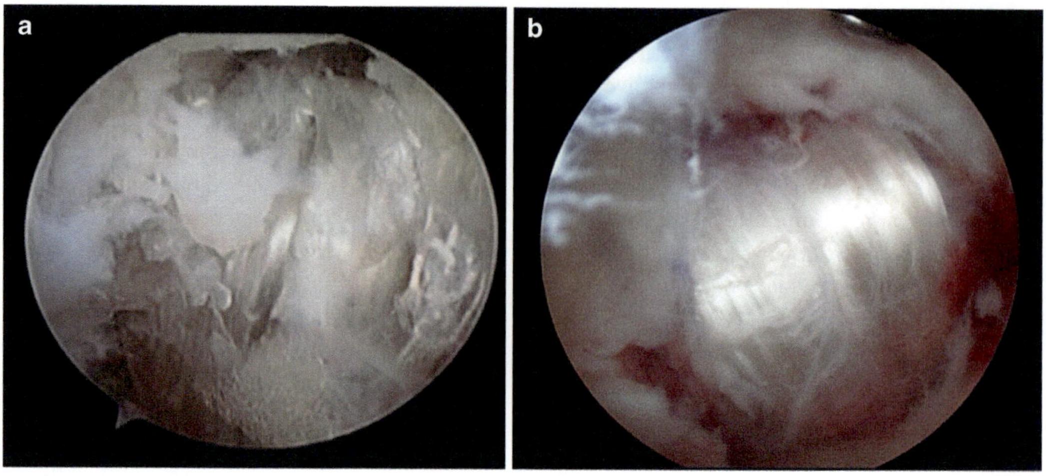

Fig. 3.5 (**a, b**) Arthroscopic picture of reconstructed PCL graft to show eccentricity. (**a**) PCL femoral tunnel, which was made with a round reamer and a round dilator. There was a gap between the tunnel margin and the graft. (**b**) PCL femoral tunnel, which was made with a rounded rectangular dilator. There was less of a gap between the tunnel margin and the graft. Compared to the round reamer tunnel, there was less gap between the tunnel and the graft

group (average side-to-side difference for anterior tibial translation, 0.6 ± 0.8 mm vs. 1.6 ± 1.4 mm; $P < 0.01$; average Lysholm score, 98.5 ± 2.1 vs. 97.5 ± 3.5; $P < 0.01$).
3. Differences in rotational laxity between the groups were significant (negative pivot shift, 94.3% vs. 92.3%; $P < 0.01$).
4. The bone tunnel enlargement ratio was significantly lower in the RFTR group (73 ± 38% vs. 107 ± 41%; $P < 0.01$).
5. The amount of length change of the grafts was 3.4 ± 0.9 mm with the anatomic rectangular tunnel technique(ART), which is more similar to the normal ACL length change.
6. A rounded-rectangular tibial tunnel was able to better cover the native ACL tibial footprint and significantly lower the risk of iatrogenic injury to the ARLM attachment than a round tibial tunnel during ACL reconstruction in a cadaver study

In our senior author's experiences, ACL reconstruction with a rounded rectangular dilator had an IKDC objective score of 89.4% (43 out of 48 patients), and ACL reconstruction using a round reamer and dilator had an IKDC score of 88.9 % (96 out of 108 patients). The rounded rectangular tunnel group was slightly better than the round dilator group. Nowadays, the rounded rectangular tunnel group was better than a round tunnel, with the same side-to-side differences in the maximal manual test in the KT 1000 arthrometer. The disadvantage of using a rounded rectangular dilator was a little bit longer operation time.

3.4 Advantages of Arthroscopic Anterior Cruciate Ligament Reconstruction with Remnant Preservation Using the Outside-In Technique

The conventional transtibial technique has been criticized by many authors because of the difficulty associated with anatomic femoral tunnel placement in anterior cruciate ligament (ACL) reconstruction. Therefore, tibial tunnel-independent drilling has attracted interest in recent years for anatomic ACL reconstruction. Among various tibial tunnel-independent drilling techniques, the anteromedial portal and outside-in (OI) techniques appear suitable for centering the graft within the ACL femoral insertion.

Several studies have investigated the femoral OI drilling technique with respect to anatomic restoration of the morphologic length, width, area, and angular orientation of the ACL femoral footprint. With the OI technique, the disadvantages include the need for a lateral incision on the distal aspect of the thigh and the risk of graft abrasion at the rough intra-articular edges of the tunnel. Recently, the OI technique has gained popularity with the introduction of retractable retrograde cutting drills and the modification of the technique. Typically, the anterior side of the ACL footprint is relatively easily observed through routine anterior portals. However, viewing the posterior side of the ACL footprint is difficult with these portals, especially during remnant-preserving ACL reconstruction. Therefore, the posterolateral (PL) portal with a 70° scope could be effective to observe the posterior side of the ACL femoral footprint. The OI femoral tunnel procedure appears to be a more reliable and precise method for achieving anatomic ACL reconstruction, and it also helps preserve the remnant bundle.

3.5 Surgical Technique of ACL Reconstruction Using the Outside-In Technique

An arthroscopic examination was performed through the anterolateral (AL) visualization portal and anteromedial (AM) working portal. After the diagnostic arthroscopy, all meniscal injuries were treated before ACL reconstruction. For all hamstring autografts, the semitendinosus and gracilis tendons, which had been harvested by using a tendon stripper, were prepared with three-strand semitendinosus and two-strand gracilis tendons (Fig. 3.6) (Video 3.3). The remaining fibers of the ACL remnant were preserved as much as possible throughout the entire procedure. To preserve the remnant ACL bundle with minimal damage as much as possible, it is very helpful to use the PL (posterolateral) portal with a 70° arthroscope for the creation of a femoral tunnel at an anatomic position (Fig. 3.7) (Video 3.4). For visualization of the ACL femoral footprint, the arthroscope was inserted through the AM portal and reached the PL compartment through the interval between the ACL and the lateral femoral condyle. After making a PL portal, the 70° arthroscope was then inserted through the PL portal and advanced to reach the posterior aspect of the intercondylar notch. With this approach, the posterior margin of the ACL femoral footprint could be clearly observed. Under visualization through the PL portal, the ACL femoral drilling guide (Arthrex, Naples, FL) was introduced through the AL portal or AM portal. The guide pin was inserted at the 4- to 5-mm anterior-distal area from the posterior proximal margin of the articular cartilage. After changing the Flip Cutter (Arthrex, Naples, FL) from a guide pin, retro-reaming was then performed to about 25 mm of the tunnel length corresponding to the measured diameter of the graft. A wire loop and No. 1-0 Maxon (Covidien, Mansfield, MA) were inserted through the femoral tunnel for passage of the graft and remnant bundle with three PDS sutures.

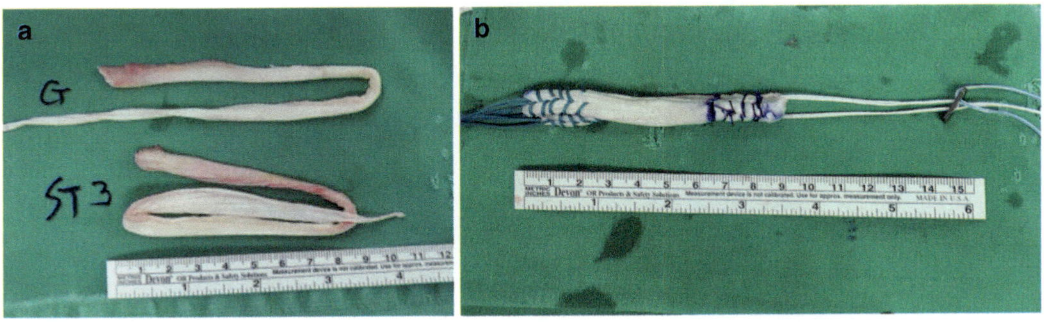

Fig. 3.6 (**a**) The semitendinosus and gracilis tendons were seen with three-strand semitendinosus (ST3) and two-strand gracilis (G) tendons. (**b**) Five-strand hamstring autografts were prepared with the TightRope for femoral fixation

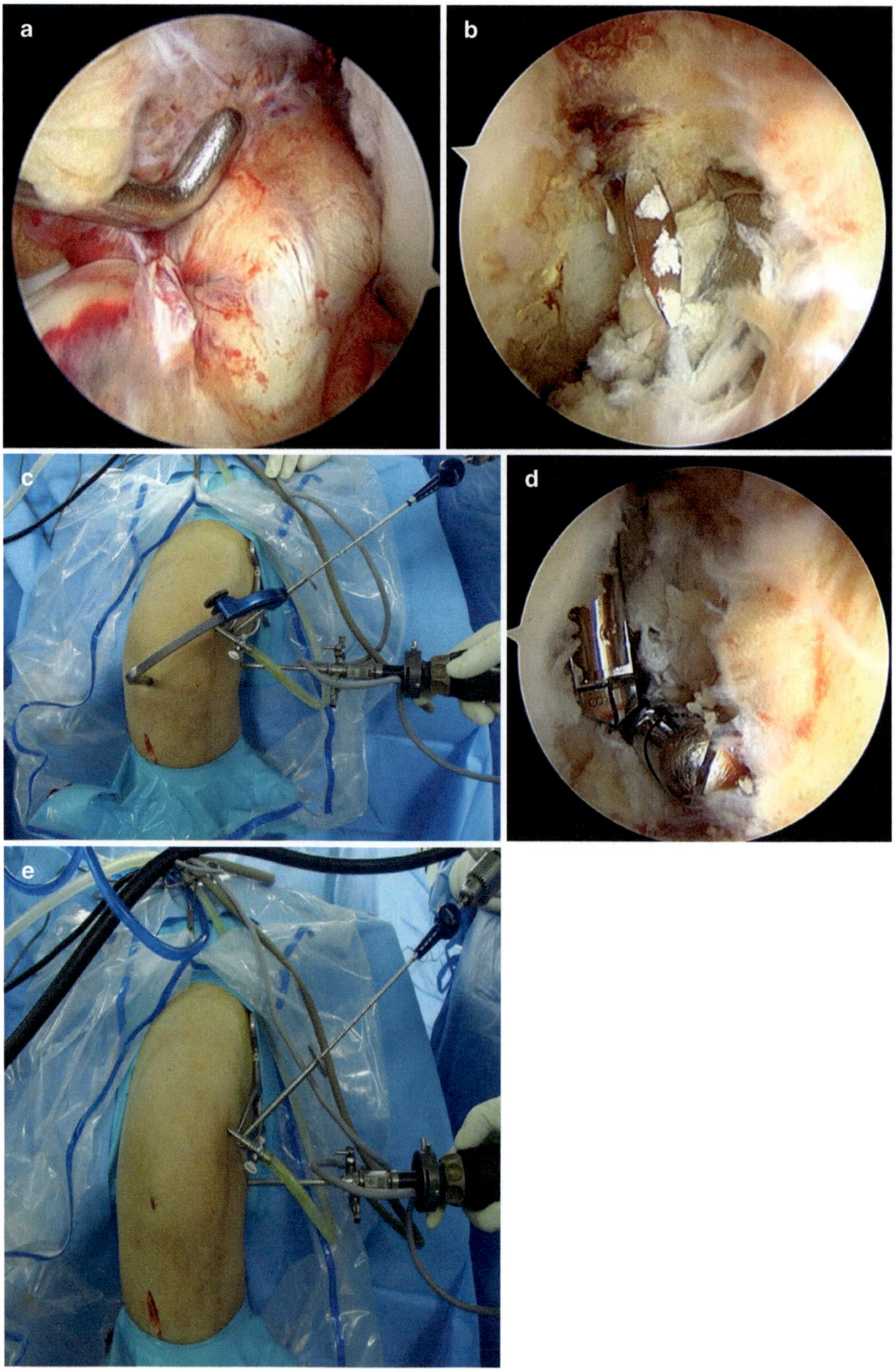

Fig. 3.7 (**a**) Acute rupture of the anterior cruciate ligament, (**b, c**) femoral guide with guide pin viewing from the posterolateral portal with 70° arthroscope, (**d, e**) retro-reaming with flip cutter viewing from posterolateral portal with 70° arthroscope

For formation of the tibial tunnel, a guide pin was inserted to the center of the ACL tibial insertion using an ACL tibial guide with a 55° angle, with preservation of the remnant bundle. Reaming of the tibial side was also adjusted according to the graft diameter. For the remnant preservation, a 45-degree curved suture hook (Linvatec, Largo, FL) with No. 0 PDS (Ethicon, Somerville, NJ) was introduced through the AM portal (Fig. 3.8) (Video 3.5). The sharp tip penetrated the remnants of the ACL near the proximal end, and the free end of the suture in the intercondylar notch was grasped and brought up to the AM portal. This step was repeated until three sutures were placed. After passing the graft with wire loop, the suture ends of the remnant tissue were simultaneously pulled past the passing suture through the tibia and out the femur. The button was pulled through the femur until it exited the lateral cortex, and the graft was advanced by tensioning on the TightRope (Arthrex, Naples, FL) shortening strands. Finally, a tie was made between the sutures of the remnant tissue and shortening strands of the TightRope. Finally, the tibial side was fixed with the same method. A bone tunnel formed at the anatomical location of the ACL femoral origin was checked on the X-ray and 3D CT image taken after surgery (Fig 3.9).

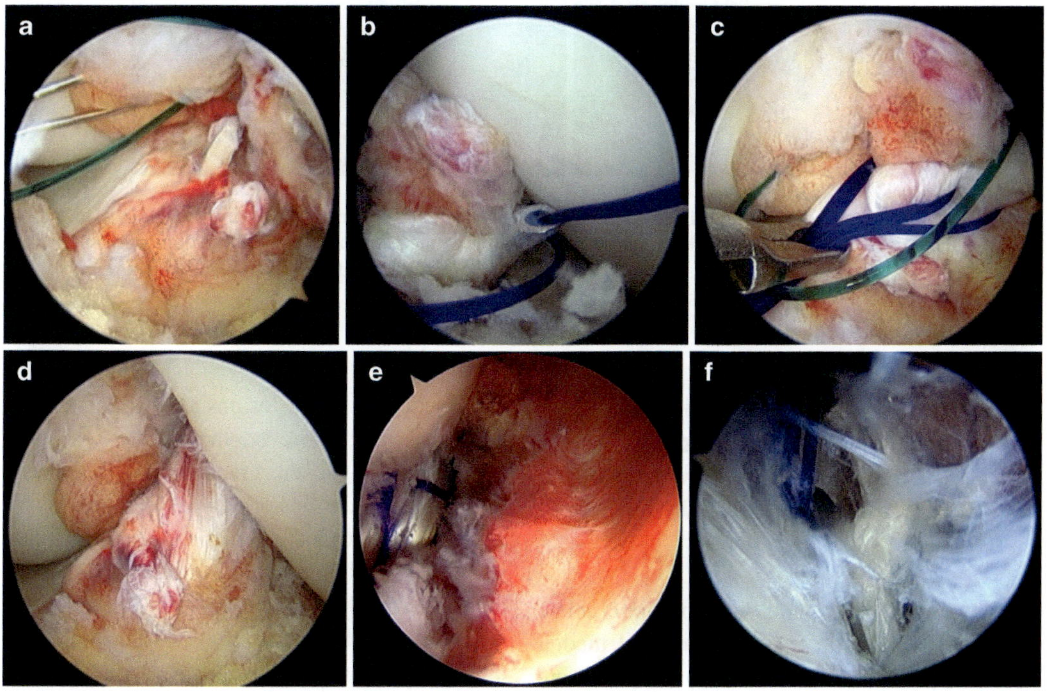

Fig. 3.8 (**a**) Tibial guide pin with remnant bundle preservation, (**b, c**) passing three sutures of the remnant tissue using a 45° curved suture hook, (**d**) graft and remnant ACL passing viewing from anterolateral portal, (**e**) graft and remnant ACL viewing from PL portal, and (**f**) direct viewing the TightRope and PDS sutures

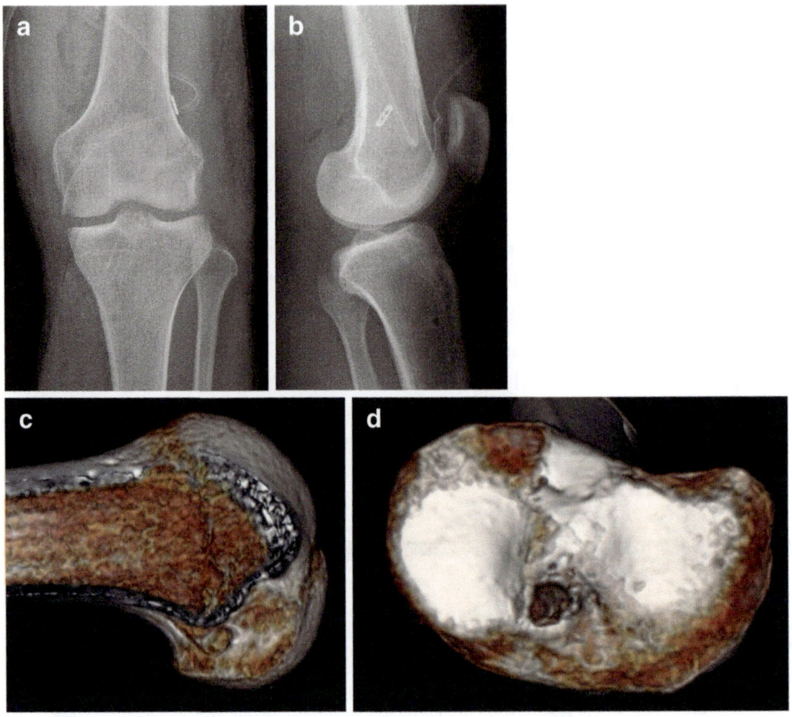

Fig. 3.9 (**a, b**) X-ray findings showed the tunnel positions and the position of the TightRope button. (**c**) On the lateral femoral side of three-dimensional computed tomography, the locations of the transtibial and tibial-independent femoral tunnels are shown. (**d**) On the top view of the proximal tibia, the locations of the transtibial and tibial-independent tibial tunnels are shown

3.6 Arthroscopic All-Inside Suture Repair of Medial Meniscus Lesion in Anterior Cruciate Ligament-Deficient Knees

Up to two-thirds of patients with anterior cruciate ligament (ACL) rupture have combined medial meniscus posterior horn (MMPH) tears. Among these, peripheral lesions in the meniscocapsular zone, known as ramp lesions, are reported as the most common meniscal lesion associated with ACL injury. Biomechanical studies have indicated that injury to the posterior meniscocapsular zone further increases anterior tibial translation and external rotation when combined with ACL injuries. Moreover, previous clinical studies demonstrated that repairing these lesions has a potential advantage in the restoration of knee biomechanics after ACL treatment. Thus, it is important to identify these lesions and to repair them when possible; however, these lesions are frequently misdiagnosed, given the low sensitivity of imaging modalities or clinical examinations.

Arthroscopic and magnetic resonance imaging (MRI) findings of the ramp lesion in ACL-deficient knee have been reported. These lesions are hard to find because of poor visualization of the MMPH meniscocapsular junction. Previous studies have shown that magnetic resonance imaging (MRI) has a sensitivity of only 69–89% for detecting meniscal tears in patients with acute or chronic ACL tears. To find the lesions properly, the posterior compartment should be visualized with sequential arthroscopic examination. The prevalence of MMPH ramp lesions has been variously reported at a range 9.3–16.6%. Recent studies were found higher prevalence, up to 34.5% after systematic arthroscopic evaluation, a rate that was relatively higher than in previous studies. Because careful systematic arthroscopic evaluations and suspicions are important when searching for ramp lesions, posteromedial inspection using a 70° arthroscope has improved the diagnostic accuracy for ramp lesion without direct exploration through the posteromedial portal.

The development of all-inside meniscus repair devices has been a turning point in the advancement of arthroscopic technique due to simplicity of implant insertion and the reduction in surgery time. Although these devices are easy to use, a repair technique with suture device was reported to have higher failure risk due to incorrect deployment of anchor of suture devices, especially chronic situations. All-inside suturing of peripheral longitudinal MMPH tears using a posteromedial (PM) portal is a very efficient and safe technique that provides anatomic coaptation of the torn meniscal fragment, easy placement of vertically oriented suture, and strong fixation while minimizing the risk of neurovascular or chondral injury. We have previously reported an arthroscopic modified all-inside Morgan suture technique using 2 PM portals for repair of MMPH tears. However, we have recently begun to perform arthroscopic all-inside sutures for MMPH tears through a single PM portal. Our suturing technique allows greater freedom in suture hook maneuvering by creating a single posterior portal without using a cannula. This technique allows excellent visualization of the posterior compartment, anatomic coaptation of the torn meniscus, and strong knot tying while avoiding inadvertent injury to the remnant meniscus and articular cartilage.

3.7 Surgical Technique of All-Inside Suture Repair

The indication for this repair technique is both longitudinal tears being within 5 mm of the peripheral rim and greater than 1 cm in size at the posterior horn of both menisci. Placement of an arthroscopic all-inside vertical suture using a suture hook appears to be safe and effective, and a high rate of meniscal healing can be expected in patients with tears located in MMPH.

The standard anterolateral and anteromedial portals are used for comprehensive examination with a 30° arthroscope and a probe. If an MMPH tear is suspected from the preoperative MRI or during arthroscopic examination, or if the ACL ligament was torn totally, the posterior compartment is approached by passing the 30° arthroscope from the anterolateral portal through the intercondylar notch between the medial femoral condyle and the posterior cruciate ligament (PCL). This is first facilitated by placing the anterior portals close to the margins of the patellar tendon. Afterward, a standard PM portal is created under direct arthroscopic visualization. This makes instruments, such as the suture hook, easier to move and manipulate. Using a probe, the posterior compartment is examined thoroughly (Fig. 3.10, Video 3.6). Switching the scope to the PM portal, the posterior horn is reexamined. After establishing a suture plan, a 70° arthroscope is reinserted to the anterolateral portal and placed through the intercondylar notch to view the posterior compartment.

While viewing from the anterolateral portal through the intercondylar notch using a 70° arthroscope, a shaver or rasp is introduced through the PM portal without a cannula for debridement of both tear sides of the tear (Fig. 3.11). A 45° curved suture hook (Linvatec, Largo, FL) loaded with a polydioxanone synthetic (PDS) No. 0 (Ethicon, Somerville, NJ) is inserted through the standard PM portal. A suture hook loaded with PDS No. 0 is introduced to the PM portal, and then a suture passage is made starting from the inner tear penetrating the most central fragment from inferior to superior (Fig. 3.12). During this procedure, care must be taken not to damage the cartilage of the femoral condyle, as the sharp tip of the hook passes close to the condyle during this procedure. Both ends of PDS No. 0 are taken out with a suture retriever through the PM portal. The superior end of the suture is marked with a straight hemostat, and the inferior suture end is left alone. A suture hook loaded with Nylon is then inserted through the

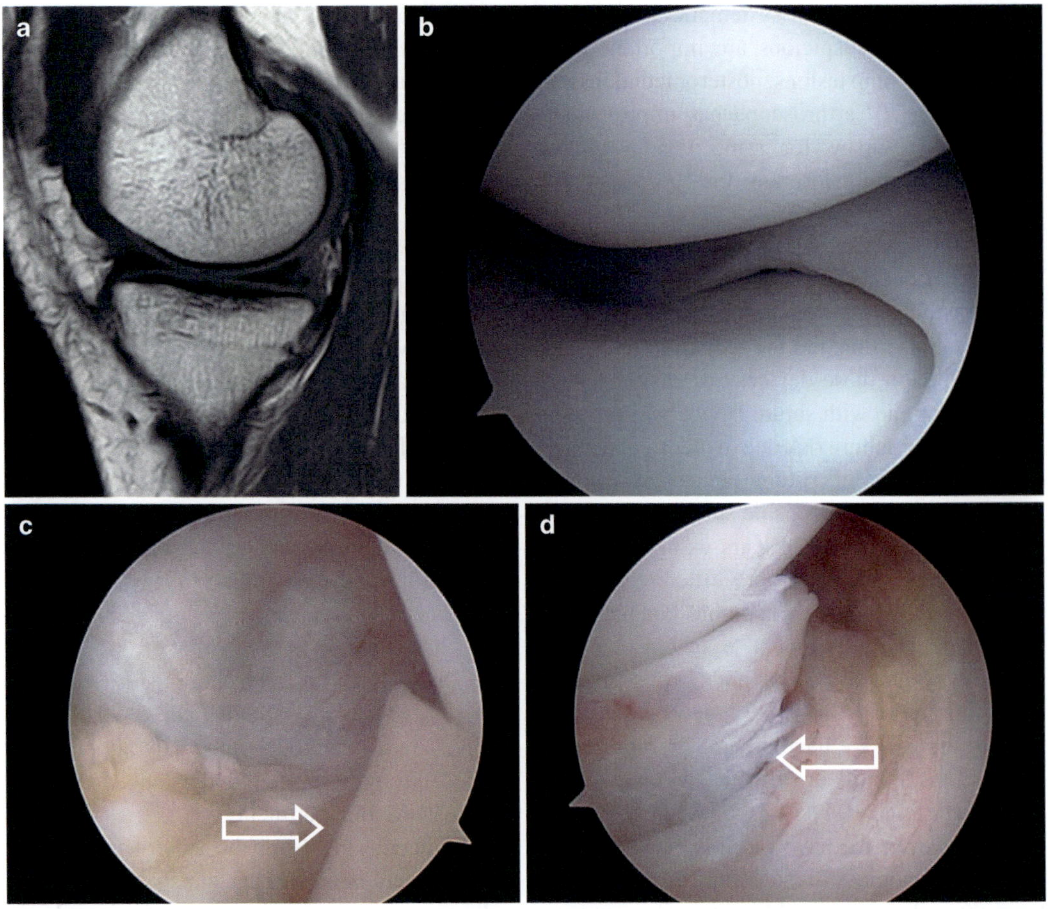

Fig. 3.10 (**a**) The sagittal MRI finding shows a longitudinal tear of the posterior horn of the medial meniscus (arrow). (**b**) The peripheral tear of the posterior horn cannot be seen from the anterior portal. (**c**) The longitudinal tear of the posterior horn (arrow) is seen from a 30° arthroscope inserted from the anterolateral portal to the posteromedial compartment. (**d**) The posteromedial portal verifies that the lesion is definitely

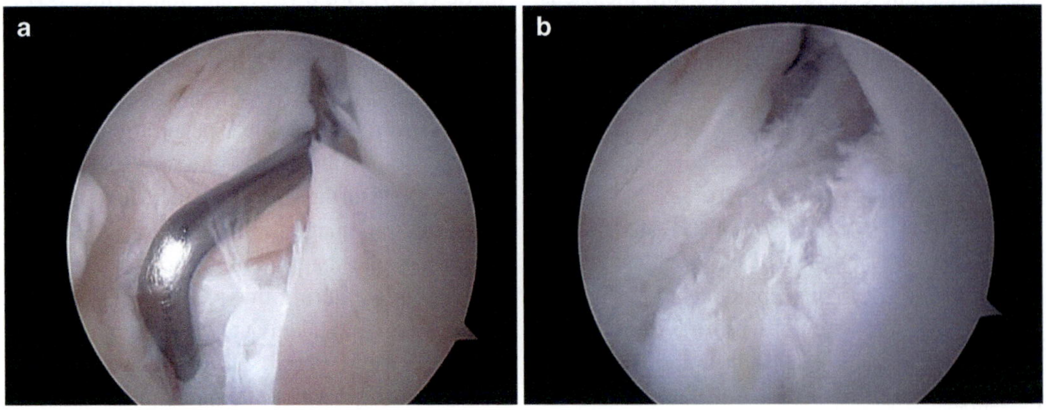

Fig. 3.11 (**a**) The tear pattern is clearly seen after changing to a 70° arthroscope, (**b**) both sides of the tear is debrided by a shaver inserted from the posteromedial portal

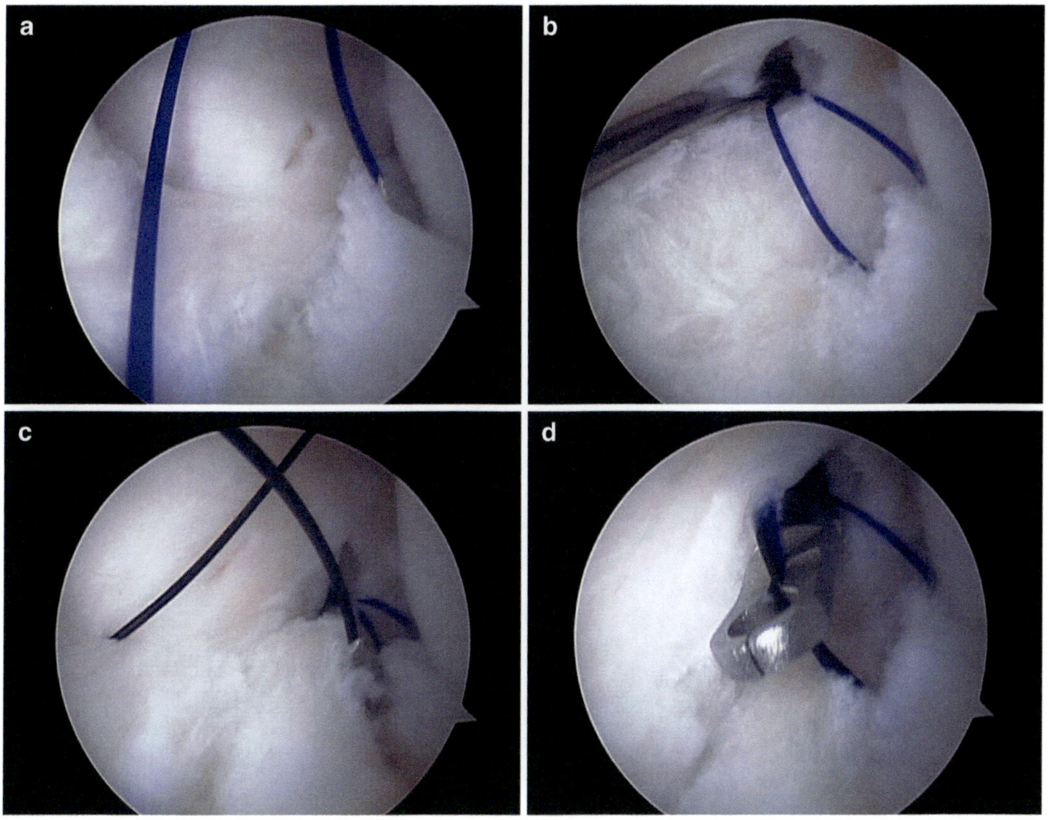

Fig. 3.12 (**a**) A suture hook loaded with PDS No. 0 is introduced to the PM portal, and then a suture passage is made starting from the inner tear, penetrating the most central fragment from inferior to superior. (**b**) From above, the cannula, 45° suture hook, and suture retriever are observed (**b**). Both ends of PDS No. 0 are taken out with a suture retriever through the PM portal. (**c**) A suture hook loaded with Nylon is then inserted through the PM portal and used to penetrate the peripheral rim at the capsular side from the superior to inferior surface in the same manner. (**d**) Both suture materials are held together and retrieved out of the posteromedial portal by the suture retriever through the cannula

PM portal and used to penetrate the peripheral rim at the capsular side from the superior to inferior surface in the same manner. After both ends of Nylon are taken out of the PM portal with a suture retriever, the superior end of the suture is marked with a straight hemostat. The inferior side of the PDS and Nylon are held together and retrieved out of the PM portal using the suture retriever at the same time to avoid soft tissue interposition between both limbs. The inferior side end of Nylon is then tied with the inferior side of the end of PDS, and the hemostat holding the superior end of Nylon is then pulled. The PDS is subsequently passed through both sides of the meniscal tear as the Nylon is changed for the PDS No.0 from the tibial to the femoral surface. Both ends of PDS are held together and retrieved at the same time through the PM portal using a suture retriever (Fig. 3.13). A SMC (Samsung Medical Center) knot is tied and slid with a knot pusher, with additional securing half-hitch sutures. An additional 2 or 3 half-hitch knots with alternating posts on reverse throws are made, and the reduction is carefully inspected arthroscopically. For good coaptation and stable fixation of the torn meniscus, we advise placing three to four sutures with a 4–5 mm interval. If the tear is extended to the mid-body, our modified inside-out technique or meniscal fixators are used in combination with all-inside suturing. If the patient has ACL insufficiency, ACL reconstruction is performed after the meniscal repair.

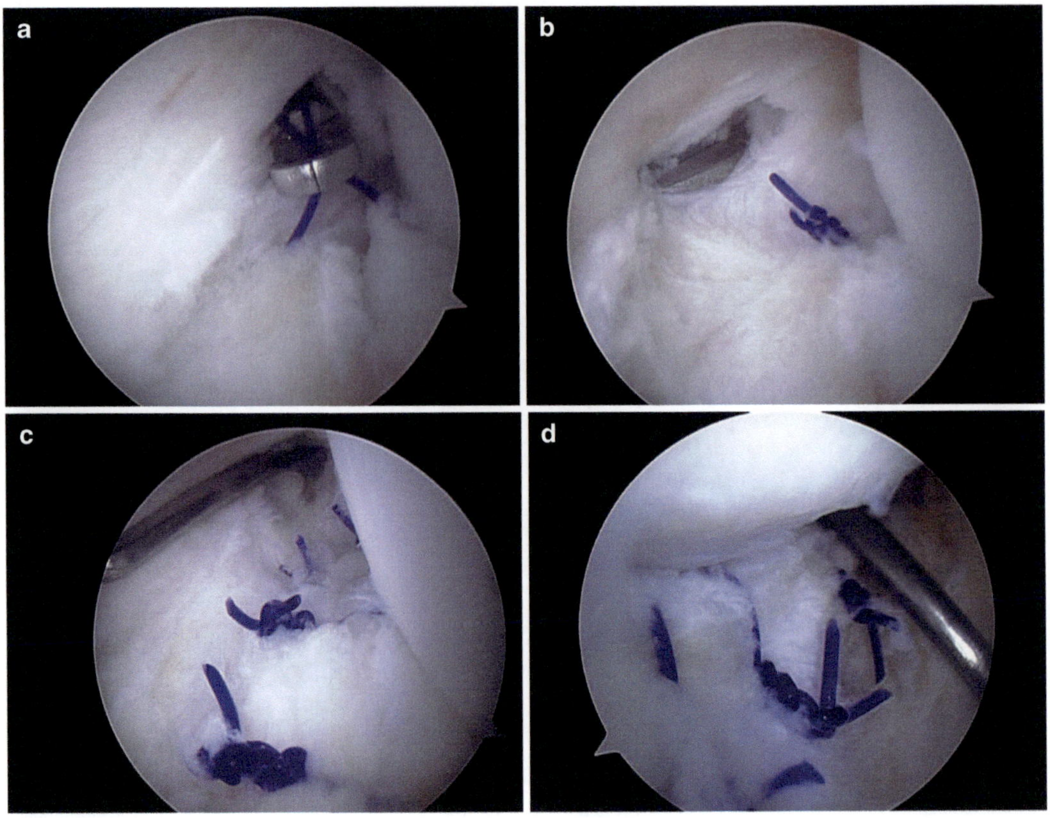

Fig. 3.13 (**a**) Both ends of PDS are held together and retrieved at the same time through the PM portal using a suture retriever. (**b**) The 30° arthroscope inserted from the posteromedial portal shows three vertical sutures at the longitudinal tear of the posterior horn of the medial meniscus. (**b**) A SMC (Samsung Medical Center) knot is tied and slid with a knot pusher. The 70° arthroscope, inserted from the anterolateral portal to the posteromedial compartment, shows the same findings. (**c, d**) Four vertical stitches were seen from the 70° arthroscope, inserted from the anterolateral portal to the posteromedial compartment and the posteromedial portal

We evaluated 83 patients who were included for this study at the author's institution; 52 patients (group 1) had ramp lesions without tear extension, and 31 patients (group 2) had ramp lesions with tear extension. On the basis of postoperative MRI scans, 67 patients (80.7%) were categorized as the completely healed group, and 16 patients (19.3%) were categorized as the not healed group (partially healed or failure/additional tears). There were no significant differences in postoperative outcomes between the completely healed group and the not healed group, as well as the rate of preoperative midbody tear extension. The second-look arthroscopy was performed on 41 patients (49.4%), and there were significant differences in findings between MRI and arthroscopy. The major differences between MRI and arthroscopy findings originated from the finding of partially healed patients; 14/17 (82.4%) of partially healed patients in MRI were categorized as completely healed patients in arthroscopic findings.

3.8 Arthroscopic All-Inside Repair for Lateral Meniscus Root Tear in Patients Undergoing Concomitant Anterior Cruciate Ligament Reconstruction

A lateral meniscus posterior horn (LMPH) root tear can occur in conjunction with an ACL ruptures and may be associated with the extrusion of the lateral meniscus. A LMPH root tear is defined as a tear that occurs less than 1 cm from the posterior insertion. It was reported that lateral meniscus tears, including posterior horn tears, stable radial flap tears, and peripheral or posterior third tears that do not extend further than 1 cm in front of the popliteus tendon, can be treated successfully with abrasion and trephination or by being left in situ.

The LMPH is inserted in both the bone and the meniscofemoral ligament (MFL). Double attachments of the root are observed in the posterior horn of the lateral meniscus, with the anterior portion attached to the tibial intercondylar eminence and the posterior portion to the femoral medial condyle through the meniscofemoral ligaments. Therefore the possibility exists that displaced posterior lateral meniscus root tears may be overlooked as a posterior-based flap tear even if the bony attachment has been completely transected. The confusion between a complete radial tear and a flap tear of the posterior root likely occurs because of a residual meniscofemoral attachment. In this situation, partial meniscectomy of the torn portion of the meniscus may lead to poor clinical results because of the failure of the hoop strain mechanism. This chapter is to document the classification of the LMPH root tear according to our experiences and describe a LMPH root repair technique using a modified all-inside suture technique (Figs. 3.14 and 3.15).

All incomplete radial tears or longitudinal tears around the posterior horn not in the root area within 1 cm from the bony insertion were excluded. Accordingly, the arthroscopic findings were categorized into four types by both the radial and longitudinal tear components, which extend to the attachment of the MFL: (1) radial tear with oblique flap, (2) longitudinal cleavage between the bony insertion and MFL insertion, (3) acute T-type, and (4) chronic inner loss-type (Fig. 3.16). Four types required similar

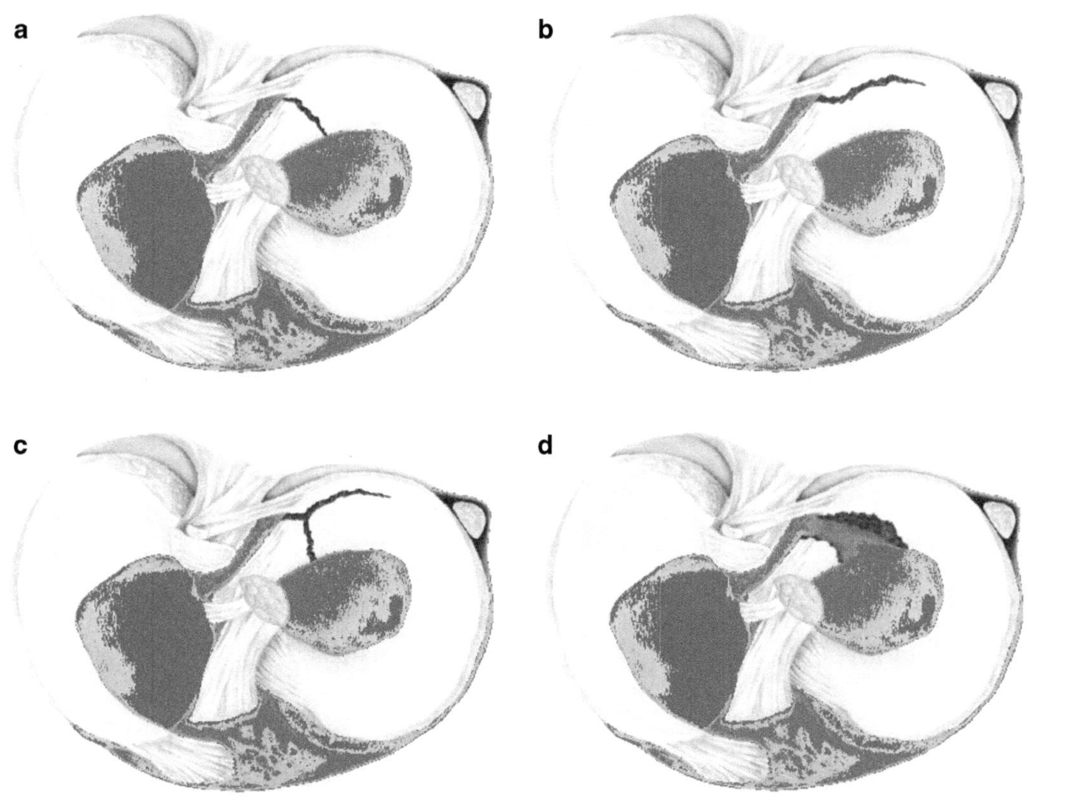

Fig. 3.14 Classification for the root tear of the lateral meniscus posterior horn. (**a**) Radial tear with oblique flap. (**b**) Longitudinal cleavage between the bony insertion and the meniscofemoral ligament insertion. (**c**) Acute T-type. (**d**) Chronic inner loss-type

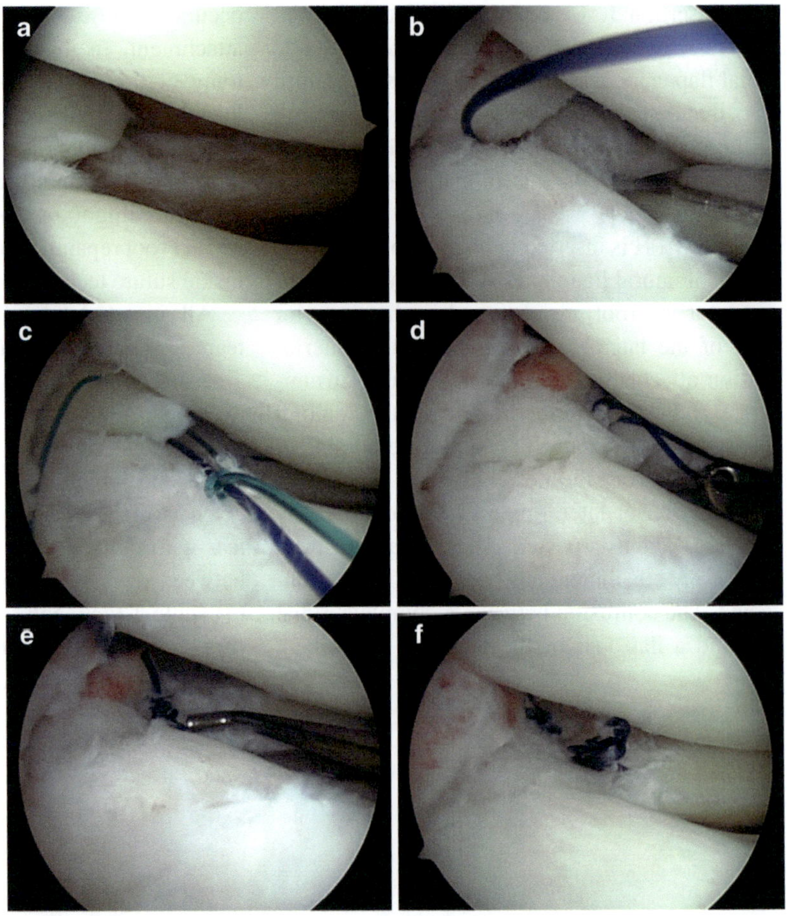

Fig. 3.15 (**a**) The arthroscope shows the radial tear in the root of the lateral meniscus posterior horn. (**b**) The suture hook loaded with PDS is inserted through the lateral side from the superior to the inferior surface. (**c**) The bottom side end of MAXON is tied with the bottom side of the end of PDS and the hemostat holding the superior end of the MAXON is pulled. (**d**) The PDS is subsequently passed through both sides of the meniscal tear as the MAXON is changed for the PDS. (**e**) The sliding knot is used for knot tying. (**f**) The arthroscope shows two vertical sutures at the radial tear of the posterior horn of the lateral meniscus

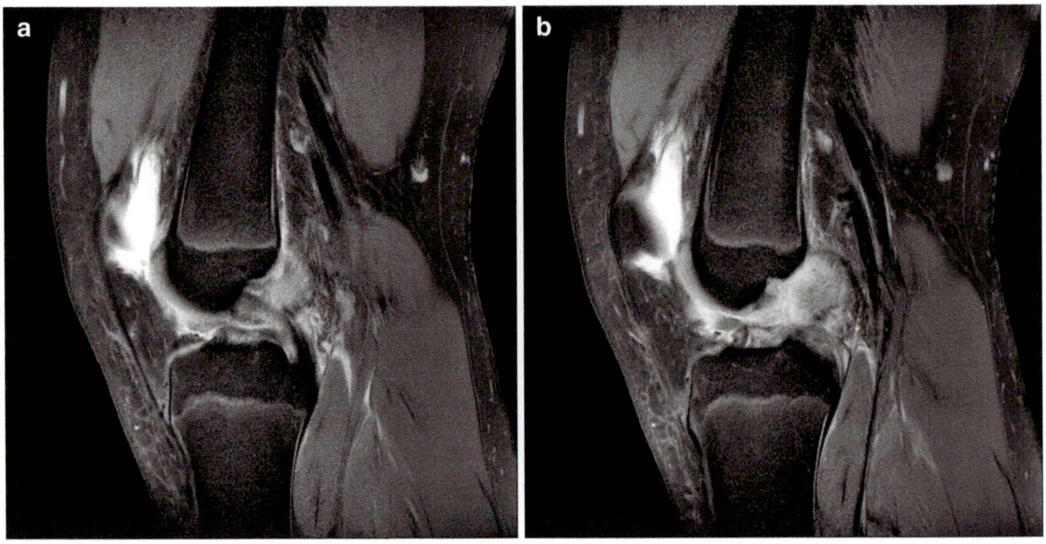

Fig. 3.16 (**a**, **b**) We can find ACL torn at the proximal substance after the first time injury (Taekwondo)

arthroscopic repair techniques, except for longitudinal cleavage and the T-shape tear, which need the repair of the longitudinal component using an additional PL portal. In the chronic inner loss-type, we think that it is necessary to repair the remaining meniscus to the flap of bony insertion to prevent the extrusion of the meniscus.

3.9 Surgical Technique

A diagnostic arthroscopic examination of the knee is performed using the standard AL and AM portals. While viewing with arthroscopy through the AM portal, the tear site is evaluated with a probe inserted through the AL portal with the knee in a "figure-four" position. Gentle debridement is performed at the tear site using a motorized shaver. A vertical suture can be inserted in top-to-bottom fashion or vice versa, according to which approach is more feasible. A straight suture hook loaded with PDS No. 0 is introduced through the AL portal and then penetrates at 3–5 mm lateral to the torn edge of the LMPH from a superior to inferior direction. Both ends of PDS No. 0 are taken out with a suture retriever through the AL portal. The superior end of the suture is marked with a straight hemostat, and the inferior suture end is left alone. The suture hook loaded with MAXON 2-0 is inserted through the AL portal and used to penetrate the posterior tibial attachment of the LM in the same manner (Fig. 3.15, Video 3.7). The bottom side of the PDS and MAXON are held together and retrieved out of the AL portal using the suture retriever at the same time to avoid soft tissue interposition between both ends. As before, the bottom end of MAXON 2-0 is tied with the bottom end of the PDS. The hemostat holding the superior end of MAXON is then pulled, bringing the PDS suture across the tear from the tibial to femoral surface. Both ends of PDS are retrieved through the AL portal and tied using a SMC sliding knot. One or two sutures are placed according to the tear length and approximation.

From 2003 to 2007, 27 (7%) of a consecutive series of 388 anterior cruciate ligament reconstructions had a concomitant LMPH root tear in the author's institution. Of the patients, 25 (92.6%) were followed up for more than 1 year. There was no postoperative effusion, joint-line tenderness, or positive McMurray provocation testing observed at the last follow-up. In comparison between preoperative and follow-up MRI, sagittal extrusion improved significantly, although no statistically significant improvement was observed in the coronal plane. Posterior lateral meniscus root tears were classified based on arthroscopic findings: type I, oblique flap; type II, T shape; type III, longitudinal cleavage; or type IV, chronic inner loss. A type I tear was found in seven patients, type II in 4, type III in 4, and type IV in 10. After repair of posterior lateral meniscus root tears, MRI showed that the displaced lateral meniscus was reduced, mainly in the sagittal plane. We introduced the repair of radial tear using the all-inside technique (Fig. 3.16).

We would like to present our case of the repair of a chronic radial tear of the lateral meniscus (lateral subluxation in the MRI film) using the inside-out technique due to narrowing of the knee joint space (Figs. 3.45, 3.46, and 3.47).

3.10 Cases of ACL Reconstruction

Case 1: ACL Combined MM Tear, Young Age

An 11-year-old male patient presented to the outpatient clinic. He had no previous history of knee problems. He injured his left knee while practicing Taekwondo, jumping, and falling. He was treated conservatively with a cylindrical cast. One year after the injury, he felt instability in the left knee and a worsening of the pain when he almost fell on a pavement block. There were no specific findings on plain radiographs taken immediately after reinjury, and physical examination revealed Lachman test grade 2, pivot shift test grade 1, varus stress test grade 2, dial test positive, posterolateral drawer test grade 2 (Fig. 3.17).

KT-2000 arthrometer maximum manual test (MMT); 8 mm right, 13 mm left were checked (Figs. 3.18, 3.19, 3.20, and 3.21)

We excised the flap-like area, and a small horizontal tear was visible.

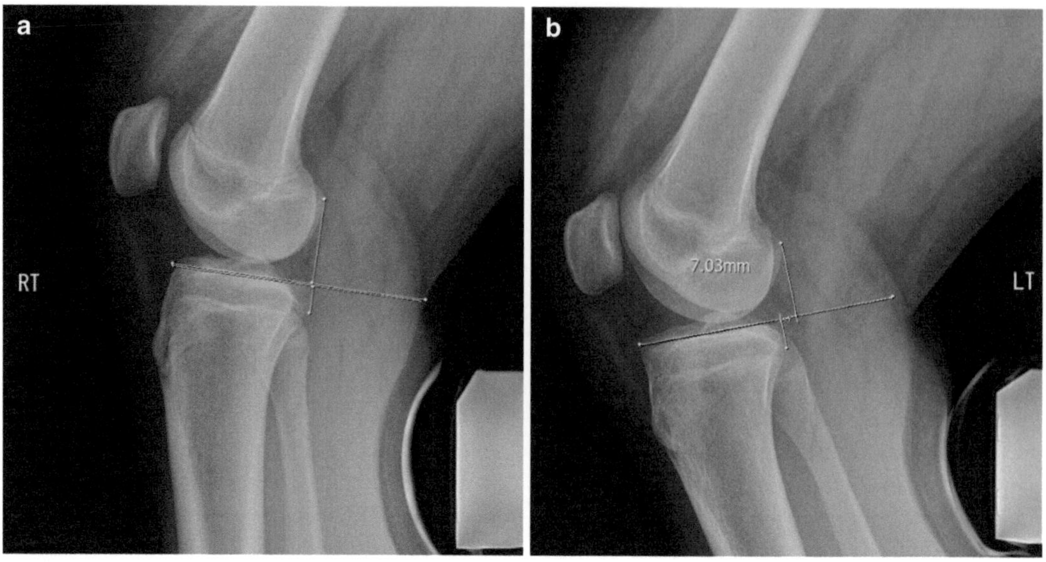

Fig. 3.17 (a, b) After 2nd time injury, a 7 mm side-to-side difference was checked compared to the unaffected side in the pull stress test imaging

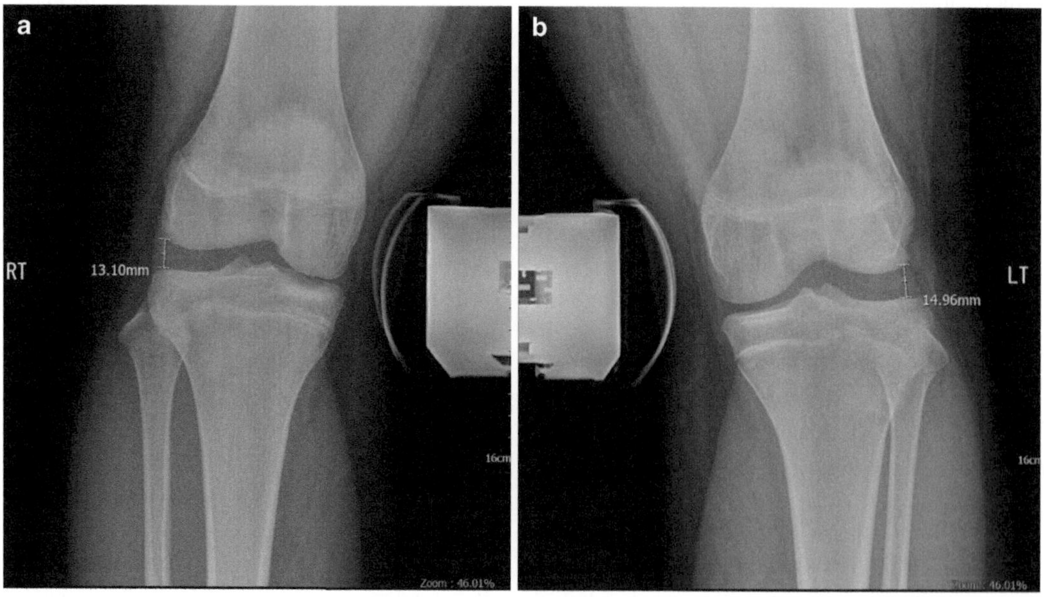

Fig. 3.18 (a, b) 0° flexion view and varus stress view; the lateral joint space slightly widened at the left knee

We repaired it again and inserted a fibrin clot. As can be seen in Figures e, f, g, and h in adults, we have to repair injured menisci as much as possible, even radial tears (Figs. 3.22, 3.23, 3.24, and 3.25).

There was no laxity on the anterior drawer test and Lachman test on physical examination. KT-2000 arthrometer maximum manual test (MMT); 9 mm right, 10–11 mm left were checked (Figs. 3.26, 3.27, and 3.28).

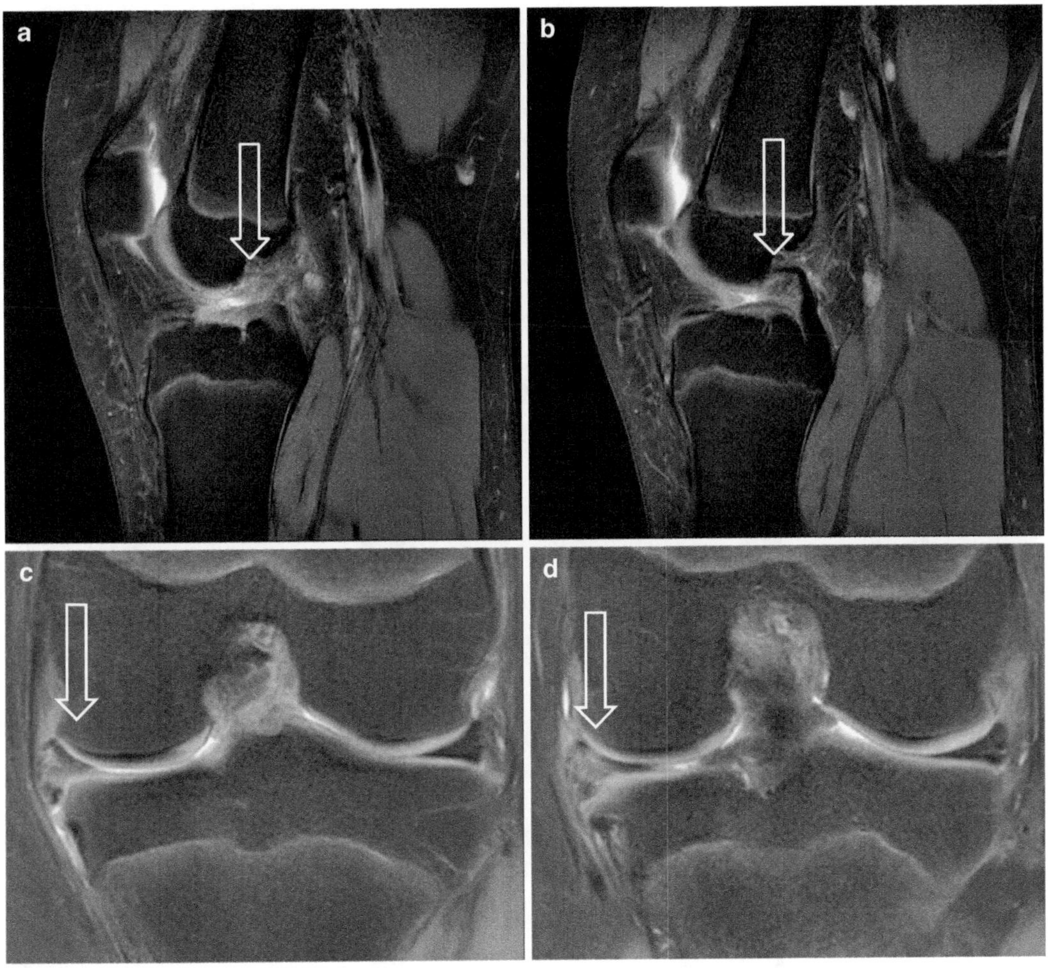

Fig. 3.19 (**a, b**) We can find a complete ACL tear. (**c, d**) Complete ACL tear and medial meniscal complex tears

Males with a skeletal age of 15 years or older and females of 13 years or older are ideal candidates for transphyseal ACL reconstruction because the risk of growth failure is minimal. Children with significant residual growth (skeletal age males ≤12 years and females ≤10 years) appear to be at greater risk of growth failure, so we generally recommend physeal-sparing techniques for these younger patients.

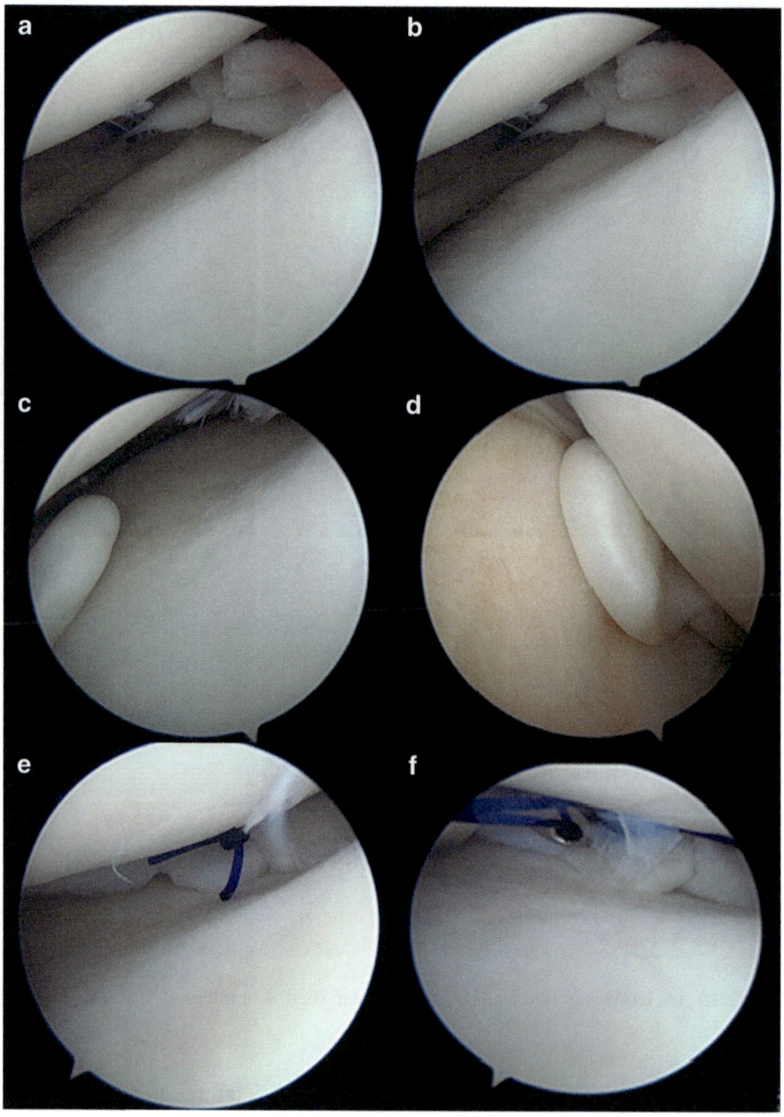

Fig. 3.20 These are the arthroscopic findings. (**a**, **b**) The torn medial meniscus looks impossible to repair, even remodeling at the torn site (**c**, **d**), but he is young, 12 years old boy; therefore, the senior author repaired it arthroscopically as much as possible. As you can see in the figure (**e**, **f**), even the tear looks impossible to repair; we tried to repair as much as possible as we can. Even though the tear locates at the white-white zone, if we repair it with the patient, it can be healed. Even in adults, we have to repair the injured meniscus, radial tear, whatever

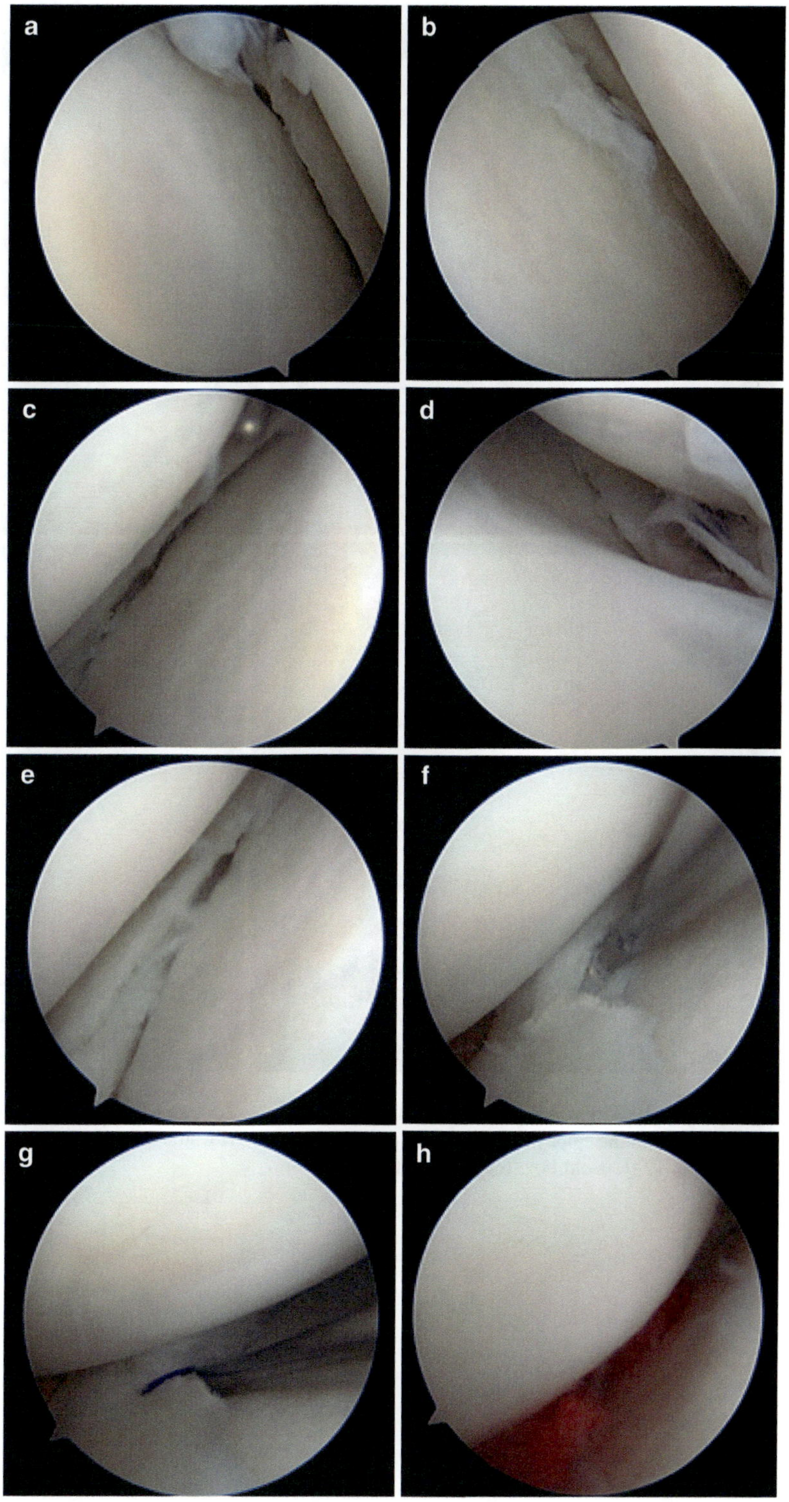

Fig. 3.21 These are the arthroscopic findings. (**a–d**) 19 months after the initial arthroscopic repair, the torn meniscus had healed except for a small flap-like area at the anterior (**e–h**)

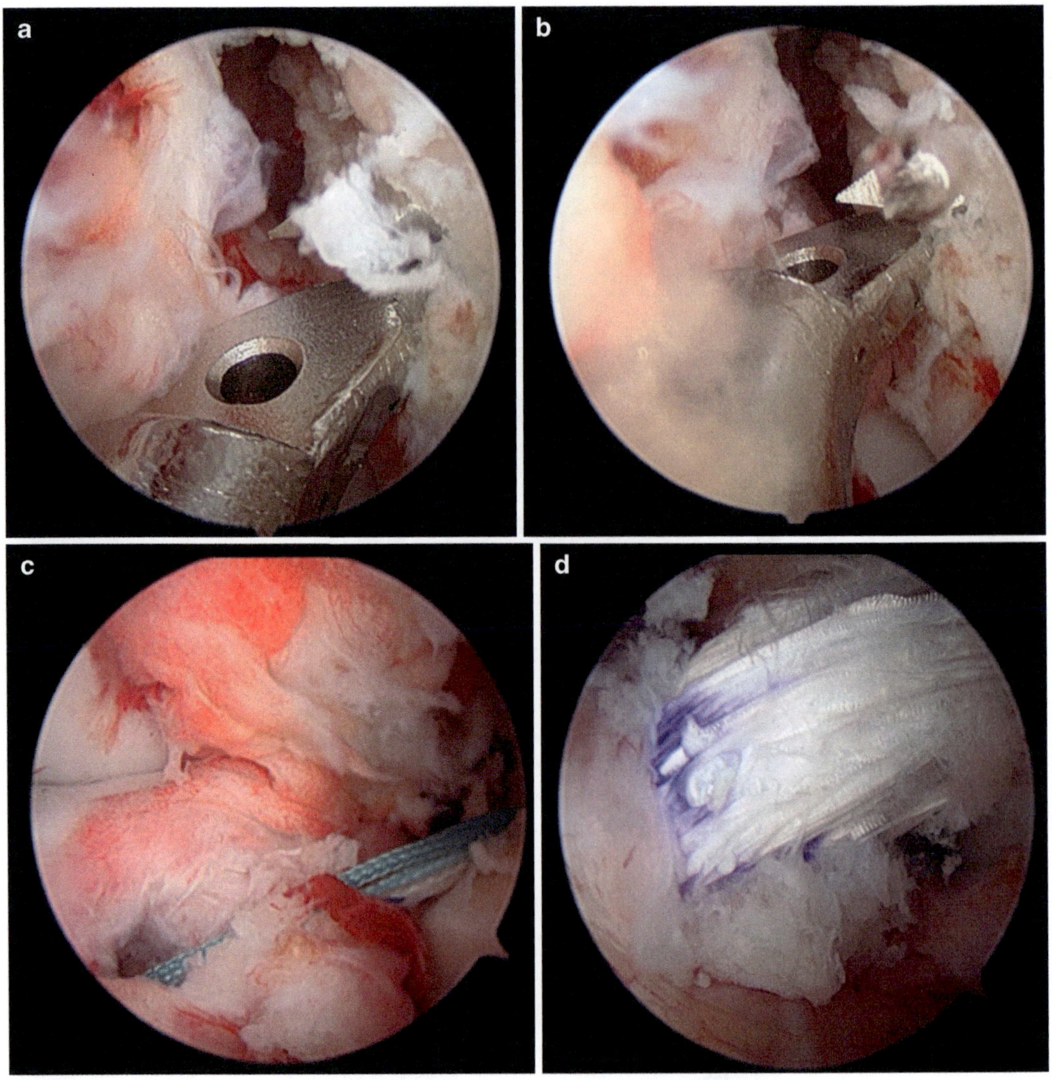

Fig. 3.22 (**a–b**) Arthroscopic ACL reconstruction using an angle guide at the epiphysis to avoid the physeal injury in the same 12-year-old boy. (**c**) ACL graft pulled from tibial tunnel to femoral tunnel using tight rope RT (**d**) ACL graft after fixation

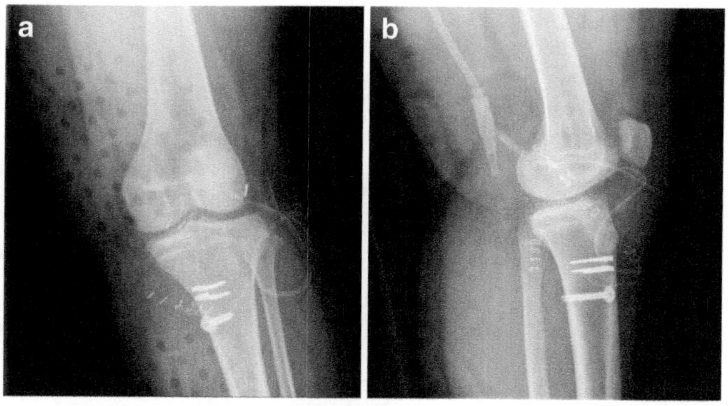

Fig. 3.23 (**a**, **b**) Arthroscopic ACL reconstruction was done through the epiphyseal femoral tunnel and transphyseal tibial and PLCS through the fibular head tunnel

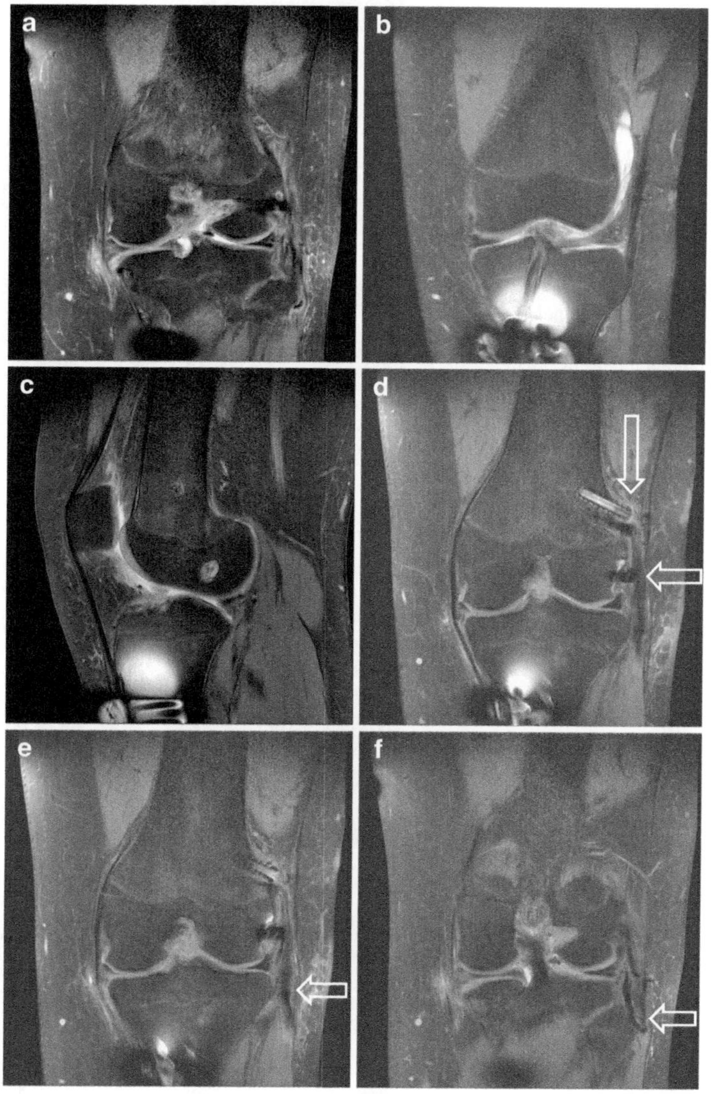

Fig. 3.24 (**a**, **c**) Five and a half months after ACL reconstruction, femoral trans-epiphyseal tunnel and tibial trans-physeal tunnel (**b**) and PLCS through fibular head tunnel to lateral metaphyseal tunnel with tibialis allograft (**d**–**f**) and medial meniscus repair

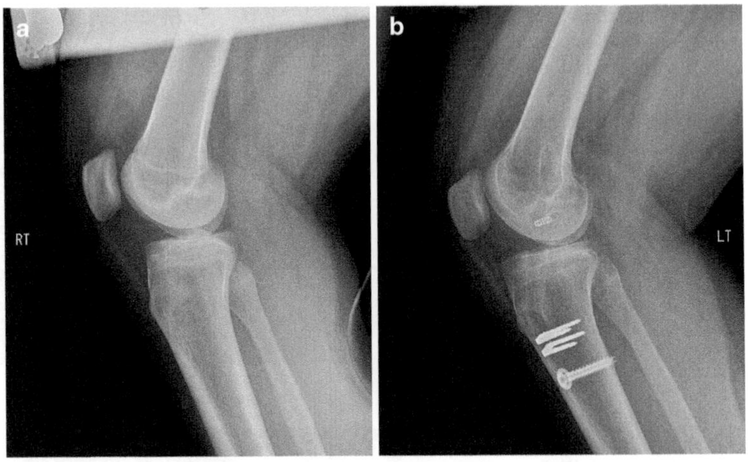

Fig. 3.25 (**a**, **b**) Follow-up pull stress radiographs showed a marked decrease in the side-to-side difference

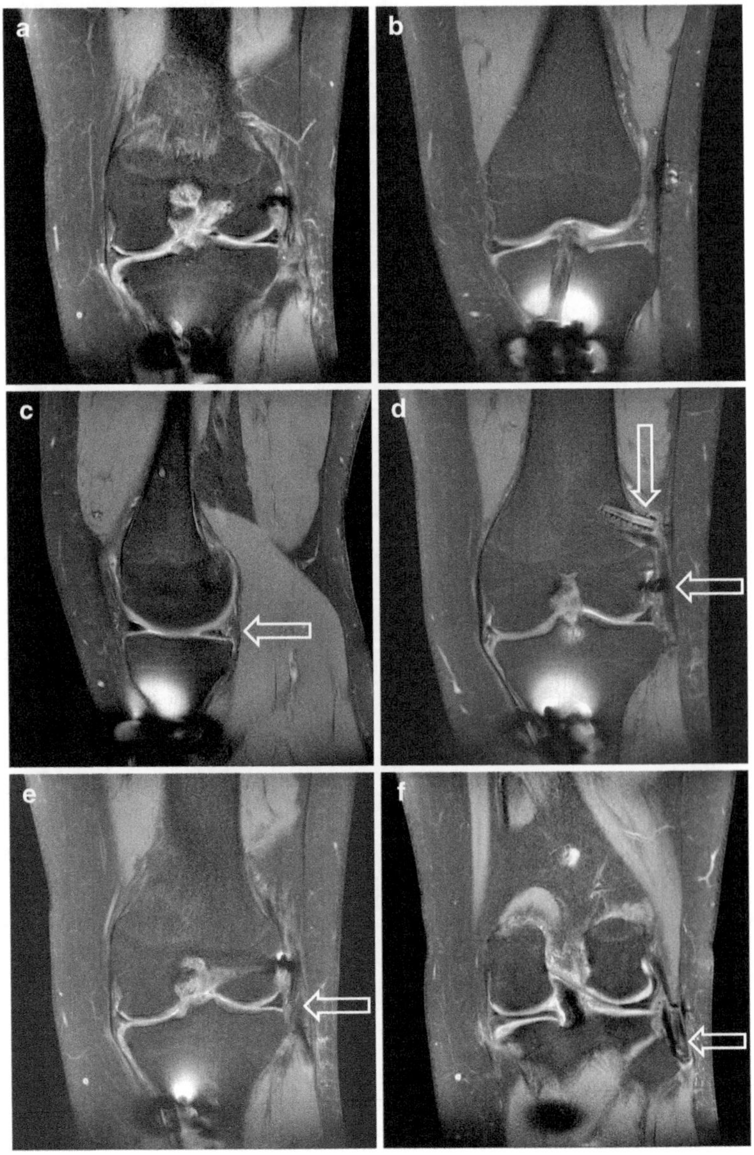

Fig. 3.26 (**a**) 1 year after ACL reconstruction, femoral trans-epiphyseal tunnel and (**b**) tibial trans-physeal tunnel and PLCS through fibular head tunnel to lateral metaphyseal tunnel with tibialis allograft and medial meniscus repair: Reconstructed ACL graft was passed through the epiphysis, not violating the growth plate. (**c**) Repaired posterior meniscus was shown. (**d**) PLCS: femoral tunnel at the femoral metaphyseal area to avoid growth plate injury. (**e, f**) Reconstructed posterolateral corner sling (PLCS) for the PLRI was shown

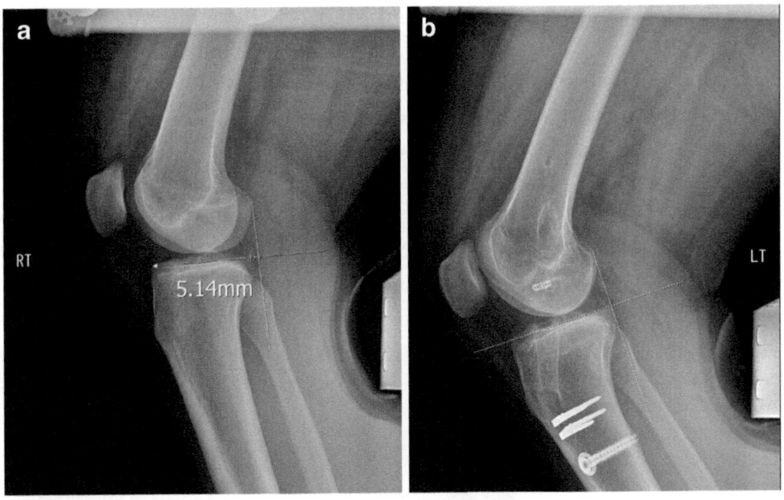

Fig. 3.27 (**a**, **b**) This is an image of pull stress view 1 year after surgery. Side-to-side difference was less than 1 mm, which means there was nearly no difference between left and right knees

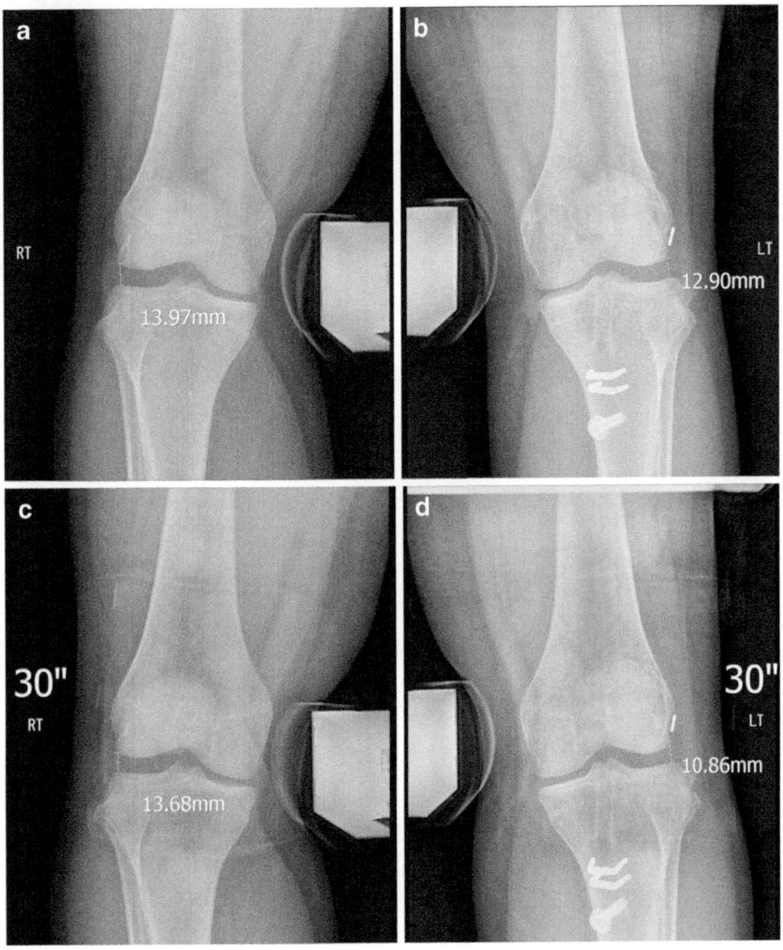

Fig. 3.28 (**a**, **b**) 0° varus stress view; (**c**, **d**) 30° flexion view; 1 year after surgery: lateral joint space slightly widened at unaffected knee which showed stabilized affected knee, there was no varus instability

Case 2: ACL Rupture with LCL and MCL Rupture

A 21-year-old male patient injured his left knee 6 months ago when he tripped on the stairs. The pain was tolerable at first but became worse. The Lachman test, pivot shift test, and varus and valgus test were positive, while the dial test and posterolateral drawer test were negative on physical examination. KT-2000 arthrometer maximum manual test (MMT): 8 mm right and 16 mm left were checked (Figs. 3.29, 3.30, 3.31, 3.32, 3.33, 3.34, 3.35, and 3.36).

On the second look, arthroscopy during metal removal, well-synovialization of ACL was found (Figs. 3.37 and 3.38a, b).

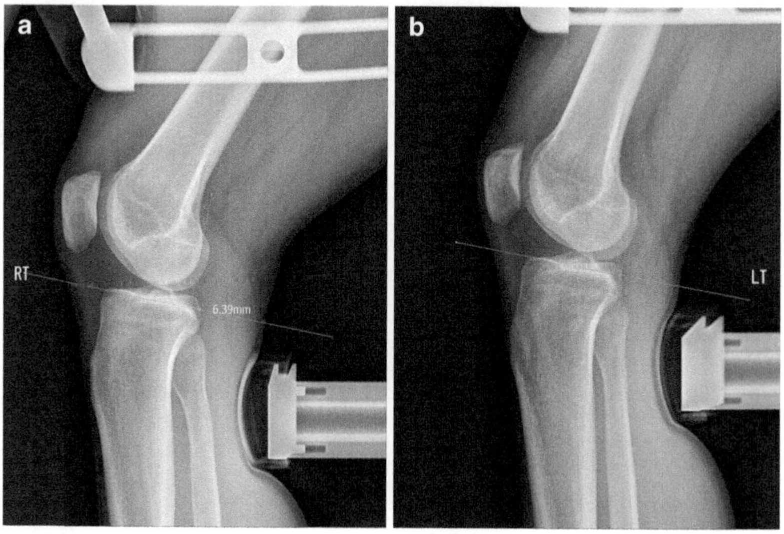

Fig. 3.29 (**a, b**) 6.3 mm side-to-side difference was checked compared to the unaffected side in the pull stress test imaging

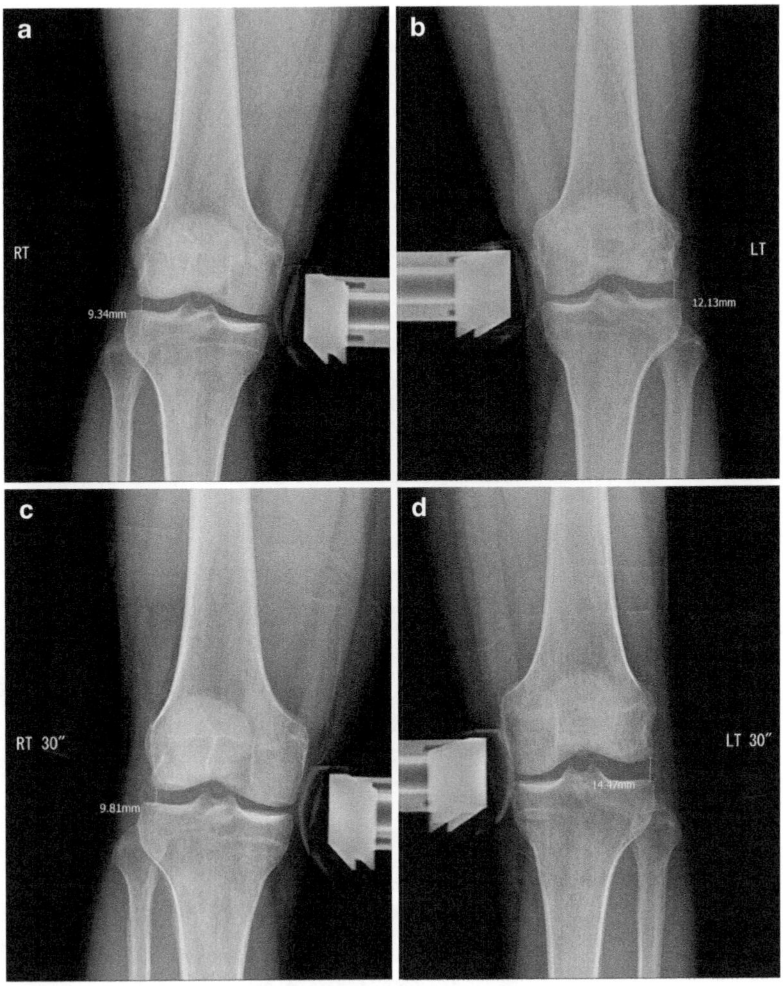

Fig. 3.30 (**a**, **b**) 0° varus stress view; (**c**, **d**) 30° flexion varus stress view, left knee lateral joint space is wider than the right knee

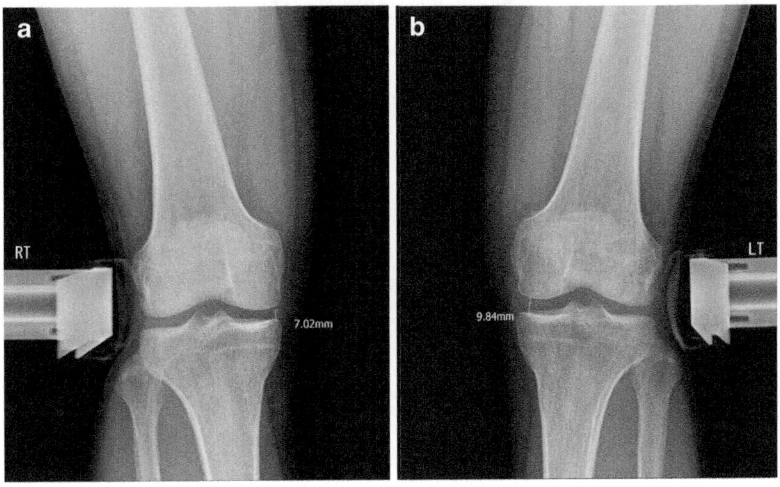

Fig. 3.31 (**a**, **b**) 0° valgus stress view; left knee medial joint space is wider than right knee

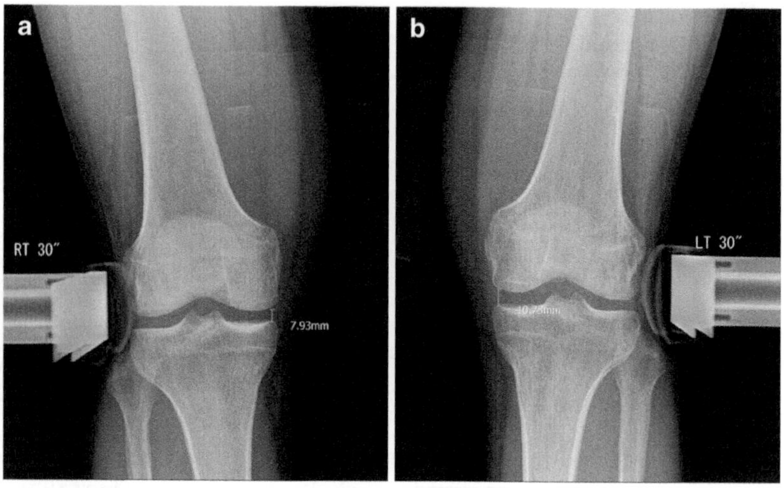

Fig. 3.32 (**a**, **b**) 30° flexion , valgus view; left knee medial joint space is wider than right knee

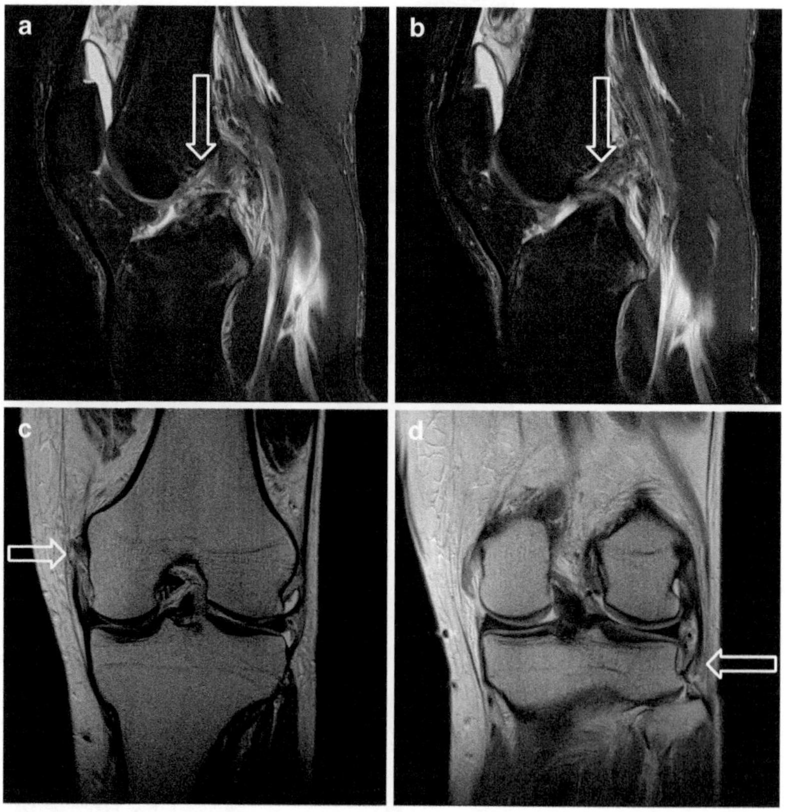

Fig. 3.33 (**a**, **b**) We found ACL rupture, (**c**) medial collateral ligament, and (**d**) lateral collateral ligament injury on MRI. Therefore, we performed ACL & LCL reconstruction and MCL repair

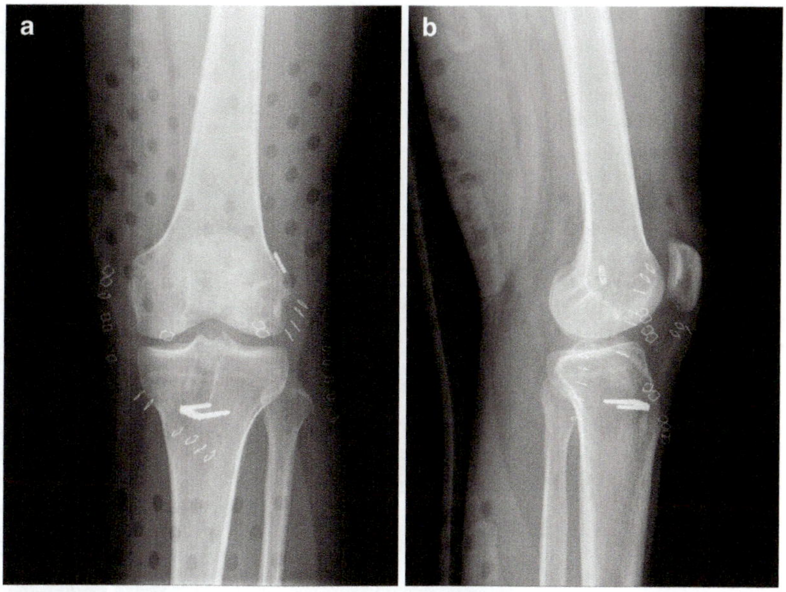

Fig. 3.34 (**a, b**) These are the postoperative images

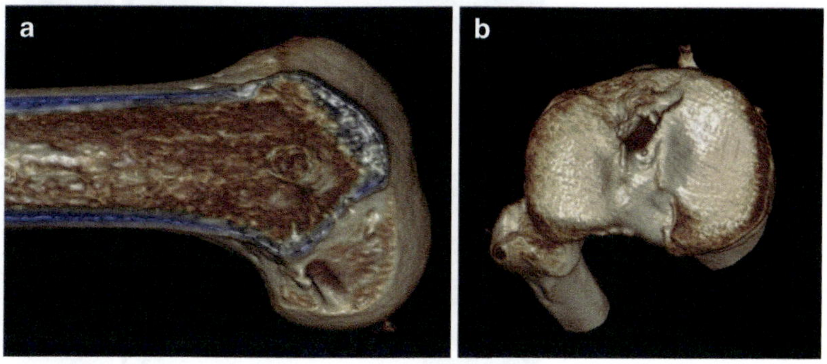

Fig. 3.35 (**a, b**) Post-OP 3D CT showing good location of the rectangular tunnel of the femur and tibia. A well-aligned rectangular tunnel was found

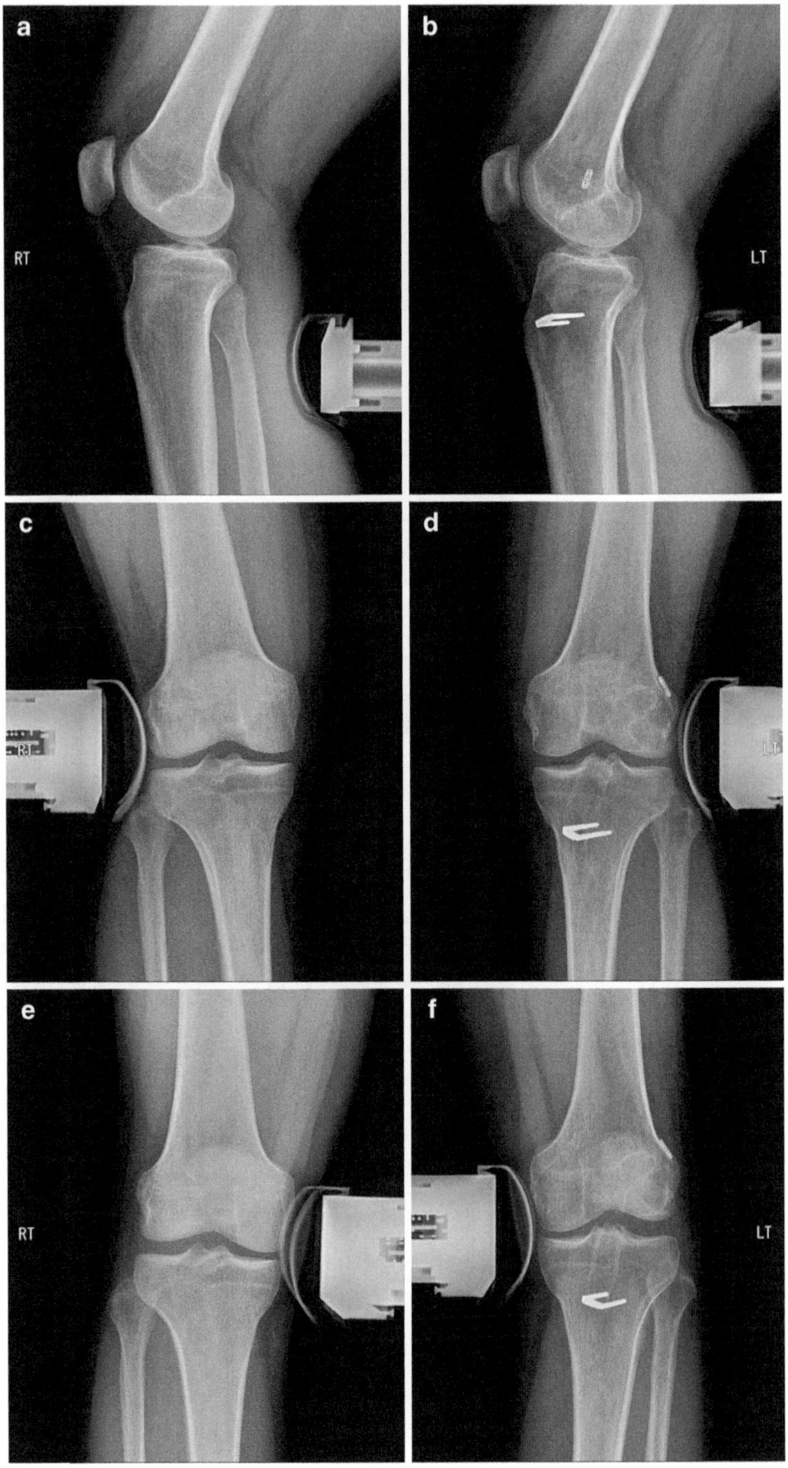

Fig. 3.36 13 months after ACL & LCL reconstruction, MCL repair. (**a**, **b**) Pull view, (**c**, **d**) valgus stress view, and (**e**, **f**) varus stress view of both knees were taken. There is no instability in varus and valgus stress view. KT-2000 arthrometer maximum manual test (MMT); 8.5 mm right and 8.5 mm left were checked on physical examination

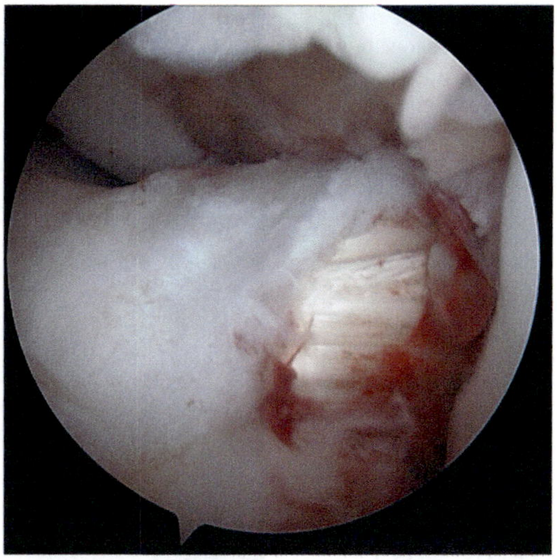

Fig. 3.37 Represents the arthroscopic findings after ACL reconstruction, with the remnant of the ACL being pulled out with sutures

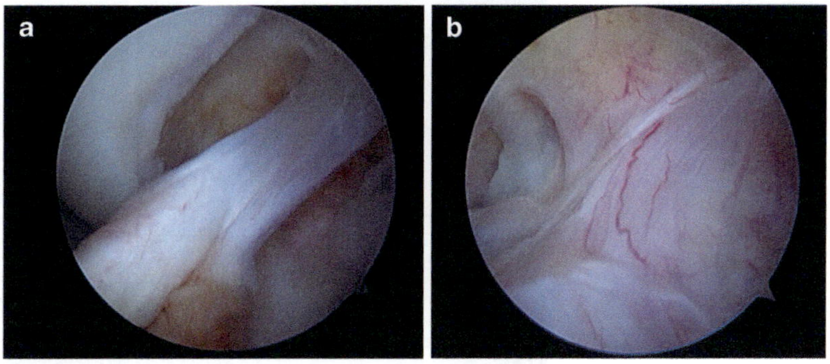

Fig 3.38 Well-synovialized ACL graft was found in second-look arthroscopy (post-op 1 year). (**a**) Ligamentum mucosum-like shape was shown (white arrow). (**b**) Well-synovialized ACL graft was shown in second look arthroscopy (post-op 1 year)

Case 3: ACL Rupture with Lateral Meniscus Bucket Handle Tear, Displaced

A 36-year-old male patient with a history of ACL reconstruction on his right knee injured his left knee 1 week ago. The pain was tolerable at first but became worse. Lachman test, pivot shift test, and varus and valgus test were positive, while dial test and posterolateral drawer test were negative on physical examination. KT-2000 arthrometer maximum manual test (MMT): 9 mm right, 13 mm left were checked (Figs. 3.39, 3.40, and 3.41).

In such cases, repair of the meniscus must be performed as soon as possible.

Therefore, we performed ACL reconstruction and lateral meniscus repair (Figs. 3.42, 3.43, and 3.44).

KT-2000 arthrometer maximum manual test (MMT); 10 mm right, 10 mm left (Fig. 3.45).

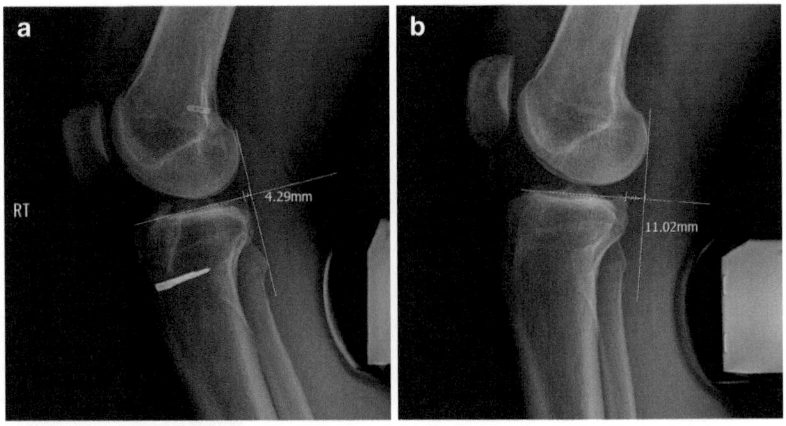

Fig. 3.39 (**a, b**) 6–7 mm side-to-side difference was checked compared to the unaffected side in the pull stress test imaging

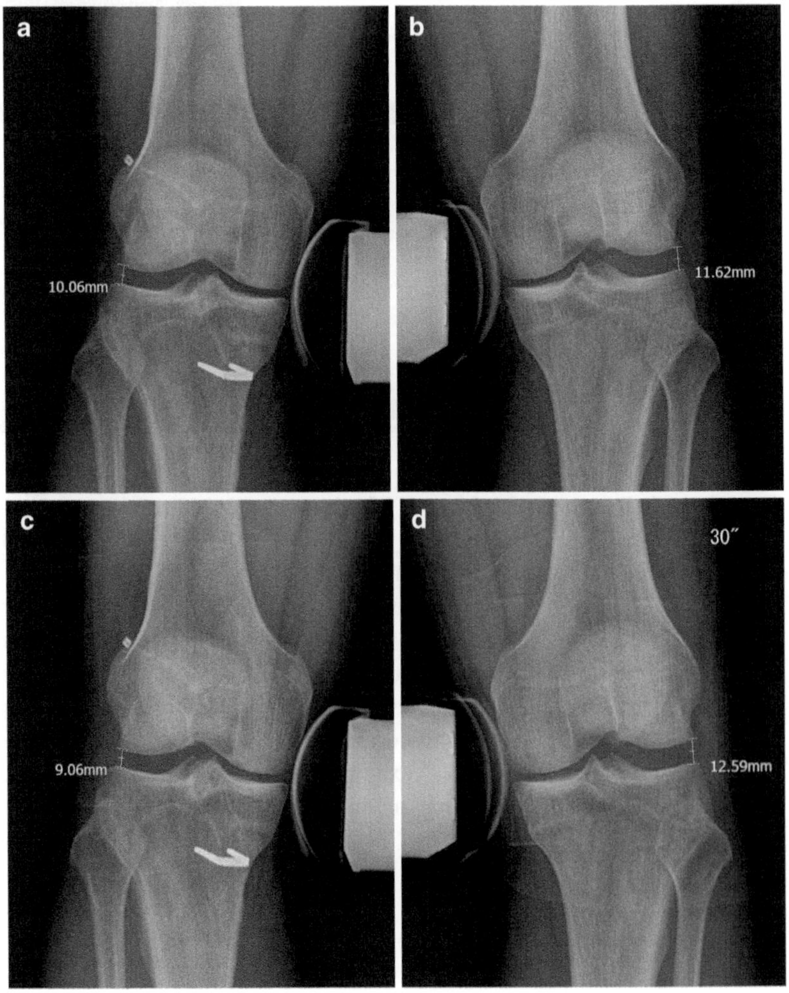

Fig. 3.40 (**a, b**) 0° varus stress view (**c, d**) 30° flexion, varus stress view; left knee lateral joint space is wider than right knee

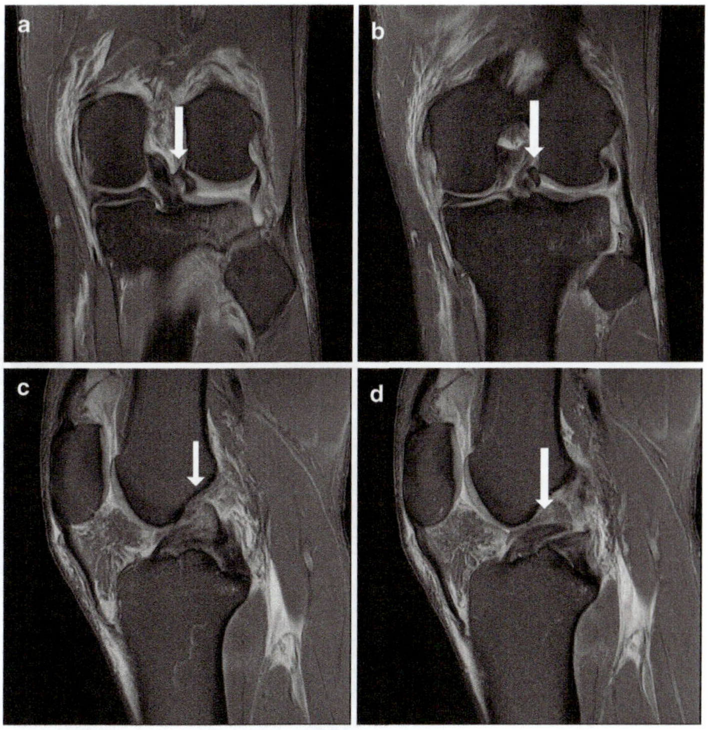

Fig. 3.41 (**a**, **b**) We found ACL rupture, a displaced bucket handle tear of the lateral meniscus on MRI coronal view, and a displaced fragment of the lateral meniscus in the intercondylar space. (**c**, **d**) Sagittal view

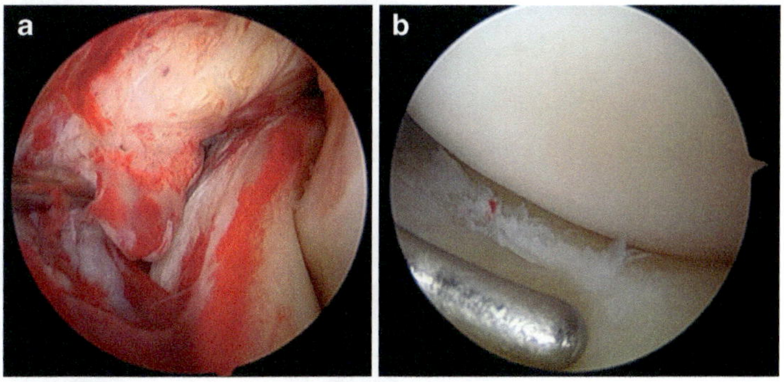

Fig. 3.42 (**a**, **b**) Intraoperative arthroscopic finding showing a displaced bucket handle tear of the lateral meniscus

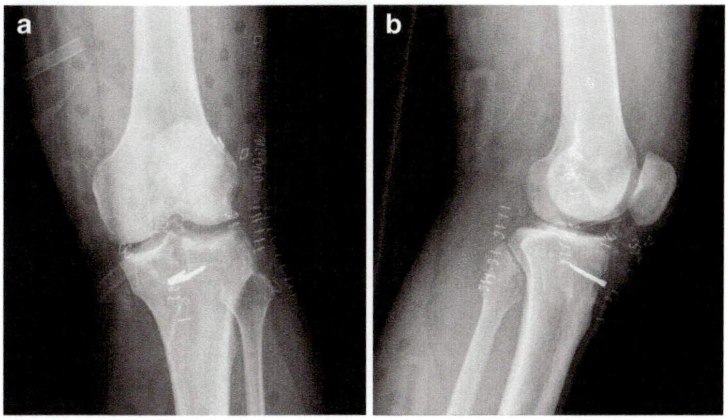

Fig. 3.43 (**a**, **b**) These are the postoperative simple X-ray images

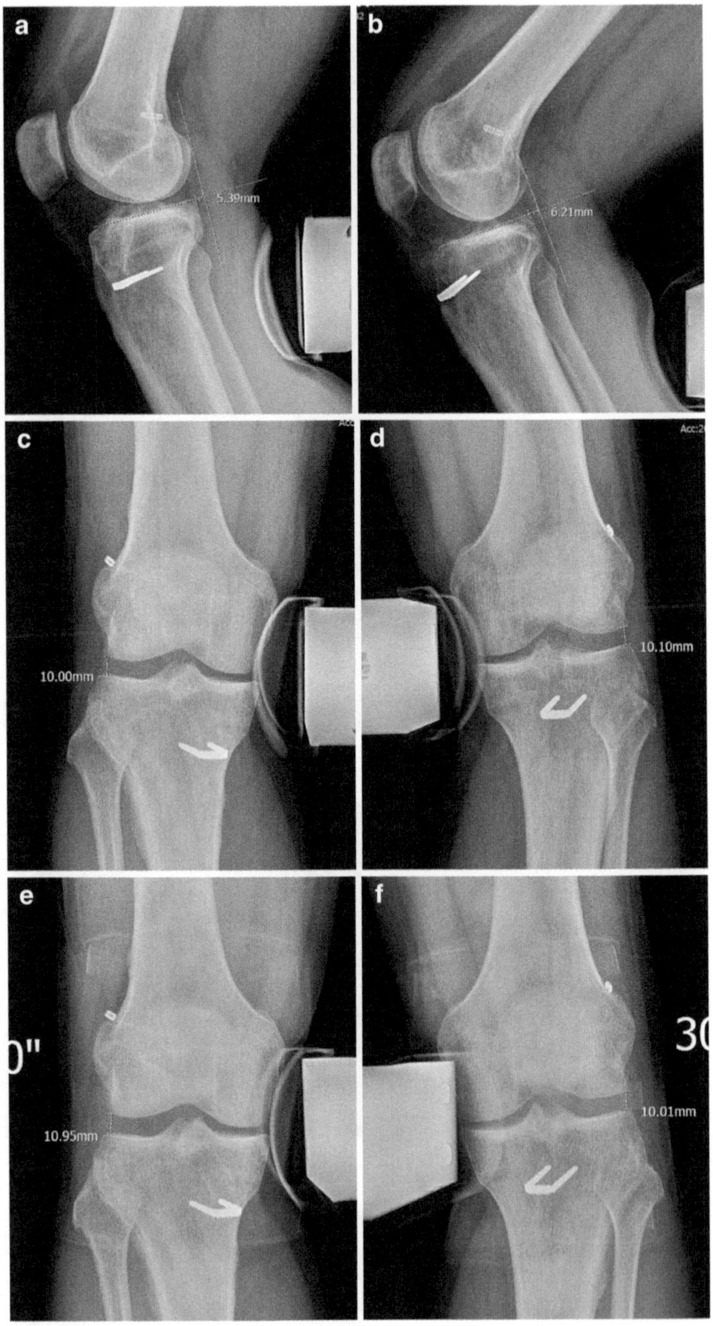

Fig. 3.44 Twelve months after ACL reconstruction and lateral meniscus repair. (**a**, **b**) Pull view (**c**, **d**) 0 varus stress, (**e**, **f**) 30° flexion varus stress view of the both knee. There is no instability were checked at stress view and on physical examination

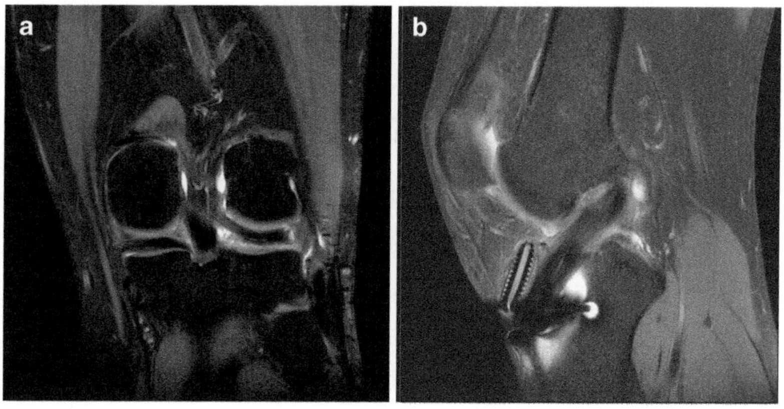

Fig. 3.45 (a, b) 12 months after ACL reconstruction and lateral meniscus repair, an F/U MRI was also taken, showing a well-preserved ACL graft and lateral meniscus

Case 4: Subluxated Lateral Meniscus with Radial Tear

In the text, we introduced the repair of radial tear using the all-inside technique. In this case, the senior author would like to introduce to you our case of the repair of a radial tear of the lateral meniscus using the inside-out technique due to narrowing of the knee joint space.

A 21-year-old male patient with no history of knee problems presented to the outpatient clinic complaining of pain in his right knee. He had an injury to his right knee during a soccer game. Plain radiographs taken immediately after the injury were unremarkable, and physical examination revealed a positive McMurray's test and lateral joint line tenderness (Figs. 3.46, 3.47, and 3.48).

The patient's right knee pain improved significantly with a negative McMurray test and lateral joint line tenderness. After 5 months postoperatively, a follow-up MRI was taken, showing the partially healed state of the lateral meniscus (Fig. 3.47a–d).

Patient's right knee pain improved a lot with a negative McMurray test and lateral joint line tenderness.

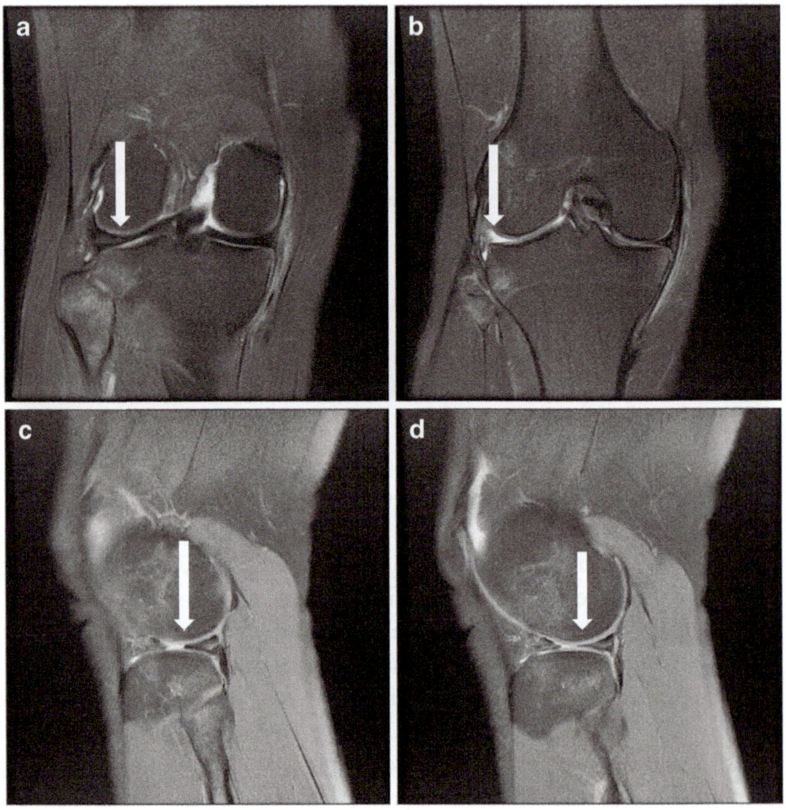

Fig. 3.46 (**a**, **b**) MRI findings showed a subluxed lateral meniscus and accompanied horizontal tear at the posterior horn, combined with a radial tear at the midbody of the lateral meniscus: coronal image of lateral meniscus radial tear with subluxation. (**c**, **d**) Sagittal image of the lateral meniscus, a blunt shape, which means a radial tear was shown

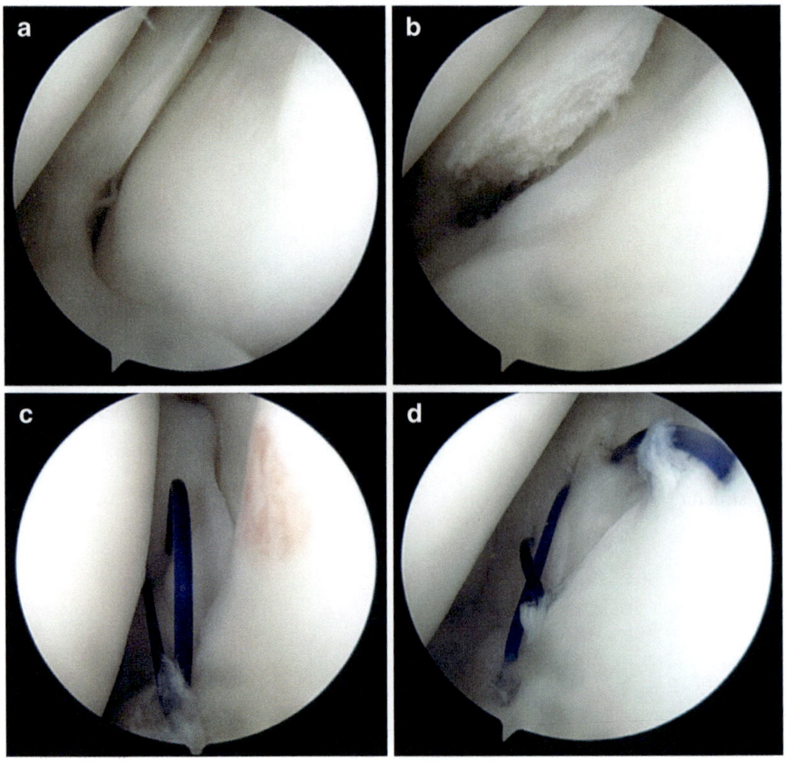

Fig. 3.47 These are the intraoperative arthroscopic findings. (**a**) Arthroscopic findings also showed some connection between the radial tear site of the lateral meniscus. (**b**) After resecting some healing tissue, which was elongated and caused subluxation of the middle body of the lateral meniscus, including radial tear. (**c**, **d**) We performed meniscus repair using the inside-out technique with No. 1-0 PDS

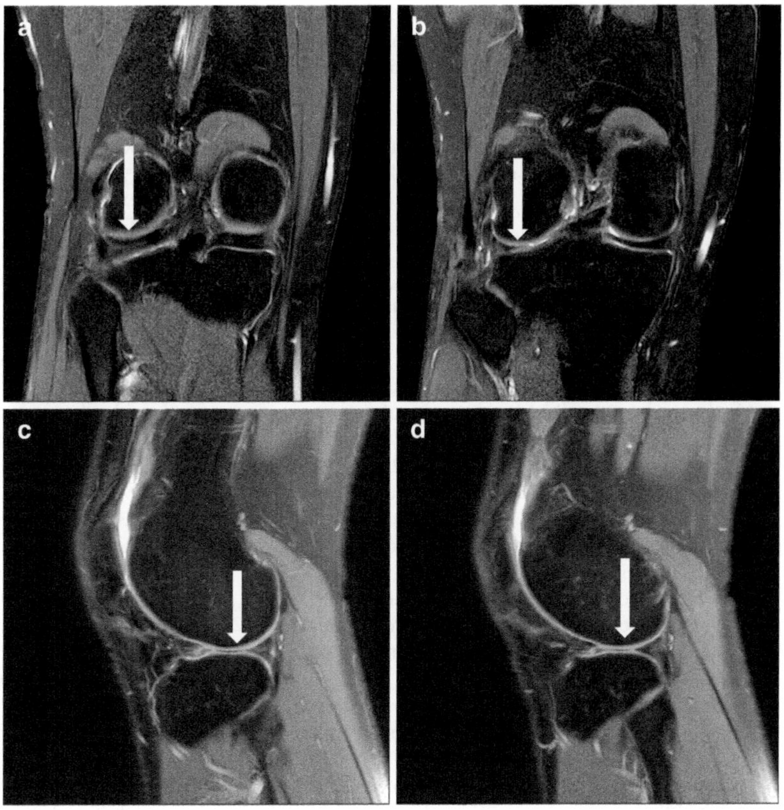

Fig. 3.48 (**a–d**) After 5 months postoperatively, a follow-up MRI was performed, showing a partially healed condition of the lateral meniscus. There was no subluxation of the lateral meniscus in the anteroposterior view

Further Reading

1. Kim SH, Jung YB, Song MK, et al. Comparison of double bundle anterior cruciate ligament (ACL) reconstruction and single-bundle reconstruction with remnant pull-out suture. Knee Surg Sports Traumatol Arthrosc. 2014;22:2085–93.
2. van Eck CF, Lesniak BP, Schreiber VM, Fu FH. Anatomic single- and double-bundle anterior cruciate ligament reconstruction flowchart. Arthroscopy. 2010;26:258–68.
3. Tashman S, Collon D, Anderson K, Kolowich P, Anderst W. Abnormal rotational knee motion during running after anterior cruciate ligament reconstruction. Am J Sports Med. 2004;32:975–83.
4. Van der Watt L, Khan M, Rothrauff BB, et al. The structure and function of the anterolateral ligament of the knee: a systematic review. Arthroscopy. 2015;31:569–582.e563.
5. Park YB, Lee HJ, Ro DH, Lee GY, Kim S, Kim SH. Anterolateral ligament injury has a synergic impact on the anterolateral rotatory laxity in acute anterior cruciate ligament-injured knees. Knee Surg Sports Traumatol Arthrosc. 2019;27:3334–44.
6. Ahn JH, Patel NA, Lin CC, Lee TQ. The anterolateral ligament of the knee joint: a review of the anatomy, biomechanics, and anterolateral ligament surgery. Knee Surg Relat Res. 2019;31:12.
7. Mochizuki T, Muneta T, Nagase T, Shirasawa S, Akita KI, Sekiya I. Cadaveric knee observation study for describing anatomic femoral tunnel placement for two-bundle anterior cruciate ligament reconstruction. Arthroscopy. 2006;22:356–61.
8. Iwahashi T, Shino K, Nakata K, et al. Direct anterior cruciate ligament insertion to the femur assessed by histology and 3-dimensional volume-rendered computed tomography. Arthroscopy. 2010;26:S13–20.
9. Smigielski R, Zdanowicz U, Drwiega M, Ciszek B, Ciszkowska-Lyson B, Siebold R. Ribbon like appearance of the midsubstance fibres of the anterior cruciate ligament close to its femoral insertion site: a cadaveric study including 111 knees. Knee Surg Sports Traumatol Arthrosc. 2015;23:3143–50.
10. Smigielski R, Zdanowicz U, Drwiega M, Ciszek B, Williams A. The anatomy of the anterior cruciate ligament and its relevance to the technique of reconstruction. Bone Joint J. 2016;98-B(8) https://doi.org/10.1302/0301-620X.98B8.37117. Instructional review: Knee Published Online:1 Aug 2016

11. Noailles T, Boisrenoult P, Sanchez M, Beaufils P, Pujol N. Torsional appearance of the anterior cruciate ligament explaining "ribbon" and double-bundle concepts: a cadaver-based study. Arthroscopy. 2017;33:1703–9.
12. Tashiro Y, Lucidi GA, Gale T, et al. Anterior cruciate ligament tibial insertion site is elliptical or triangular shaped in healthy young adults: high-resolution 3-T MRI analysis. Knee Surg Sports Traumatol Arthrosc. 2018;26:485–90.
13. Siebold R, Schuhmacher P, Fernandez F, et al. Flat midsubstance of the anterior cruciate ligament with tibial "C"-shaped insertion site. Knee Surg Sports Traumatol Arthrosc. 2015;23:3136–42.
14. Guenther D, Irarrázaval S, Nishizawa Y, et al. Variation in the shape of the tibial insertion site of the anterior cruciate ligament: classification is required. Knee Surg Sports Traumatol Arthrosc. 2017;25:2428–32.
15. Nakase J, Toratani T, Kosaka M, et al. Technique of anatomical single bundle ACL reconstruction with rounded rectangle femoral dilator. Knee. 2016;23:91–6.
16. Shino K, Mae T, Tachibana Y. Anatomic ACL reconstruction: rectangular tunnel/bone-patellar tendon-bone or triple-bundle/semitendinosus tendon grafting. J Orthop Sci. 2015;20:457–68.
17. Takata Y, Nakase J, Numata H, Oshima T, Tsuchiya H. Computed tomography value and tunnel enlargement of round and rounded rectangular femoral bone tunnel for anterior cruciate ligament reconstruction. Arch Orthop Trauma Surg. 2016;136:1587–94.
18. Herbort M, Tecklenburg K, Zantop T, et al. Single-bundle anterior cruciate ligament reconstruction: a biomechanical cadaveric study of a rectangular quadriceps and bone patellar tendon-bone graft configuration versus around hamstring graft. Arthroscopy. 2013;29:1981–90.
19. Lee BH, Bansal S, Park SH, Wang JH. Eccentric graft positioning within the femoral tunnel aperture in anatomic double-bundle anterior cruciate ligament reconstruction using the transportal and outside-in techniques. Am J Sports Med. 2015;43:1180–8.
20. Taketomi S, Inui H, Sanada T, Yamagami R, Tanaka S, Nakagawa T. Eccentric femoral tunnel widening in anatomic anterior cruciate ligament reconstruction. Arthroscopy. 2014;30:701–9.
21. Okimura S, Shino K, Nakagawa S, Iuchi R, Take Y, Mae T. Minimal tibial tunnel enlargement after anatomic rectangular tunnel anterior cruciate ligament reconstruction with bone-patellar tendon-bone graft. J Orthop Sci. 2020;25:635–9.
22. Shino K, Nakata K, Nakamura N, et al. Rectangular tunnel double-bundle anterior cruciate ligament reconstruction with bone-patellar tendon-bone graft to mimic natural fiber arrangement. Arthroscopy. 2008;24:1178–83.
23. Tachibana Y, Mae T, Shino K, et al. Femoral tunnel enlargement after anatomic anterior cruciate ligament reconstruction: bone-patellar tendon-bone/single rectangular tunnel versus hamstring tendon/double tunnels. J Orthop Sci. 2018;23:1011–8.
24. Suzuki T, Shino K, Nakagawa S, et al. Early integration of a bone plug in the femoral tunnel in rectangular tunnel ACL reconstruction with a bone-patellar tendon-bone graft: a prospective computed tomography analysis. Knee Surg Sports Traumatol Arthrosc. 2011;19:S29–35.
25. Suzuki T, Shino K, Otsubo H, et al. Biomechanical comparison between the rectangular-tunnel and the round-tunnel anterior cruciate ligament reconstruction procedures with a bone-patellar tendon-bone graft. Arthroscopy. 2014;30:1294–302.
26. Tachibana Y, Shino K, Mae T, Iuchi R, Take Y, Nakagawa S. Anatomical rectangular tunnels identified with the arthroscopic landmarks result in excellent outcomes in ACL reconstruction with a BTB graft. Knee Surg Sports Traumatol Arthrosc. 2019:2680–90.
27. Hayashi H, Kurosaka D, Saito M, et al. Positioning the femoral bone socket and the tibial bone tunnel using a rectangular retro-dilator in anterior cruciate ligament reconstruction. PLoS One. 2019;14:e0215778.
28. Kim SH, Park YB, Ham DW, Lim JW, Lee HJ. Stress radiography at 30 degrees of knee flexion is a reliable evaluation tool for high-grade rotatory laxity in complete ACL-injured knees. Knee Surg Sports Traumatol Arthrosc. 2020;28:2233–44.
29. Lee HJ, Park YB, Kim SH. Diagnostic value of stress radiography and arthrometer measurement for anterior instability in anterior cruciate ligament injured knees at different knee flexion position. Arthroscopy. 2019;35:1721–32.
30. Collins NJ, Misra D, Felson DT, Crossley KM, Roos EM. Measures of knee function: International Knee Documentation Committee (IKDC) Subjective Knee Evaluation Form, Knee Injury and Osteoarthritis Outcome Score(KOOS), Knee Injury and Osteoarthritis Outcome Score Physical Function Short Form (KOOS-PS), Knee Outcome Survey Activities of Daily Living Scale (KOS-ADL), Lysholm Knee Scoring Scale, Oxford Knee Score (OKS),Western Ontario and McMaster Universities Osteoarthritis Index (WOMAC), Activity Rating Scale (ARS), and Tegner Activity Score (TAS). Arthritis Care Res. 2011;63(Suppl 11):S208–28.
31. Feucht MJ, Mauro CS, Brucker PU, Imhoff AB, Hinterwimmer S. The role of the tibial slope in sustaining and treating anterior cruciate ligament injuries. Knee Surg Sports Traumatol Arthrosc. 2013;21:134–45.
32. Jung YB, Jung HJ, Siti HT, et al. Comparison of anterior cruciate ligament reconstruction with preservation only versus remnant tensioning technique. Arthroscopy. 2011;27:1252–8.
33. Mariscalco MW, Flanigan DC, Mitchell J, et al. The influence of hamstring autograft size on patient-reported outcomes and risk of revision after anterior cruciate ligament reconstruction: a Multicenter

Orthopaedic Outcomes Network (MOON) Cohort Study. Arthroscopy. 2013;29:1948–53.
34. Oshima T, Nakase J, Numata H, Takata Y, Tsuchiya H. The cross-sectional shape of the fourfold semitendinosus tendon is oval, not round. J Exp Orthop. 2016;3:28.
35. Kim SH, Seo JH, Kim DA, Lee JW, Kim KI, Lee SH. Steep posterior lateral tibial slope, bone contusion on lateral compartments and combined medial collateral ligament injury are associated with the increased risk of lateral meniscal tear. Knee Surg Sports Traumatol Arthrosc. 2021;9:021–06504.
36. Wang HD, Gao SJ, Zhang YZ. Hamstring autograft versus hybrid graft for anterior cruciate ligament reconstruction: a systematic review. Am J Sports Med. 2020;48:1014–22.
37. Nakase J, et al. Clinical study of anatomical ACL reconstruction using a rounded rectangular dilator. BMC Musculoskelet Disord. 2021;22:38.
38. Kim BS, Kim JH, Park YB, RO DH, Jung YB, Pujol N, Kim SH. No differences in clinical outcomes between rectangular and round tunnel techniques for anterior crucial ligament reconstruction. Arthroscopy. 2022;38:1–11.
39. Shao JY, Zhang JH, Ao YF. Better coverage of the ACL tibial footprint and less injury to the anterior root of the lateral meniscus using a rounded-rectangular tibial tunnel in ACL. Reconstruction: a cadaveric study. Orthop J Sports Med. 2022;10(3)
40. Ahn JH, Bae TS, Kang KS, Kang SY, Lee SH. Longitudinal tear of the medial meniscus posterior horn in the anterior cruciate ligament-deficient knee significantly influences anterior stability. Am J Sports Med. 2011;39(10):2187–93.
41. Ahn JH, Kim SH, Yoo JC, Wang JH. All-inside suture technique using two posteromedial portals in a medial meniscus posterior horn tear. Arthroscopy. 2004;20(1):101–8.
42. Ahn JH, Lee YS, Chang JY, Chang MJ, Eun SS, Kim SM. Arthroscopic all inside repair of the lateral meniscus root tear. Knee. 2009;16(1):77–80.
43. Ahn JH, Lee YS, Yoo JC, Chang MJ, Koh KH, Kim MH. Clinical and second-look arthroscopic evaluation of repaired medial meniscus in anterior cruciate ligament-reconstructed knees. Am J Sports Med. 2010;38(3):472–7.
44. Ahn JH, Lee YS, Yoo JC, Chang MJ, Park SJ, Pae YR. Results of arthroscopic all-inside repair for lateral meniscus root tear in patients undergoing concomitant anterior cruciate ligament reconstruction. Arthroscopy. 2010;26(1):67–75.
45. Kim SH, Seo HJ, Seo DW, Kim KI, Lee SH. Analysis of risk factors for ramp lesions associated with anterior cruciate ligament injury. Am J Sports Med. 2020;48(7):1673–81.
46. Kim SH, Seo JH, Kim DA, Lee JW, Kim KI, Lee SH. Steep posterior lateral tibial slope, bone contusion on lateral compartments and combined medial collateral ligament injury are associated with the increased risk of lateral meniscal tear. Knee Surg Sports Traumatol Arthrosc. 2022;30(1):298–308.

ACL Reconstruction with Anterolateral Ligament (ALL) Reconstruction or Lateral-Extra-Articular Tenodesis (LET)

4

Abstract

Graft ruptures are a major concern after anterior cruciate ligament(ACL) reconstruction. Reported rates vary from 1.4% to 18%, reflecting that the cause of re-ruptures is multifactorial. Graft choice has been extensively studied as a potential prognosticator of re-ruptures after primary reconstruction, but despite several randomized controlled trials and meta-analyses, no major difference has been demonstrated between the most common autograft types utilized. There were many attempts to prevent failure by drilling a more anatomic position of the femoral tunnel using either anteromedial or outside-in techniques or using the double-bundle technique. However, the majority of studies revealed that none of these methods reduced the rate of revision surgery. It is for this reason that there is currently great interest in the role of the anterolateral structures of the knee in controlling rotatory laxity and their ability to share loads with the ACL graft.

Several studies concluded that anatomical single-bundle reconstruction fails to confer control of rotational stability and does not reduce the risk of knee arthritis. Recently, light has been thrown on the ALL and its precise anatomy, which contributes to the rotator stability. Many surgeons now have many interests in ALL reconstruction and lateral extra-articular tenodesis (LET).

Many studies attempted to compare several outcomes between ACL reconstruction, ACL and ALL reconstruction, ACL reconstruction and LET procedure. Mogos et al. performed a prospective RCT, including 57 patients, to compare two groups (group 1, isolated ACL reconstruction; group 2, ACL reconstruction combined with ALL reconstruction). They found out that although there were no significant differences in anterior laxity, group 2 was statistically superior to group 1 in the residual pivot shift test and IKDC objective score. Also, there were no significant differences in associated lesions or complications between the two groups.

Porter et al. compared outcomes between the isolated ACL reconstruction group and the ACL reconstruction with LET group after 2 years of follow-up. The study revealed that the recurrence rate of the former one was lower than the other ($P < 0.001$). Also, although not statistically significant, residual pivot shift was lower in ACL reconstruction with the LET group.

Some authors say differently about performing LET with ACL reconstructions. Castoldi et al. performed an RCT, including 79 ACL rupture patients. After an average of 19.4 years of follow-up, the study compared

Y. B. Jung et al., *Treatment of the Cruciate Ligaments Injuries*,
https://doi.org/10.1007/978-981-95-9039-1_4

several outcomes between two groups (group 1, isolated ACL reconstruction; group 2, combined ACL reconstruction and LET). They found out that there were no significant differences in long-term outcomes but rather an increased risk of developing lateral compartment OA.

There are many complications, including infection, stiffness, arthrofibrosis, reoperation for removal of metal work, and over-constraint.

To evaluate the result of ALL reconstruction, Sonnery et al. performed an RCT, including 224 patients with a mean follow-up of 12.3 months. A significantly higher rate of reoperation for cyclops syndrome was noted in the isolated ACLR group compared with the combined ACL þ ALLR group (8.9% vs 0%, respectively; P ¼ 0.0012). No significant differences were found in

the frequency of graft rupture (ACLR, 5.4%; ACL þ ALLR, 0.9%; P ¼ 0.1191), range of motion deficits, pain, or reoperation for meniscectomy between groups. No cases of postoperative infection, venous thromboembolism, or arthrofibrosis were seen. Subjective IKDC (81.2 vs 86.8; $P = 0.0048$), Lysholm (88 vs 92; $P = 0.0131$), and some components of the KOOS were significantly better in the combined ACL and ALLR group.

Keywords

ACL reconstruction • Anterolateral ligament Lateral extra-articular

4.1 Principles of Treatment of Anterior Cruciate Ligament and Additional Anterolateral Augmentation

When ACL (anterior cruciate ligament) reconstruction is combined with lateral augmentation, such as lateral extra-articular tenodesis (LET) or anterolateral ligament (ALL) reconstruction, the main goal is to provide multi-planar stability to the knee. This combined approach aims to improve outcomes by addressing not just anterior-posterior stability (provided by the ACL) but also rotational stability (augmented by the lateral procedure).

The anterolateral ligament (ALL) is a ligament on the outside of the knee that contributes to rotational stability. It was anatomically defined fairly recently in the context of knee ligaments and is thought to work synergistically with the anterior cruciate ligament (ACL) to prevent abnormal rotation and translation of the tibia relative to the femur. ALL reconstruction aims to restore the stabilizing function of the native ALL, and this is often performed in conjunction with ACL reconstruction, particularly in patients with high rotational instability.

The principle behind ALL reconstruction is similar to that of other ligament reconstructions: to replace the damaged ligament with graft tissue that can eventually incorporate into the joint and provide stability.

Lateral extra-articular tenodesis (LET) is a surgical procedure often performed in conjunction with anterior cruciate ligament (ACL) reconstruction to improve knee stability, particularly in individuals with high rotational laxity or those who are at higher risk for graft failure. The procedure aims to reduce anterolateral rotational instability of the knee.

The main principle behind LET is to tighten the lateral (outer) structures of the knee to help control excessive rotational movement and augment the newly reconstructed ACL or the native ACL if it is still intact. This is often done using part of the iliotibial band (ITB) or another tendon graft.

4.2 Surgical Technique

Two lateral extra-articular procedure techniques will be introduced, including LET and combined ACL and ALL reconstruction.

The modified Lemaire lateral extra-articular tenodesis has been shown to reduce anterolateral rotatory laxity in the ACL-reconstructed knee and, hence, may be important to help reduce failure of ACLR in young patients returning to contact pivoting sports who are at a high risk of graft failure or in the revision ACLR scenario. The following indications were developed from a recent International ALC[Anterolateral Complex] Consensus Group Meeting and represent the current thinking as to when LET may be added to ACLR: revision ACLR, high-grade rotational laxity(a grade-2 or 3 pivot shift), generalized ligamentous laxity, or genu recurvatum of >10°, a young patient (<25 years old) returning to a contact pivoting sport.

LET is divided into six steps. The first step is the completion of ACLR. Pass, tension, and fix the ACL graft in a standard manner. When the ACLR is complete, we are ready to perform LET. The next step is a lateral skin incision. Position the leg with the knee at approximately 80° of flexion. Make a minimum 6 cm longitudinal incision 1 cm posterior to the lateral femoral epicondyle, starting 2 cm proximal to Gerdy's tubercle. If greater visualization is required, particularly in patients with abundant subcutaneous tissue, extend the incision proximally. Dissect the subcutaneous fat down to the iliotibial band(ITB) and sweep the fat posteriorly to identify the posterior border of the ITB, enabling palpation of Gerdy's tubercle distally (Fig. 4.1a).

The third step is the fashioning of the ITB graft. Harvest an 8 cm long by 1 cm wide strip of ITB from the posterior half of the ITB using a double blade, ensuring that the most posterior fibers of the deep ITB (capsule-osseous layer) remain intact (Fig. 4.1b). Leave the distal attachment at Gerdy's tubercle intact. Release the deep attachments to the vastus lateralis off the proximal 6 cm of the graft and place a whipstitch with Ethibond in the free end (Fig. 4.1c).

After fashioning the ITB graft, the formation of passage of the ITB graft will be the next step. When identification of FCL by palpation is done, make small capsular incisions anterior and posterior to the proximal portion of the FCL and place Metzenbaum scissors deep to the FCL from anterior to posterior to bluntly dissect out a tract for graft passage. Attempt to remain extracapsular, while ensuring there is no iatrogenic damage to

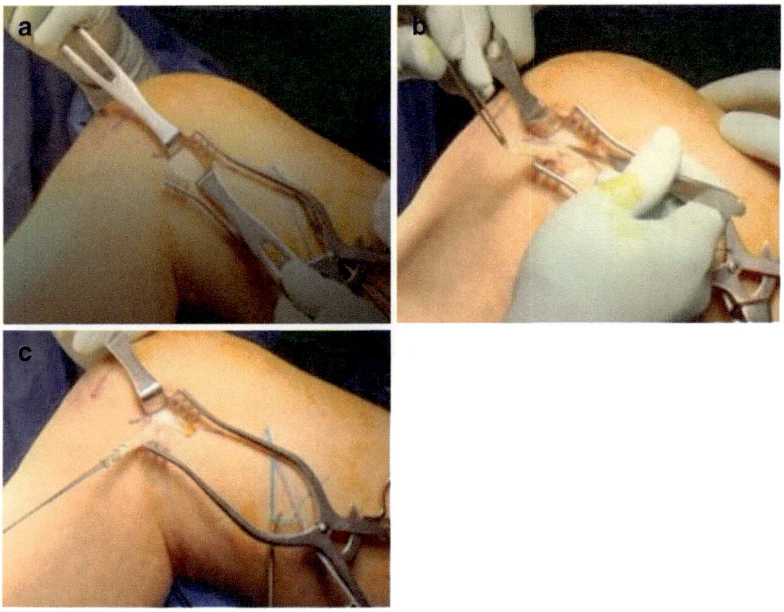

Fig. 4.1 (**a**) Lateral incision is placed just posterior to the lateral epicondyle, maintaining the knee flexed position at 90 degrees. The length of incision is approximately around 5 cm. (**b**) A strip of ITB is harvested from the middle to the posterior half of the ITB, making sure that the most posterior fibers of the deep ITB remain intact. Kaplan fiber should be preserved. The diameter of the ITB strip could be 10 mm, according to the leg size. (**c**) After releasing deep attachments to the vastus lateralis off the graft, place a whipstitch with Ethibond in the free end

the popliteus or FCL. Then, pass the ITB graft beneath the FCL from distal to proximal using a right-angled clamp. The author himself uses a slightly different method at this step. After experiencing knee stiffness, the LET author himself passes the ITB beyond the FCL rather than passing it deep to the FCL.

Fixation of the ITB graft to the femur is the fifth step. Using electrocautery, clear the lateral femoral supracondylar area of the small fat pad found proximal to the lateral head of the gastrocnemius. Cauterize the superior-lateral genicular artery, which may be found here, to avoid unwanted bleeding. (This is not necessary if not found.) Identify the attachment site just anterior and proximal to the lateral head of the gastrocnemius tendon, on the lateral metaphyseal flare of the lateral femoral condyle. Clear the periosteum using a Cobb elevator on the metaphyseal flare of the lateral femoral condyle. Insert the guide pin from lateral to medial femoral condyle (Fig. 4.2a). After forming the tunnel for the ITB graft, pass the ITB graft through the tunnel using a guide pin (Fig. 4.2b). When the graft is fixed into the tunnel, use the bio-screw for the final fixation (Fig. 4.2c). When inserting the bio-screw, maintaining the tension of the ITB graft is the crucial point.

When the above procedures are done, irrigate the wound; confirm hemostasis and closure of ITB, and closing the wound layer by layer will be the next and final step.

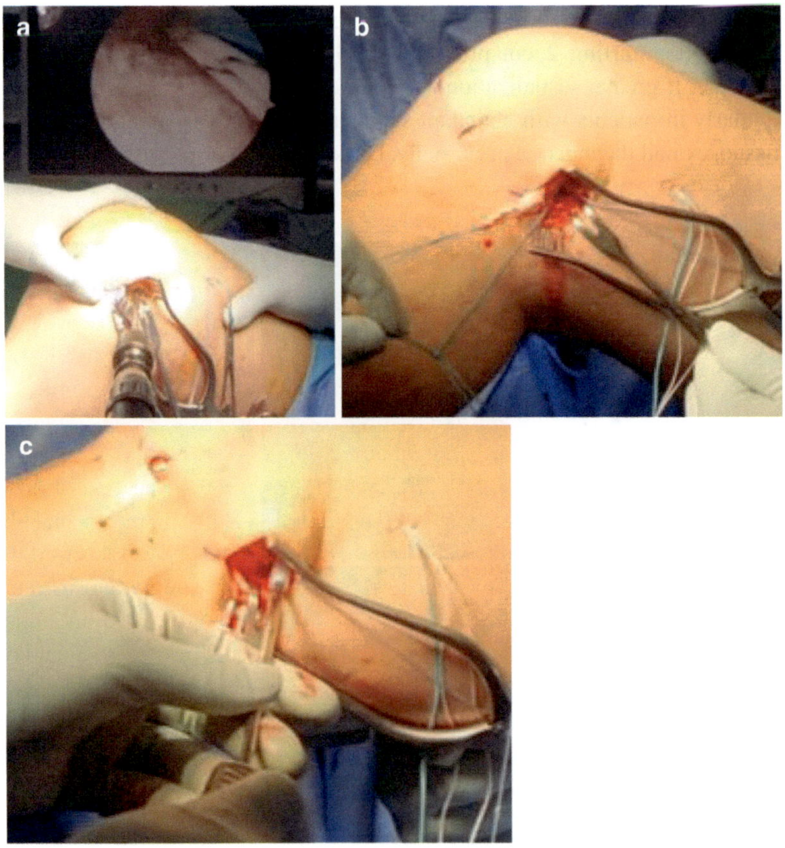

Fig. 4.2 (**a**) After identifying an adequate point of tunnel, drill the tunnel. The most appropriate position of the femoral tunnel is 1 cm proximal and 5 mm posterior to the lateral epicondyle. However, there is a risk of tunnel coalition between the ACL femoral tunnel and the lateral tenodesis femoral tunnel; the lateral tenodesis femoral tunnel could be transferred proximally with arthroscopic evaluation. (**b**) By using the guide pin, the ITB graft passes through the femoral tunnel. (**c**) After passing the ITB graft, fixation of the graft using a 7 mm bio-screw is done. The over-constrained graft should be avoided due to the increased risk of progression of osteoarthritis

Combined ACL and ALL reconstruction is a bit more complicated. The three bony landmarks are marked, namely, the head of the fibula, the Gerdy tubercle, and the lateral epicondyle (Fig. 4.3).

Two stab incisions, separated by roughly 2 cm, are made approximately 1 cm distal to the joint line between the Gerdy tubercle and the fibular head. One stab incision is made slightly posterior and proximal to the lateral epicondyle on the femur (Fig. 4.3). A 4.5-mm drill bit is then used to create a bony tunnel on the tibia, and the entrances to the tunnels are widened to ease the passage of the graft. The two tunnels are connected in a subcortical manner using a right-angled clamp. A suture or wire is then passed in a retroverted fashion to create a loop and ease graft passage (Fig. 4.4).

It is recommended that a small longitudinal incision be made on the femur to find the exact location for the femoral tunnel of ALL reconstruction and to avoid tunnel coalition between ACL and ALL femoral tunnels. The femoral tunnel for ALL was established on the 1 cm proximal and 1 cm posterior to the lateral epicondyle. During the femoral tunnel preparation, arthroscopic assessment of the ACL femoral tunnel through the anteromedial portal should be performed to avoid coalition of femoral tunnels between ACL and ACLL. If the risk of tunnel coalition seems to be high, a more proximal location of the ALL femoral tunnel would be recommended (Fig. 4.5a, b).

The femoral tunnel of ALL was established using the 7 mm reamer and fixed with a bio-screw. During fixation, the knee position was kept at 15° of flexion, and the small graspers could be used to adjust the tension of ALL graft (Fig. 4.6).

The knee is then taken through the range of motion to ensure a non-isometricity of the ALL graft that is tight in extension and slack in flexion.

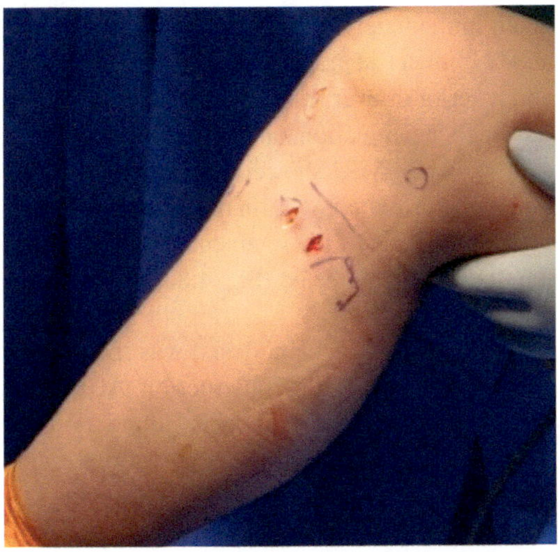

Fig. 4.3 As shown in the left knee (lateral view), three stab incisions are positioned in relation to the three bony landmarks for combined anterior cruciate ligament and anterolateral ligament reconstruction. One is placed on the femoral side, slightly proximal and posterior to the lateral epicondyle (LE). Two tibial stab incisions are subsequently positioned 8–10 mm below the joint line between the Gerdy tubercle (GT) and fibula head (FH)

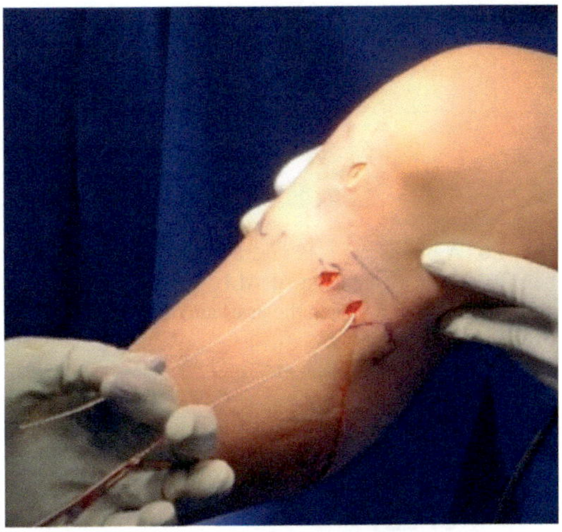

Fig. 4.4 As shown in the left knee (lateral view), two convergent bony tunnels are created through the tibial stab incision with a 4.5 mm drill. The two tunnels could be connected with a right-angled clamp. A wire is then passed in a retroverted fashion to create a loop for further anterolateral ligament graft passage

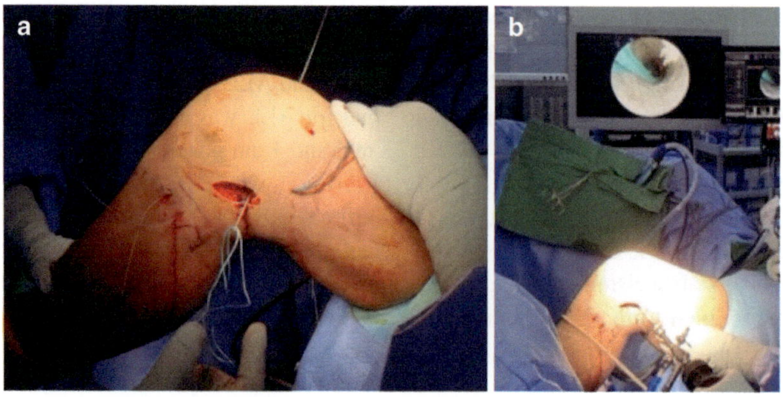

Fig. 4.5 (**a**) A femoral tunnel of anterolateral ligament reconstruction was established 1 cm proximal and 5 mm posterior to the lateral epicondyle. If finding the lateral epicondyle is difficult, it would be helpful to find the fiber of the lateral collateral ligament first. (**b**) During femoral tunnel establishment, an arthroscopic assessment of the femoral tunnel would be helpful to avoid tunnel coalition. If there is a risk of tunnel coalition, the proximal migration of the femoral tunnel could be performed due to similar isometry

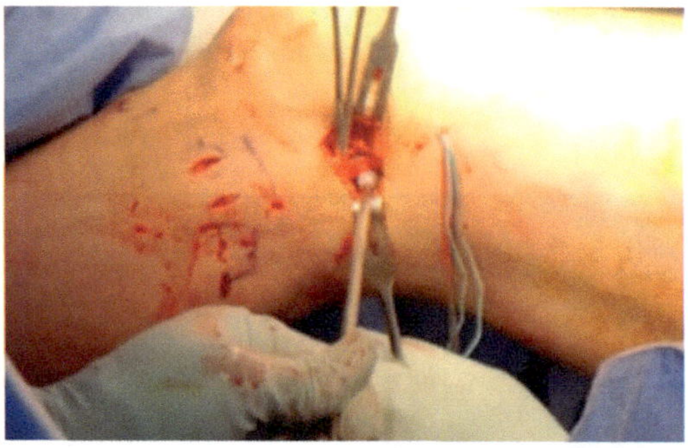

Fig. 4.6 A bio-screw was inserted into the femoral tunnel. To adjust the tension of ALL graft, small graspers could be inserted between the graft and the femur to avoid over-constraint

4.3 Cases of ACL Reconstruction with ALL Reconstruction or LET

Case 1: ACL Oval Reconstruction with LET

A 29-year-old female patient with no previous history of knee visited the outpatient department complaining of pain in her right knee. The symptoms began to occur after his left knee was twisted while doing Futsal 1 month ago. There were no specific findings on the plain radiograph taken immediately after the injury (Fig. 4.7a, b), and Lachman test grade 3, Pivot shift test grade 3, and anterior drawer test grade 2 were checked on physical examination and Telos stress view (Fig. 4.7c, d). MRI showed acute complete rupture in the proximal ACL. In the T2 signal sagittal plane, the shade of the ligament is increased and the fiber is disconnected (Fig. 4.8a, b).

Therefore, ALL tenodesis was performed along with A/S ACL reconstruction. ACL acute injury and complete tear were found on A/S, and ACL reconstruction was performed using oval-shaped tunneling (Fig. 4.9a–f) using TA tendon allograft, and ALL tenodesis was performed using a SwiveLock anchor (Figs. 4.10 and 4.11).

There was no discomfort in the patient's knee during outpatient follow-up after surgery, and laxity was not confirmed in the anterior drawer test and Lachman tests on physical examination. A 3D reconstructed femoral tunnel, an oval-shaped tunnel, was shown (Fig. 4.12a–f).

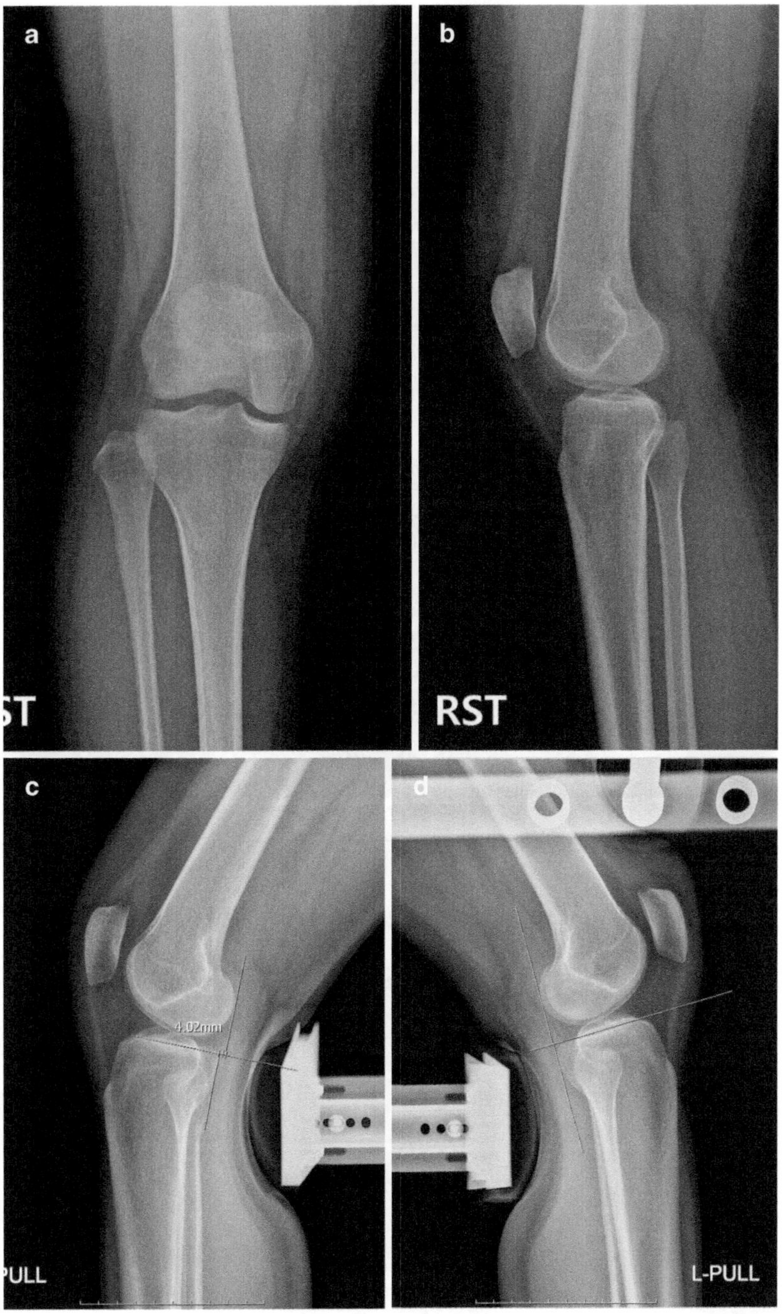

Fig. 4.7 (**a**, **b**) There were no specific findings on the plain radiograph taken immediately after the injury. (**c**, **d**) A 4 mm SSD (side-to-side difference) was checked compared to the unaffected side in the pull test imaging

Fig. 4.8 (**a**, **b**) MRI showed an acute complete rupture in the proximal ACL. (**b**) In the T2 signal sagittal plane, the shade of the ligament is increased, and the fiber connection is disconnected

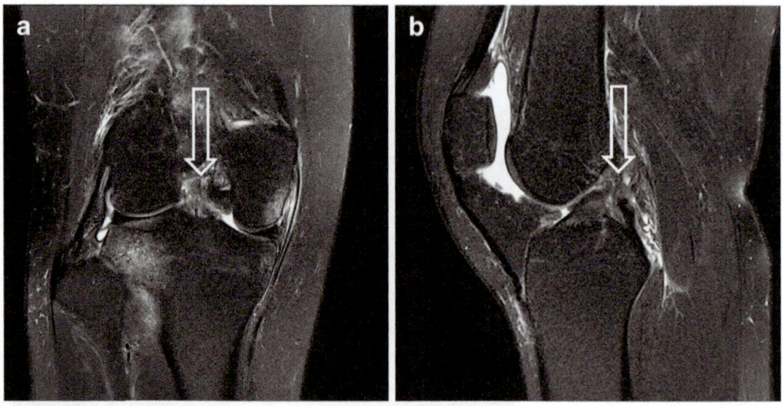

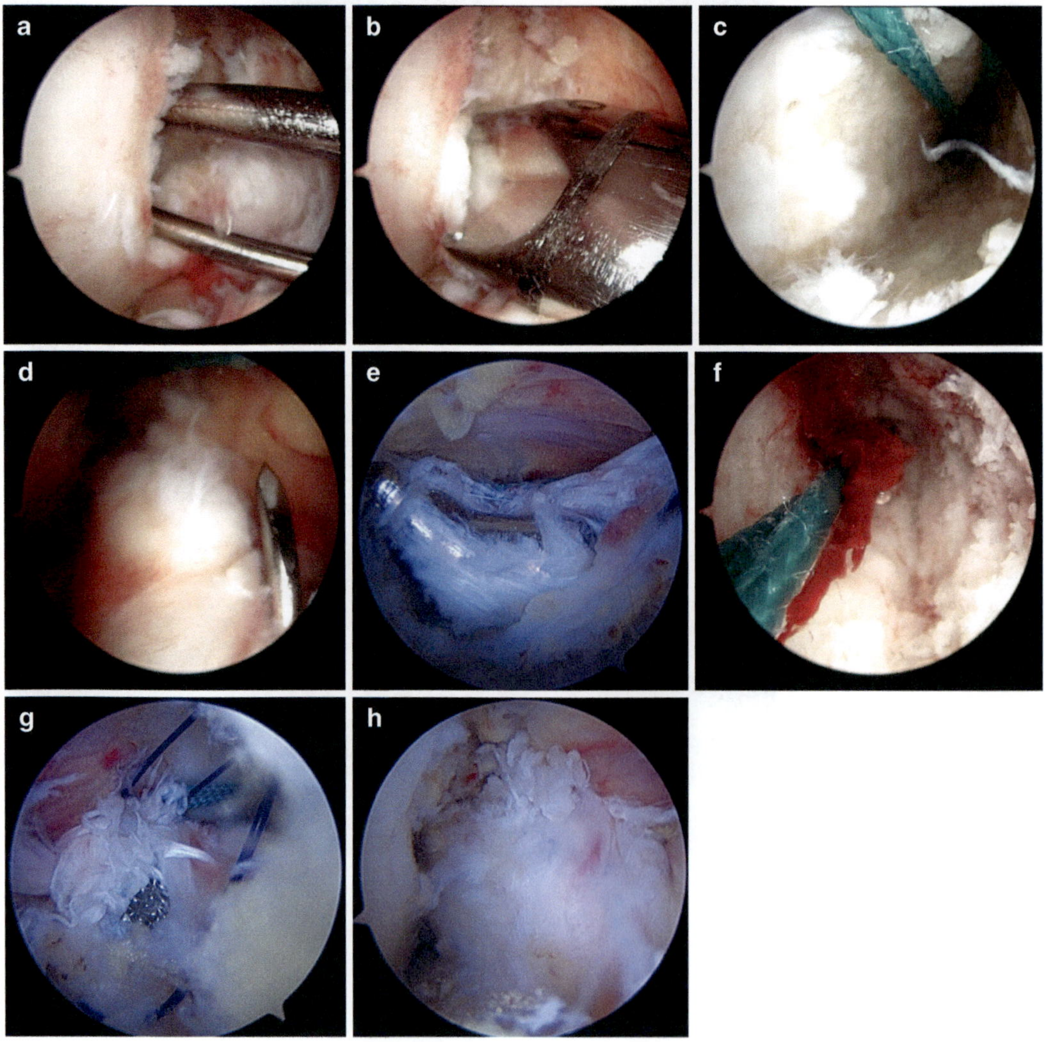

Fig. 4.9 (**a**) Formation of a femur tunnel using two guided oval-shaped dilator was shown. The additional guide pin would be helpful to locate the dilator in the appropriate direction. (**b**, **c**) Using the additional guide pin, the axes of the ACL femoral footprint and oval-shaped dilator could be aligned exactly. (**d**) Formation of a tibial tunnel using two guided oval-shaped dilators was shown. (**e**, **f**) Alike the femoral tunnel, an additional guide pin would be used to align the axes of the footprints and dilator. (**g**, **h**) ACL graft is well fixed with preservation and pullout of the ACL remnant fiber

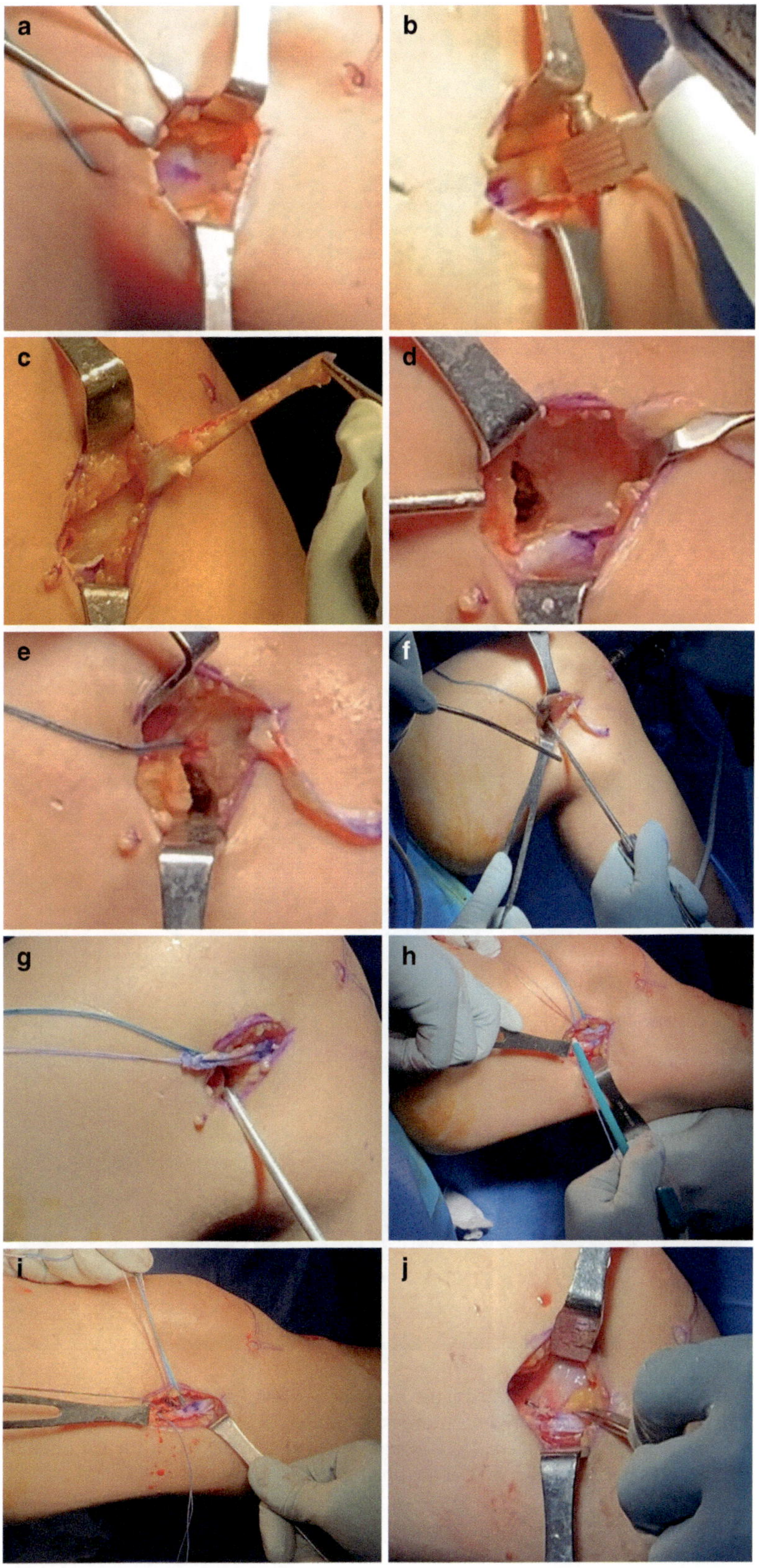

Fig. 4.10 (**a**) Intraoperative photos of the LET procedure were shown. A lateral incision is placed just posterior to the lateral epicondyle, maintaining the knee flexed position at 90°. (**b**, **c**) A strip of ITB is harvested from the middle to the posterior half of the ITB, making sure that the most posterior fibers of the deep ITB remain intact. Kaplan fiber should be preserved. The diameter of the ITB strip could be 10 mm, according to the leg size. (**d**, **e**) After releasing deep attachments to the vastus lateralis off the graft, place a whipstitch with Ethibond in the free end. (**f**–**h**) After evaluation of the risk of tunnel coalition, an anchor (SwiveLock, Arthrex) could be used to fix the femoral graft. (**i**, **j**) After finalization of the anchor fixation, a final adjustment of graft tension would be performed with an empty needle using the sliding suture of the anchor

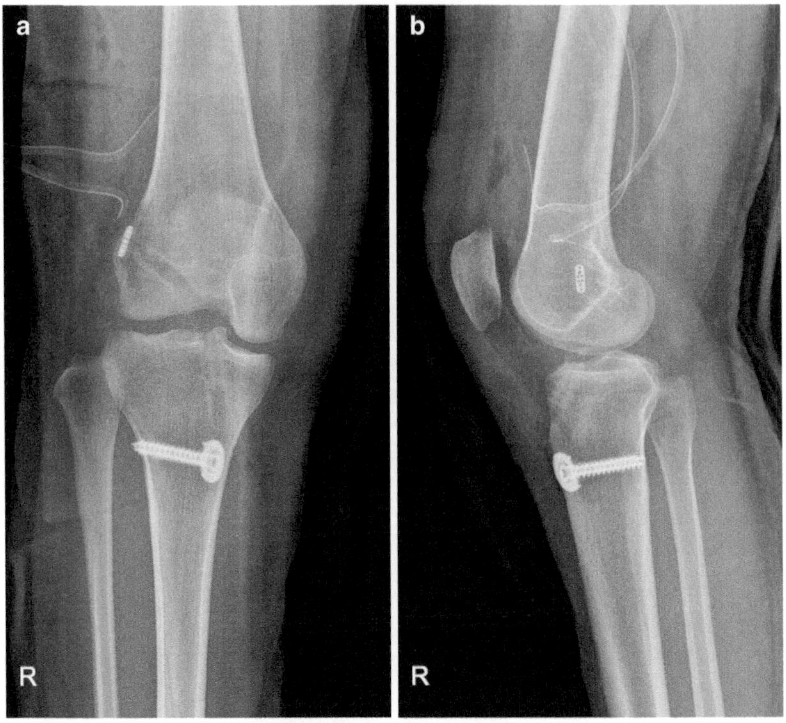

Fig. 4.11 These are the postoperative images (**a**) anterior-posterior view (**b**) lateral view

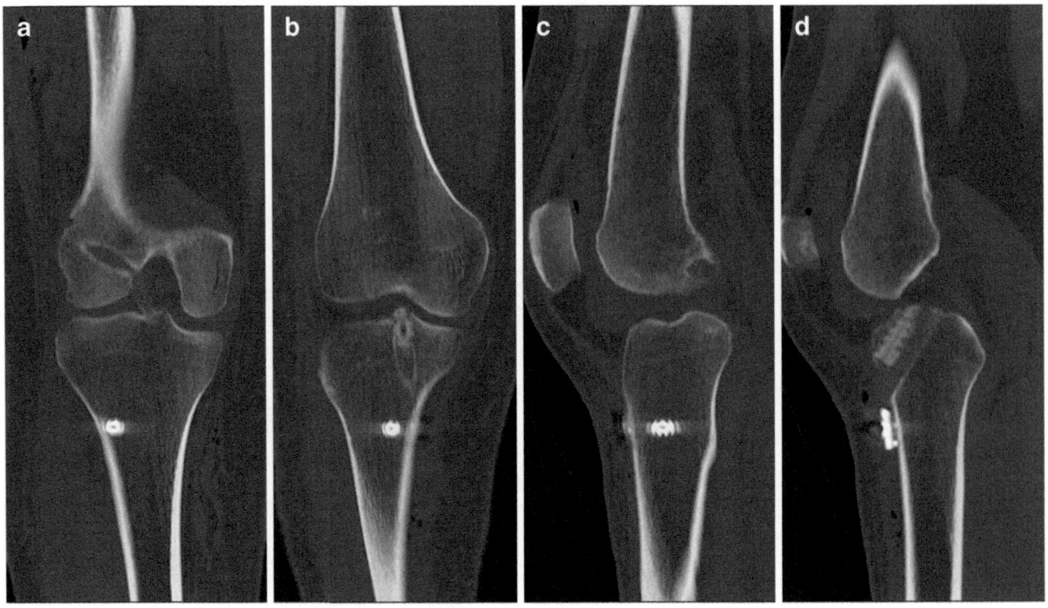

Fig. 4.12 A bone tunnel formed at the anatomical location of the ACL femoral origin was checked on the 3D CT image taken after surgery. (**a**) Coronal view of the femoral tunnel, (**b**) coronal view of the tibial tunnel, (**c**) and sagittal view of the femoral tunnel. Oval-shaped tunnel was shown (**d**) sagittal view of tibial tunnel, (**e**) 3D reconstructed tibial tunnel, oval-shaped tunnel was shown

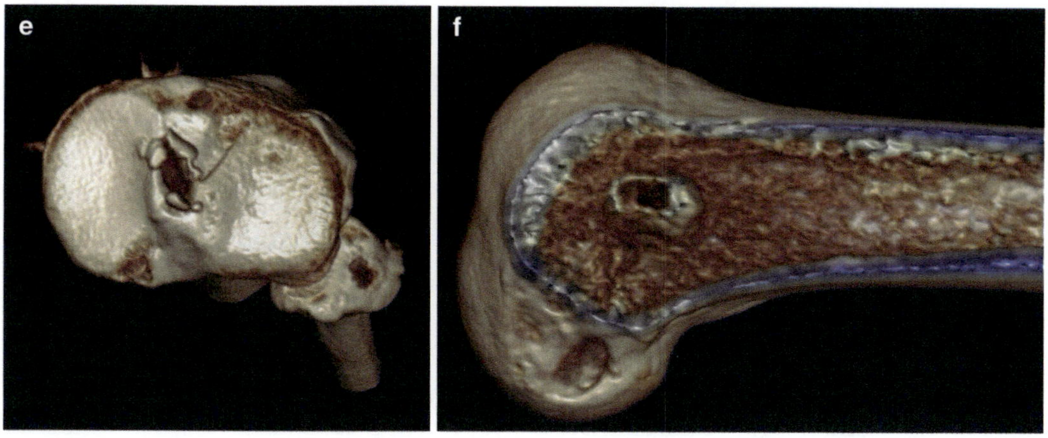

Fig. 4.12 (continued)

Case 2: ACL Oval Reconstruction with ALL Reconstruction

A 23-year-old female patient with no previous history of knee pain visited the outpatient department complaining of pain in her left knee. The patient is a Taekwondo master, and the symptoms began to occur after his left knee was twisted in the process of landing while doing Taekwondo 2 weeks ago. Lachman test grade 2, pivot shift test grade 1, and anterior drawer test grade 2 were checked on physical examination, simple radiography, and Telos stress view (Fig. 4.13a–d). The MRI showed an acute complete rupture in the proximal ACL. (B) In the T2 signal sagittal plane, the shade of the ligament is increased, and the fiber connection is disconnected (Fig. 4.14a, b).

Therefore, ALL reconstruction was performed along with A/S ACL reconstruction. ACL acute on chronic injury and complete tear were found on A/S; ACL reconstruction was performed using an oval-shaped tunneling using TA tendon allograft (Fig. 4.15a–h), and ALL recon was performed using an anchor (Figs. 4.16a–l and 4.17).

There was no discomfort in the patient's knee during outpatient follow-up after surgery, and laxity was not confirmed in the ADT and Lachman tests on physical examination and Telos stress view (Fig. 4.18a, b).

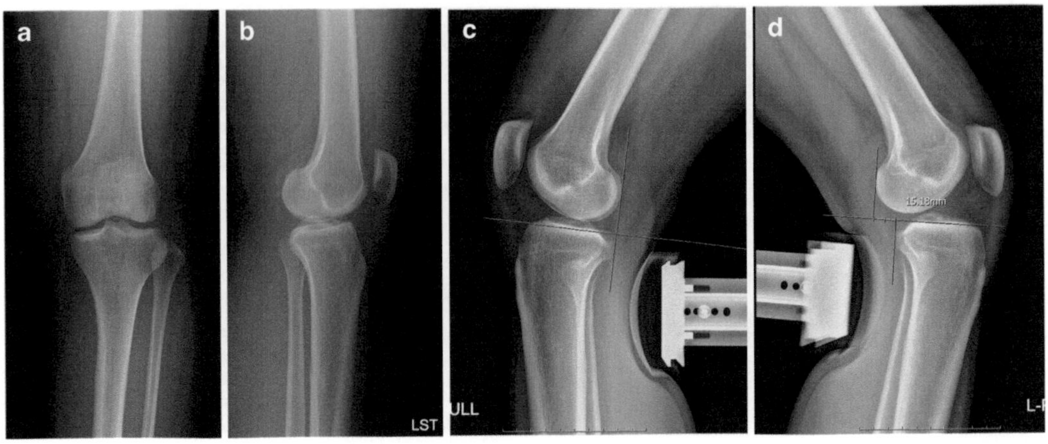

Fig. 4.13 (**a, b**) There were no specific findings on the plain radiograph taken immediately after the injury. Lachman test grade 2, pivot shift test grade 1, and anterior drawer test grade 2 were checked on physical examination. (**c, d**) A 15 mm SSD (side-to-side difference) was checked compared to the unaffected side in the pull test imaging

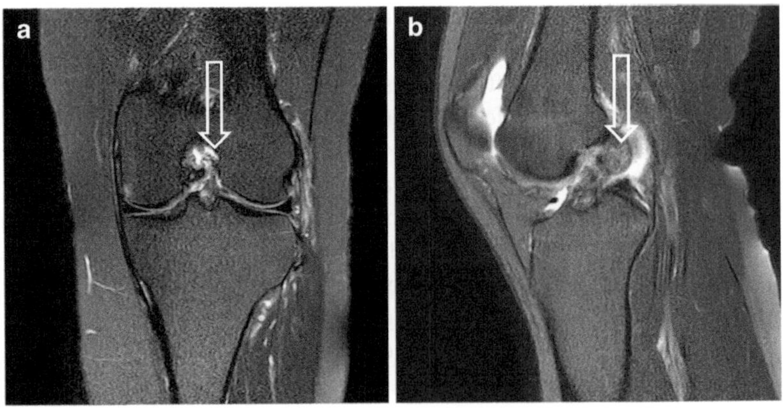

Fig. 4.14 (**a, b**) The MRI showed an acute complete rupture in the proximal ACL. (**b**) In the T2 signal sagittal plane, the shade of the ligament is increased, and the fiber connection is disconnected

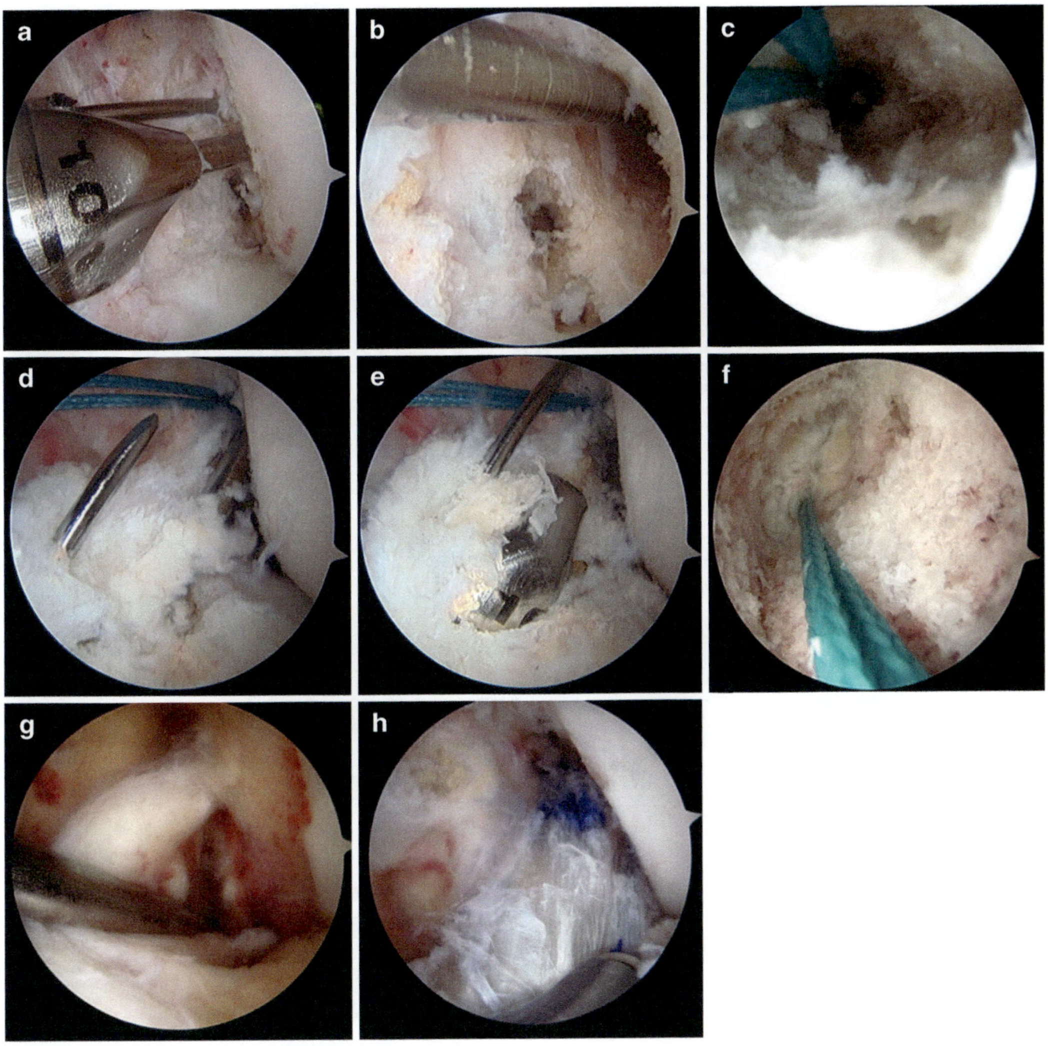

Fig. 4.15 (**a–c**) Formation of the femoral tunnel using two guided oval-shaped dilators was shown, as described previously. (**d–f**) Formation of the tibial tunnel using two guided oval-shaped dilators was shown, as described previously. (**g, h**) The preoperative and postoperative pictures of arthroscopy were shown. The twisted-ribbon-like appearance of the reconstructed ACL was shown

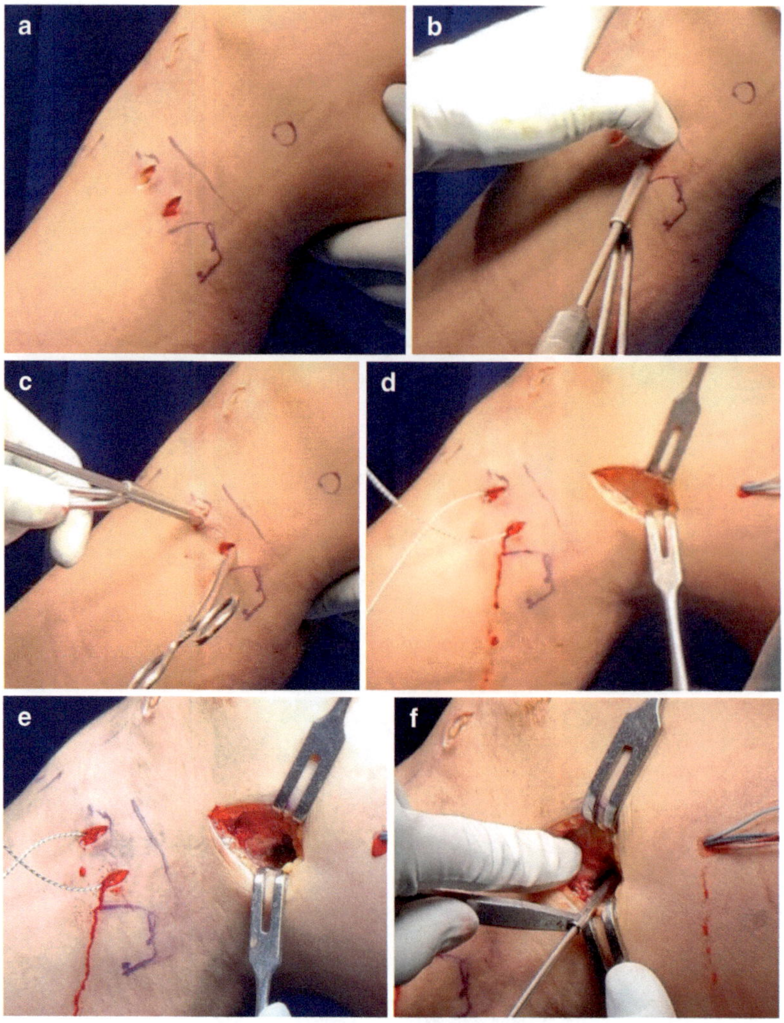

Fig. 4.16 Intraoperative photos of ALL reconstruction were shown. (**a**) As shown in the left knee (lateral view), three stab incisions are positioned in relation to the three bony landmarks for combined anterior cruciate ligament and anterolateral ligament reconstruction. One is placed on the femoral side, slightly proximal and posterior to the lateral epicondyle. Two tibial stab incisions are subsequently positioned 8–10 mm below the joint line between the Gerdy tubercle and fibula head. (**b**) Two convergent bony tunnels are created through the tibial stab incision with a 4.5 mm drill. The two tunnels could be connected with a right angled clamp. (**c**) A wire is then passed in a retroverted fashion to create a loop for further anterolateral ligament graft passage. (**d–f**) A femoral tunnel of anterolateral ligament reconstruction was established 1 cm proximal and 5 mm posterior to the lateral epicondyle. During femoral tunnel establishment, arthroscopic assessment of the femoral tunnel would be helpful to avoid tunnel coalition. If there is a risk of tunnel coalition, the proximal (upward) migration of the femoral tunnel could be performed due to similar isometry. (**g**) The diameter of the femoral tunnel would be appropriately around 7 mm, according to the graft diameter. (**h–k**) The final fixation was done using the bio-screw. (**l**) To adjust the tension of the ALL graft, small graspers could be inserted between the graft and the femur to avoid over-constraint

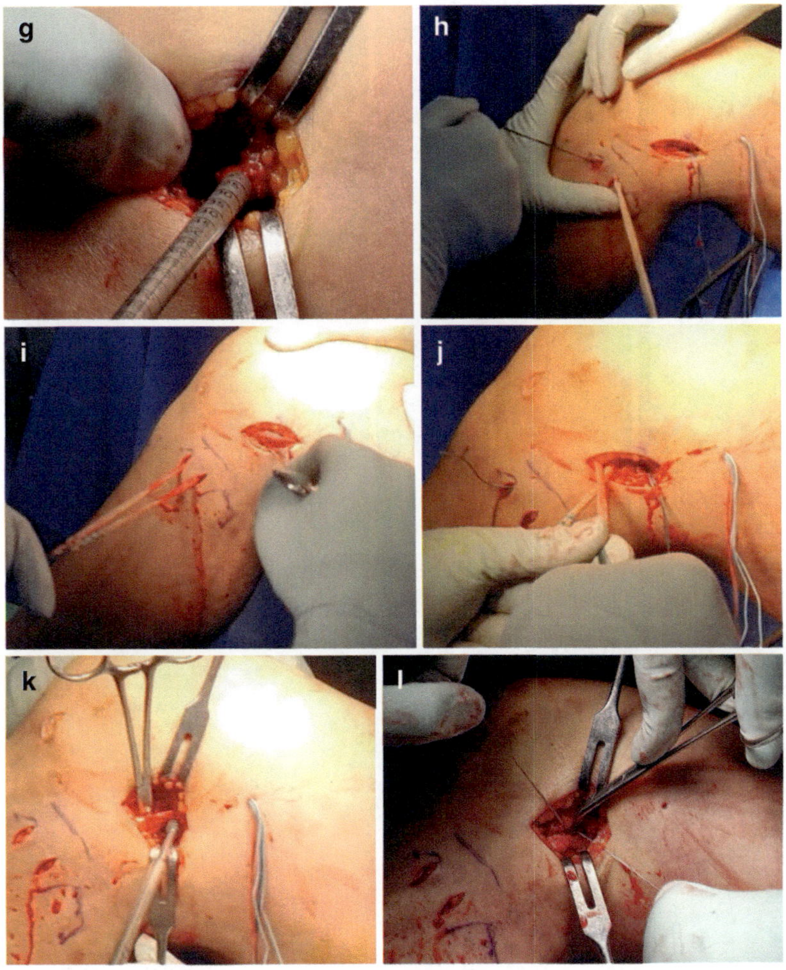

Fig. 4.16 (continued)

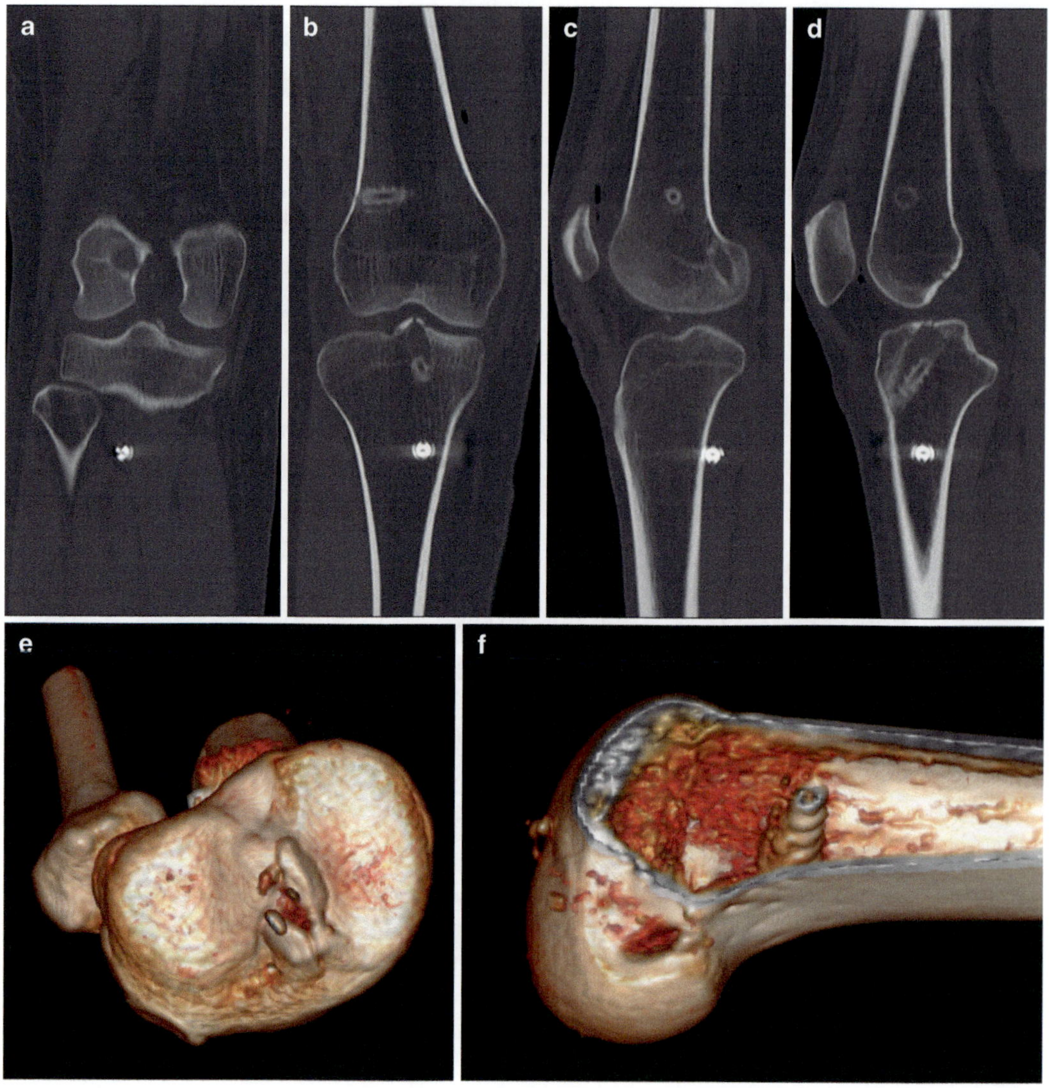

Fig. 4.17 A bone tunnel formed at the anatomical location of the ACL femoral origin was checked on the 3D CT image taken after surgery. Well-aligned footprints were shown. (**a**) Coronal view of the femoral tunnel. (**b**) Coronal view of tibial tunnel. (**c**) Sagittal view of femoral tunnel. Oval-shaped tunnel was shown. (**d**) Sagittal view of tibial tunnel. (**e**) 3D reconstructed tibial tunnel, oval-shaped tunnel was shown. (**f**) 3D reconstructed femoral tunnel, oval-shaped tunnel was shown

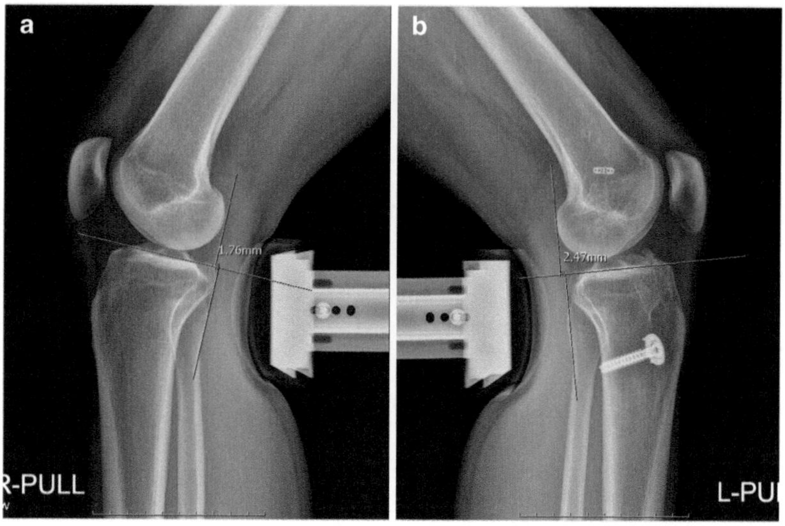

Fig. 4.18 (**a, b**) Compared to before the operation, the follow-up stress view showed a side-to-side difference (SSD) decrease (SSD, 1 mm)

References

1. Webster KE, Feller JA. Exploring the high reinjury rate in younger patients undergoing anterior cruciate ligament reconstruction. Am J Sports Med. 2016;44(11):2827–32.
2. Sonnery-Cottet, et al. Anterolateral ligament reconstruction is associated with significantly reduced ACL graft rupture rates at a minimum follow-up of 2 years. Am J Sports Med. 2017;45(7):1547–57.
3. Inghan SJM, de Carvalho RT, Martins CAQ, et al. Anterolateral ligament anatomy: a comparative anatomical study. Knee Surg Sports Traumatol Arthrosc. 2017;25(4):1048–54.
4. Vincent JP, Magnussen RA, Gezmez F, et al. The anterolateral ligament of the human knee: an anatomic and histologic study. Knee Surg Sports Traumatol Arthrosc. 2012;20(1):147–52.
5. Parsons EM, Gee AO, Spiekerman C, Cavanagh PR. The biomechanical function of anterolateral ligament of the knee. Am J Sports Med. 2015;43(3):669–74.
6. Mogos S, D'Ambrosi R, Antonescu D, Stoica I-C. Combined anterior cruciate ligament and anterolateral ligament reconstruction results in superior rotational stability compared with isolated anterior cruciate ligament reconstruction in high grade pivoting sport patients: a prospective randomized clinical trial. J Knee Surg. 2021;
7. Porter M, Shadbolt B, et al. Modified iliotibial band tenodesis is indicated to correct intraoperative residual pivot shift after anterior cruciate ligament reconstruction using an autologous hamstring tendon graft. Am J Sports Med. 2020;48(5):1069–77.
8. Castoldi M, Magnussen RA, et al. A randomized controlled trial of bone-patellar tendon –bone anterior cruciate ligament reconstruction with and without lateral extra-articular tenodesis. Am J Sports Med. 2020;48(7):1665–72.
9. O'Brien SJ, Warren RF, Wickiewicz TL, et al. The iliotibial band lateral sling procedure and its effect on the results of anterior cruciate ligament reconstruction. Am J Sports Med. 1991;19(1):21–4.

Anterior Cruciate Ligament Injury with PLRI

5

Abstract

Injuries to the posterolateral corner(PLC) structures can result in posterolateral rotatory instability (PLRI) of the knee, which is a pathological instability caused by posterolateral tibial subluxation when an external rotational force is applied to the knee joint. However, the diagnosis of PLC injury can be easily missed, unless there is a high level of clinical suspicion for possible injury to this region, so routine assessment of PLRI is necessary to make the correct diagnosis. The presence of PLRI was assessed by physical examination using the posterolateral drawer test and the dial test and by palpation of subluxation of the posterior tibial condyle by placing four small fingers on the posterolateral aspect of the popliteal fossa. Markolf et al. measured the force on a simulated intact ACL with and without the posterolateral knee structures and found that cutting the posterolateral structures increased the force on the ACL during varus loading.

LaPrade et al. examined the force on ACL grafts in cadaver knees in which the posterolateral structure had been selectively cut and found that grade III posterolateral injuries were associated with significantly increased force on ACL grafts. In addition, untreated posterolateral injuries were associated with graft failure in ACL and PCL reconstructions, highlighting the clinical importance of treating posterolateral injuries when other ligament injuries are present. More recently, anatomical reconstructions of the PLC have been shown to provide the best results when compared to other surgical techniques for the treatment of in the treatment of chronic posterolateral instability. However, a cadaveric biomechanical study by Apsingi et al. showed that anatomical PLC reconstruction did not outperform the single fibular sling technique. The varus bony malalignment and varus thrust gait should be corrected prior to surgical reconstruction of severe lateral and posterolateral ligament deficiencies. In chronic ACL defects, varus malalignment, medial meniscus loss, and partial to complete ACL insufficiency, a valgus tibial osteotomy should be performed first to avoid overloading the lateral capsular structures to be reconstructed. Therefore, patients with suspected PLC injury should be carefully monitored for limb alignment using full-length weight-bearing radiographs and changes in gait.

Keywords

PLRI · Posterolateral corner structures · Varus thrust gait · Chronic ACL deficiency

Supplementary Information The online version contains supplementary material available at https://doi.org/10.1007/978-981-95-9039-1_5.

Y. B. Jung et al., *Treatment of the Cruciate Ligaments Injuries*,
https://doi.org/10.1007/978-981-95-9039-1_5

5.1 Principles of Treatment of Anterior Cruciate Ligament and Posterolateral Instability

The importance of the posterolateral corner (PLC) structures in maintaining knee stability and their functional interaction with the cruciate ligaments has been better understood in recent years. Injuries to the PLC structures can lead to posterolateral rotatory instability (PLRI) of the knee, a pathological instability caused by posterolateral tibial subluxation when an external rotational force is applied to the knee joint.

These injuries do not usually occur in isolation but are often associated with an ACL injury. However, the diagnosis of a PLC injury can be easily neglected unless there is a high clinical suspicion for a possible injury to this region (Videos 5.1 and 5.2). Failure to diagnose and treat PLRI in patients with anterior cruciate ligament (ACL) tears can affect the success of ACL reconstruction. ACL reconstruction is a common procedure performed after ACL rupture to restore knee stability and has shown satisfactory results in recent outcome studies. However, a review of the literature has shown that 11–30% of cases have relatively poor long-term outcomes; more importantly, ACL reconstruction has been found to cause a persistent Pivot shift test positive in more than 15% of cases. Anterior cruciate ligament reconstruction is one of the most commonly performed surgical procedures in orthopedics. Failure rates for primary reconstructions are reported to be between 0.7% and 8%. Graft revision results are much less predictable, with failure rates ranging from 5% to 25%. Many authors have suggested that the main cause of ACL and PCL graft failure is unrecognized and therefore untreated posterolateral rotatory instability.

5.2 Surgical Technique

ACL Reconstruction Technique (see ACL Reconstruction Page)

The surgical technique used to repair the PLRI was a modified form of Larson's technique, called the modified posterolateral corner sling (PLCS) method, which involves passing through the fibular head tunnel. Compared to Larson's technique, we used the following modifications: (1) a separate skin incision and (2) obliquity of the fibular tunnel from the anteroinferior to the posterosuperior aspect. Two separate 2–3 cm incisions were made transversely over the lateral epicondyle and obliquely over the fibular head, respectively. For the fibular tunnel, a 5 mm or 6 mm tunnel (depending on the size of the graft) was made obliquely on the fibula from the anteroinferior to the posterosuperior aspect using the ACL guide. Protection of the peroneal nerve with a curette helps to prevent injury to the nerve during reaming of the fibula head. After confirming the isometric point, the femoral tunnel was enlarged to the diameter of the four-strand graft and chamfered with a rasp. The hamstring tendon autograft (or tibialis allograft) was first pulled out through the fibular head tunnel, and both ends of the grafts were passed under the iliotibial band in a figure of eight pattern to the femoral tunnel. The grafts were fixed to the femoral tunnel with a bioabsorbable interference screw at 8–10 lb. of tension in neutral rotation and 70* flexion of the knee after 20 repetitions of cyclic loading Fig. 5.1(a, b).

Combined chronic ACL-PLC instabilities can be successfully treated by ACL reconstruction with reconstruction of the PLC structures. The frequency with which PLC injuries accompany ACL injuries is poorly understood, but several studies have suggested that up to 11% of ACL tears are accompanied by PLC injuries. However, it is possible that combined ACL and PLC injuries are more common than combined PCL and PLC injuries because ACL injuries are much larger than PCL injuries. Our series has shown that 12.5% (54/432) of patients who underwent ACL reconstruction in the same period also had a PLC injury, which is a relatively higher rate than previously reported. Recently, we have been more carefully, routinely examining PLRI; we have found more than 15–20% cases of PLRI in combination with ACL injury or even isolated PLRI. This may reflect the fact that we are aware

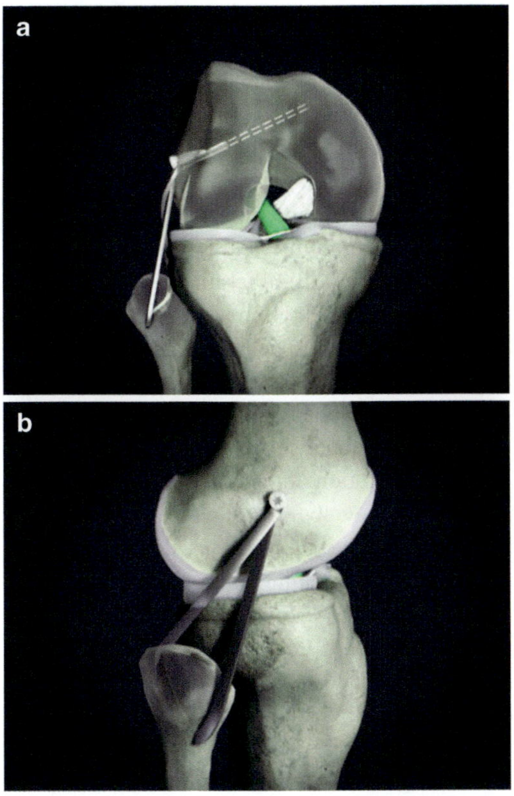

Fig. 5.1 (**a, b**) Schematic representation of the modified posterolateral corner sling passing through the fibular head tunnel and the oblique tunnel configurations used to reduce the killer turn effect. Both ends of the grafts were passed through the femoral tunnel in a figure-of-eight pattern.

that the neglecting of a PLC injury in the presence of a known ACL tear may lead to failure of the cruciate ligament reconstruction. As a result, we tend to test rigorously for the possibility of a PLC injury. It can be difficult to diagnose an injury to the structures of the PLC, and a physical examination of the PLRI illustrated the different methods. Hughston reported: "A posterolateral drawer test and an external rotation recurvatum test are useful in making the diagnosis." Loomer also reported that a physical examination with both feet externally rotated at 90* hip and knee flexion is useful. Arthroscopic examination of the posterolateral gap of the knee joint, the gap between the meniscus and the tibial plateau, and the insertion of the popliteus tendon are also useful. In the cases reported here, the presence of PLRI was assessed by physical examination using the posterolateral drawer and dial tests and by palpating for subluxation of the posterior tibial condyle by placing the examiner's four small fingers on the posterolateral aspect of the popliteal fossa. All 44 patients in this series had preoperative posterolateral instability, as evidenced by positive results on a posterolateral drawer test and a dial test performed with the knee flexed at 30* and 90*, which was 10* more external rotation than the uninjured lower extremity. Forty of the 44 knees (91%) with PLRI were successfully corrected surgically. This was demonstrated by the posterolateral drawer test. Recent biomechanical studies have shown that PLC structures functionally interact with the ACL. Markolf et al. measured the force on a simulated intact ACL with and without the posterolateral knee structures. They found that cutting the posterolateral structures increased the force on the ACL during varus loading. LaPrade et al. examined the force on ACL grafts in cadaver knees in which the posterolateral structure had been selectively cut. They found that grade III posterolateral injuries were associated with significantly increased force on ACL grafts. In addition, untreated posterolateral injuries have been associated with graft failure in ACL and PCL reconstruction, indicating the clinical importance of treating posterolateral injuries when other ligament injuries are present. Consequently, it has been recommended that injured posterolateral (PLC) structures be reconstructed at the time of ACL reconstruction. Various surgical techniques for PLC reconstruction have been reported, but most involve only partial reconstruction of the posterior structures. Hughston and Jacobson reported a method of moving the arcuate complex with bone advancement. Clancy et al. reported a method of rerouting the biceps tendon to the lateral epicondyle with excellent results in 50 cases. However, the above methods are not anatomic reconstructions, and results vary. More recently, anatomic reconstructions of the PLC have been shown to have the best results compared to other surgical methods for treating chronic posterolateral instability. However, anatomic PLC reconstruction did not perform better than the single fibular sling technique in a cadaveric biomechanical study by Apsingi et al. Experienced clinicians recommend that correction of varus malalignment and varus thrust gait should be performed prior to surgical reconstruction of severe lateral and posterolateral ligament deficiencies. One study reported on a unique group of patients with severely affected knees who had chronic ACL deficiency, varus angulation, medial meniscus loss, and partial to complete PLC insufficiency. In this condition, they recommended that a valgus tibial osteotomy be performed first in order to avoid excessive stress on the lateral capsular structures that are to be reconstructed. Therefore, patients with suspected PLC injury should be carefully monitored for limb alignment with full weight-bearing radiographs and gait changes. Several authors have agreed that the most consistently important structures for reconstruction in the posterolateral corner are the popliteus tendon, the lateral collateral ligament, and especially the popliteofibular ligament. The popliteofibular ligament also plays an important role in preventing primary external rotation, varus rotation, and excessive posterior translation, as shown in several cadaveric studies. Albright and Brown reconstructed the posterolateral ligament by passing through the lateral aspect of the tibia. However, Fanelli and Larson reported that passing through the fibular head tunnel and tunneling 1 cm anterior to the lateral epicondyle by passing the tendon medially with a lateral bio-absorbable screw fixation had better results than passing through the tibial tunnel. Of these two methods of reconstruction, the tunneling of the fibula head is technically easier and results in a better isometry than the one that passes through the lateral tunnel of the tibial plateau. We reported that PLC reconstruction with a single sling through the fibular tunnel resulted in shorter operative time and was associated with less surgical morbidity and better rotational stability compared with tibial tunnel reconstruction (Video 5.2). Although potential complications include possible fibular head fracture and peroneal nerve injury, these problems can be avoided if the surgeon takes appropriate precautions as described previously. In cases of tibiofibular joint instability, fixation of the fibular head to the anterior tibia may be considered. Alternatively, another technique should be used.

In conclusion, injuries to the posterolateral structures of the knee are frequently associated with chronic ACL deficiency. In our experience, chronic combined ACL and grade II PLRI can be successfully treated with arthroscopic ACL reconstruction and posterolateral reconstruction with a single sling through the fibular head tunnel (Modified Larson's technique). However, in a grade III PLRI case, we should use a stronger graft because anatomic reconstruction would be better. Even with anatomic reconstruction, the posterolateral stability of the knee was not sufficient.

Therefore, the authors recommend using as strong a graft as possible for LCL and PLCS through the head of the fibula and also through the tibial tunnel in grade III PLRI cases (Fig. 5.2).

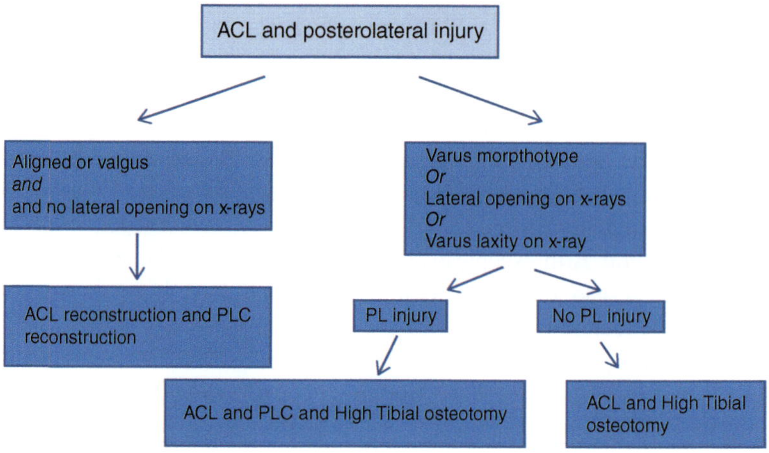

Fig. 5.2 Flowchart for the ACL and PLRI

5.3 Cases of ACL with PLRI

Case 1– ACL Reconstruction with PLC Reconstruction (Modified Larson Technique)
A 42-year-old male patient with left knee pain presented to the outpatient clinic. He injured his left knee after colliding with someone while walking in the street. There were no specific findings on plain radiographs taken immediately after the injury, and physical examination revealed Lachman test grade 2, pivot shift test grade 1, anterior drawer test grade 2, varus stress test grade 1, dial test positive, and posterolateral drawer test grade 2. The KT-2000 arthrometer maximum manual test (MMT) (7–8 mm right and 17 mm left) was checked (Figs. 5.3, 5.4, 5.5, 5.6, and 5.7).

KT-2000 arthrometer maximum manual test (MMT); 9 mm right, 11 mm left were checked.

Case 2—ACL Reconstruction with Remnant Tensioning and PLC Reconstruction
A 31-year-old male patient with right knee pain presented to the outpatient clinic with no history of knee problems. He injured his right knee while running and felt a twist in the knee. There were no specific findings on the plain radiograph taken immediately after the injury, and physical examination revealed Lachman test grade 2, pivot shift test grade 1 and anterior drawer test grade 1, varus stress test grade 1–2, dial test positive, posterolateral drawer test grade 2. KT-2000 arthrometer maximum manual test (MMT); 12–13 mm right, 9 mm left were checked (Figs. 5.8, 5.9, 5.10, 5.11, 5.12, and 5.13).

The KT-2000 arthrometer maximum manual test (MMT) of 9 mm right and 8.5 mm left was checked on physical examination.

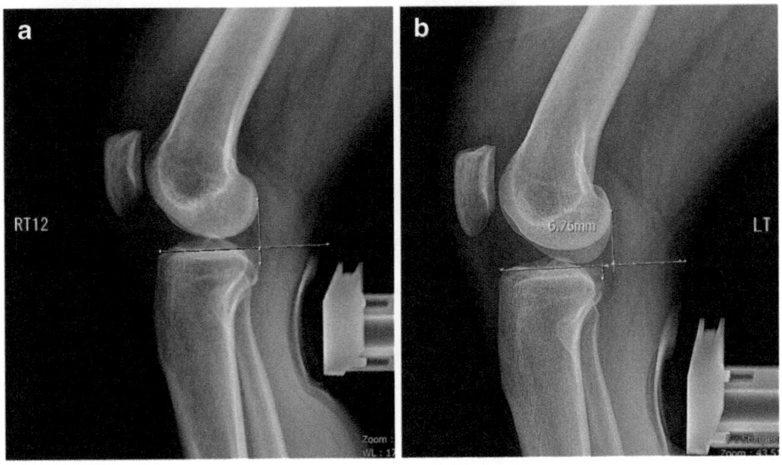

Fig. 5.3 (**a**, **b**) A 6.7 mm side-to-side difference was checked compared to the unaffected side in the pull stress test imaging.

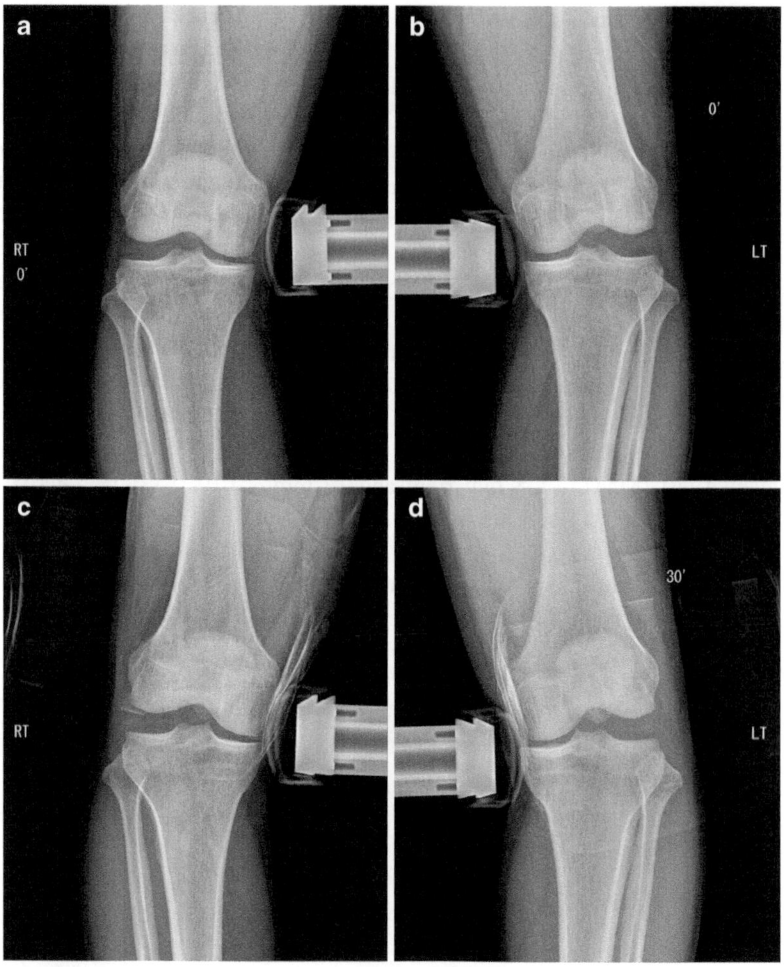

Fig. 5.4 (**a**, **b**) 0° varus view (**c**, **d**) 30° flexion, varus stress view; left knee lateral joint space is wider than that of the right knee.

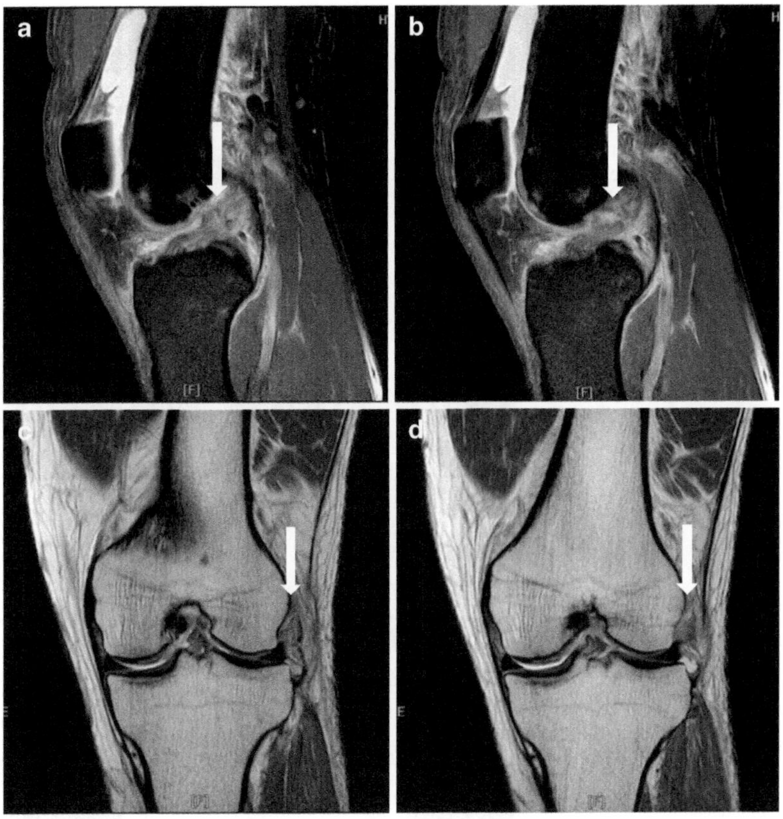

Fig. 5.5 (**a**, **b**) We can find ACL rupture at mid-substance, (**c**, **d**) the popliteofibular ligament, and lateral collateral ligament injury.

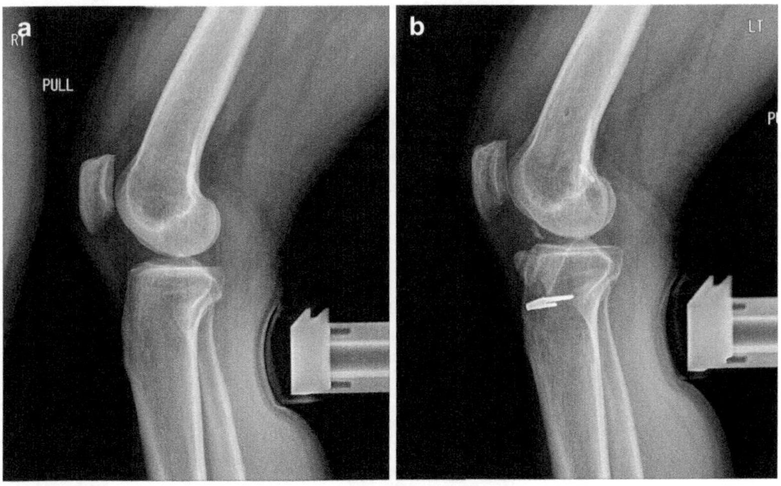

Fig. 5.6 23 months after ACL and PLCS reconstruction, (**a**, **b**) pull stress view. There is no instability in the pull stress view

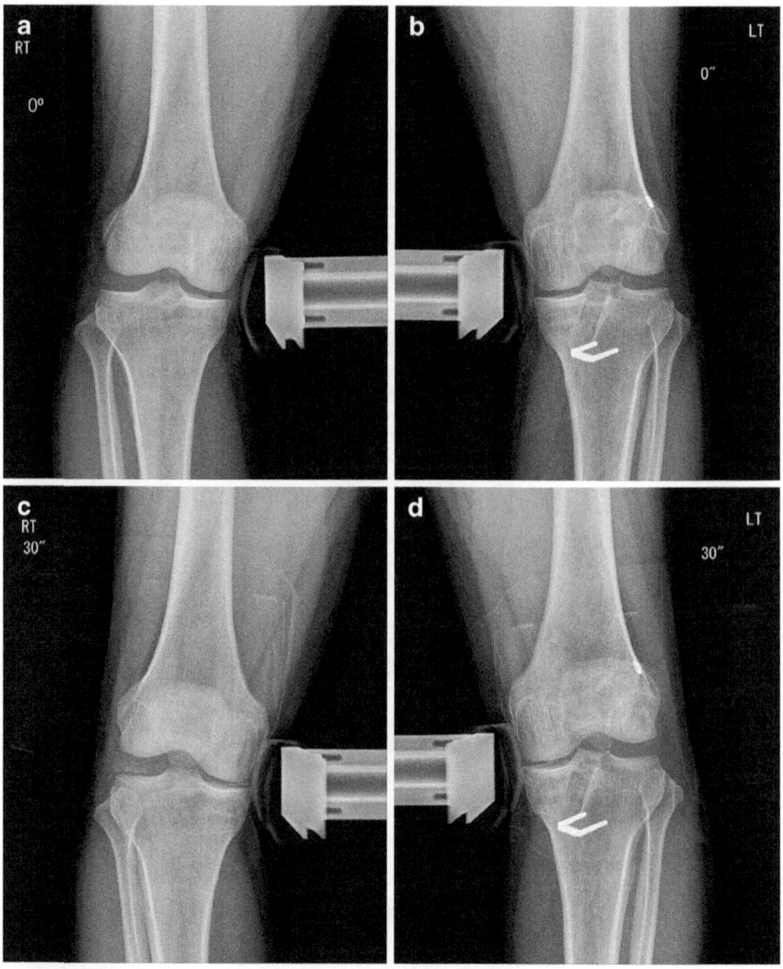

Fig. 5.7 23 months after ACL and PLCS reconstruction. (**a**, **b**) Varus stress view 0° and (**c**, **d**) 30° degree flexion of both knees. There is no instability in the varus stress view in 0° and 30° flexion

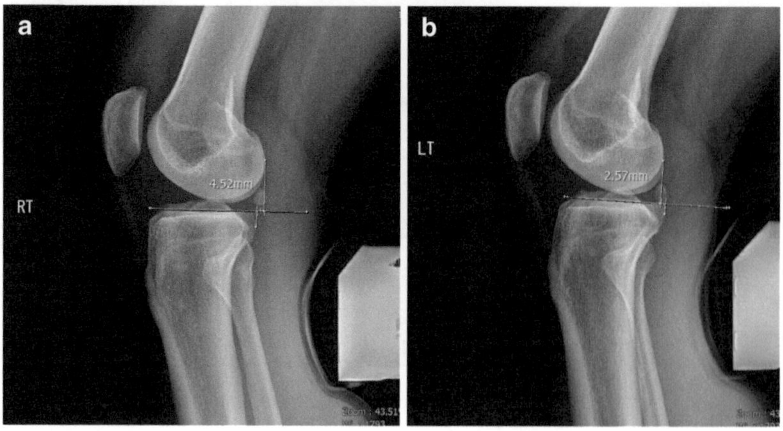

Fig. 5.8 (**a**, **b**) A 7 mm side-to-side difference was checked compared to the unaffected side in the pull stress test imaging.

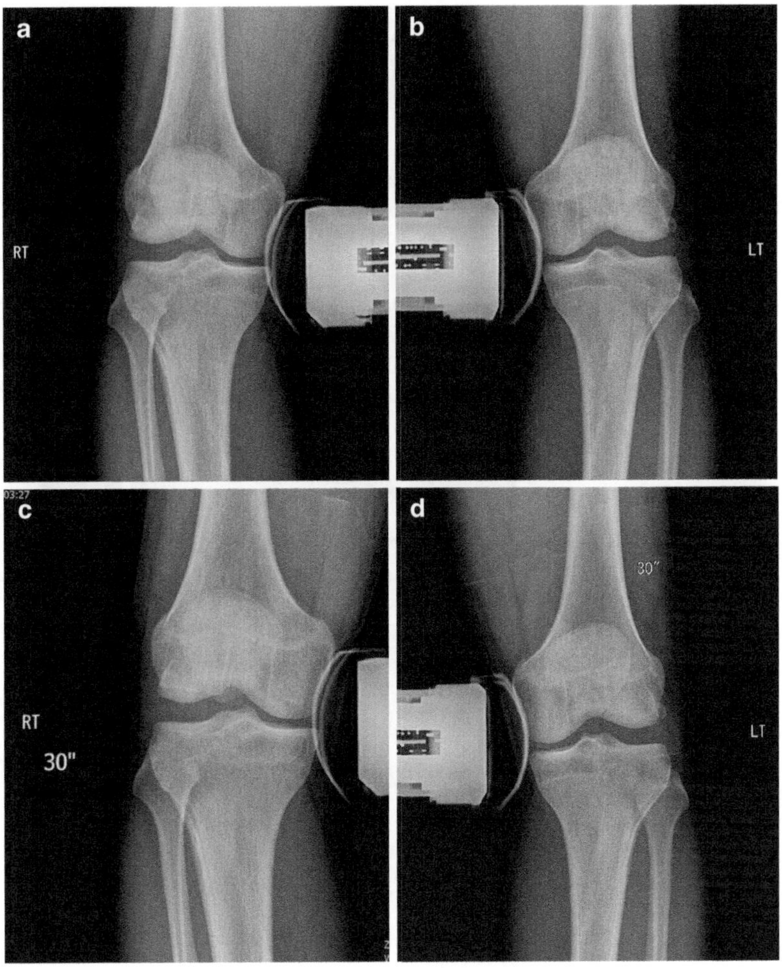

Fig. 5.9 (**a**, **b**) 0° varus stress view; (**c**, **d**) 30° flexion varus stress view; ACL and posterolateral rotatory instability grade 2, meaning varus test grade 1–2 and dial test positive, posterolateral drawer test grade 2, right lateral gap greater than left.

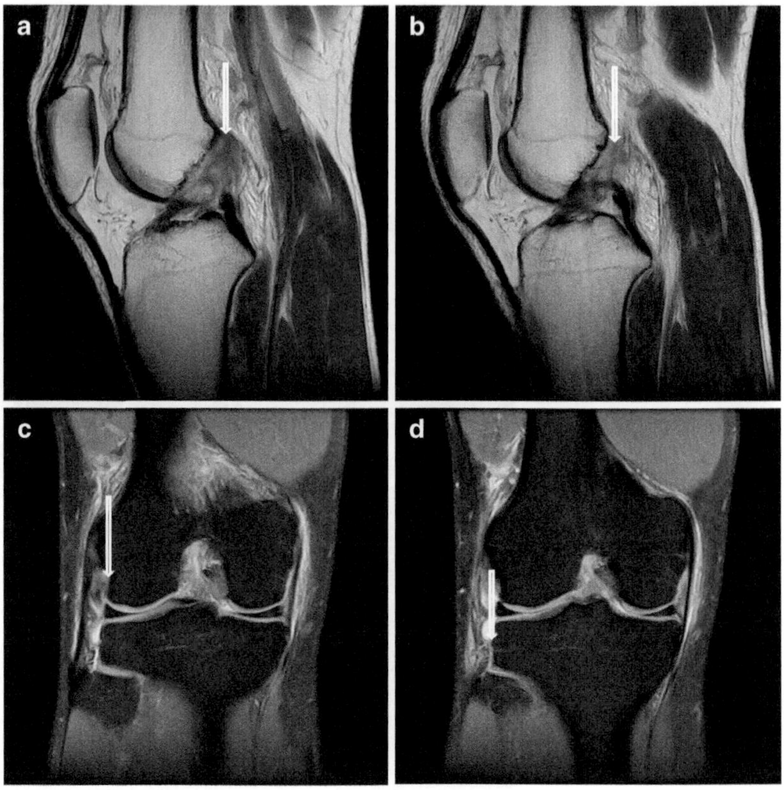

Fig. 5.10 (**a**, **b**) We can find ACL ruptured at the proximal substance (**c**, **d**) popliteal-tibial area signal intensity increased due to popliteofibular ligament injury.

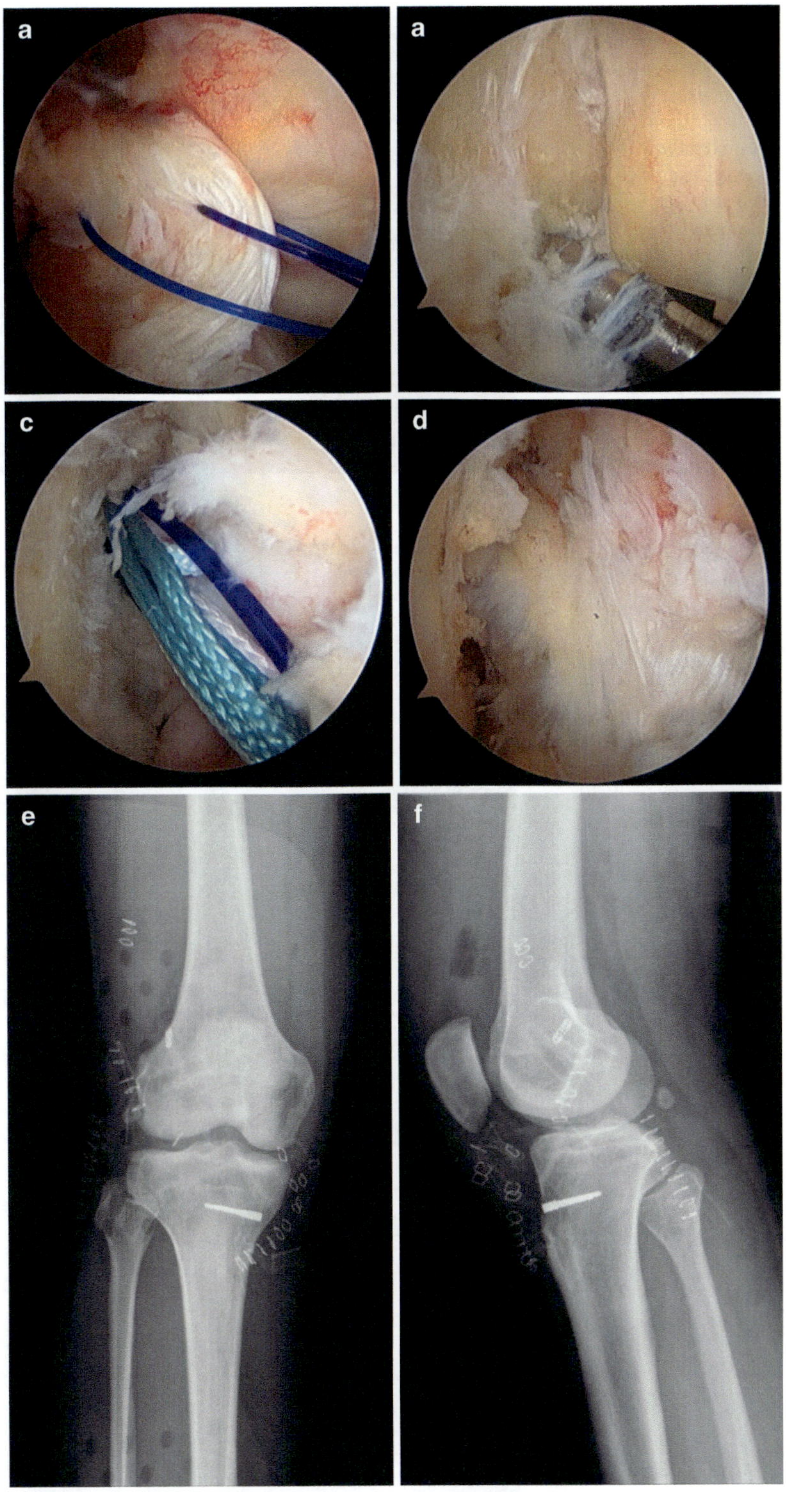

Fig. 5.11 Therefore, a modified posterolateral corner sling (PLCS) was performed along with the A/S ACL reconstruction. (**a**) ACL remnant fiber was sutured with no. 1 PDS using a suture hook. (**b**) Femoral tunnel guide insert (**c**) The ACL graft passing with ACL remnant fiber suture material pulling into the femoral tunnel (**d**) The ACL reconstruction was performed with autogenous semitendinosus and gracilis, preserving the remnant ACL, and the PLCS reconstruction was performed with tibialis allograft through the fibular head tunnel to the lateral femoral epicondyle area. (**e**, **f**) Postoperative X-ray was shown

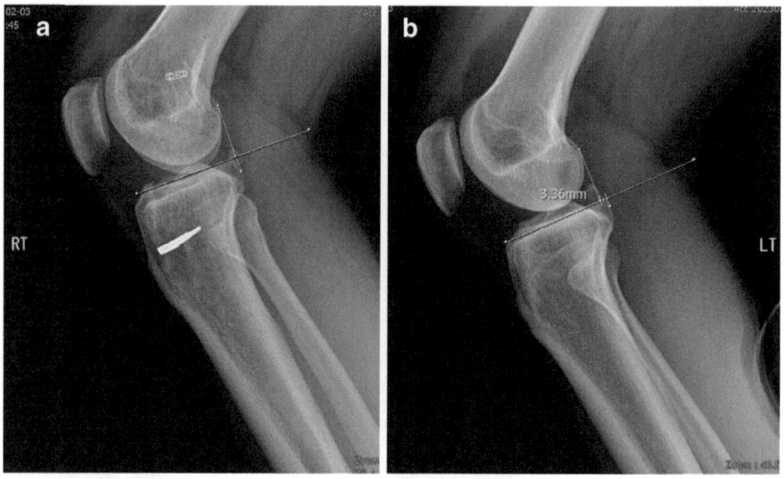

Fig. 5.12 (**a**, **b**) There was no laxity on the anterior drawer test and Lachman test on physical examination, but mild muscle weakness in the right knee at 1 year postoperatively. Follow-up pull stress radiographs showed a marked decrease in side-to-side difference. (Rather, it shows that the left side is pulled more)

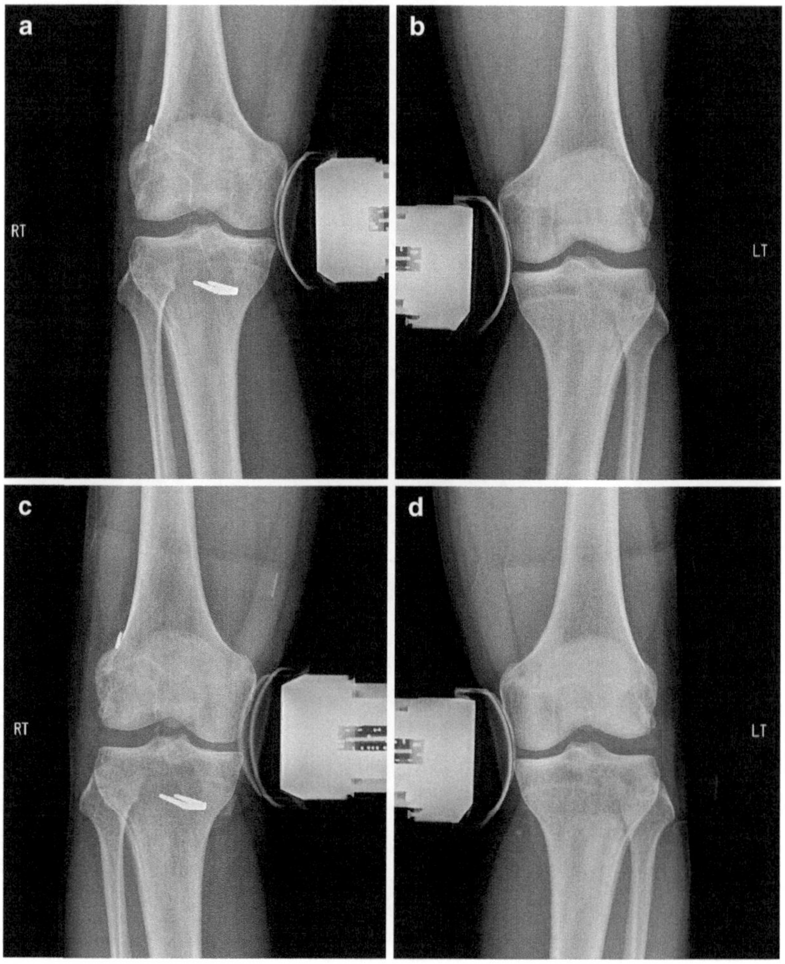

Fig. 5.13 (**a**, **b**) One year after ACL reconstruction with autogenous ST and gracilis and PLCS (with tibialis allograft) through the fibular head tunnel to the lateral femoral epicondyle area. Varus view 0°,(**c**, **d**) 30° flexion varus stress view; there is no difference between the right and left knee

Further Reading

1. Albright JP, Brown AW. Management of chronic posterolateral rotatory instability of the knee: surgical technique form the posterolateral corner sling procedure. Instr Course Lect. 1998;47:369–78.
2. Apsingi S, Nguyen T, Bull AM, Unwin A, Deehan DJ, Amis AA. A comparison of modified Larson and 'anatomic' posterolateral corner reconstructions in knees with combined PCL and posterolateral corner deficiency. Knee Surg Sports Traumatol Arthrosc. 2009;17:305–12.
3. Fanelli GC, Larson RV. Practical management of posterolateral instability of the knee. Arthroscopy. 2002;18:1–8.
4. Gollehon DL, Torzilli PA, Warren RF. The role of the posterolateral and cruciate ligaments in the stability of the human knee. A biomechanical study. J Bone Joint Surg Am. 1987;69:233–42.
5. Jung YB, Jung HJ, Kim SJ, Park SJ, Song KS, Lee YS, Lee SH. Posterolateral corner reconstruction for posterolateral rotatory instability combined with posterior cruciate ligament injuries: comparison between fibular tunnel and tibial tunnel techniques. Knee Surg Sports Traumatol Arthrosc. 2008;16:239–48.
6. Kim JG, Ha JG, Lee YS, Yang SJ, Jung JE, Oh SJ. Posterolateral corner anatomy and its anatomical reconstruction with single fibula and double femoral sling method: anatomical study and surgical technique. Arch Orthop Trauma Surg. 2009;129:381–5.
7. La Prade RF, Gilbert TJ, Bollom TS, Wentorf F, Chaljub G. The magnetic resonance imaging appearance of individual structures of the posterolateral knee. A prospective study of normal knees and knees with surgically verified grade III injuries. Am J Sports Med. 2000;28:191–9.
8. LaPrade RF, Johansen S, Wentorf FA, Engebretsen L, Esterberg JL, Tso A. An analysis of an anatomical posterolateral knee reconstruction: an in vitro biomechanical study and development of a surgical technique. Am J Sports Med. 2004;32:1405–14.
9. LaPrade RF, Resig S, Wentorf F, Lewis JL. The effects of grade III posterolateral knee complex injuries on anterior cruciate ligament graft force. A biomechanical analysis. Am J Sports Med. 1999;27:469–75.
10. Loomer RL. A test for knee posterolateral rotatory instability. Clin Orthop Relat Res. 1991;264:235–8.
11. Markolf KL, Graves BR, Sigward SM, Jackson SR, McAllister DR. How well do anatomical reconstructions of the posterolateral corner restore varus stability to the posterior cruciate ligament-reconstructed knee? Am J Sports Med. 2007;35:1117–22.
12. Maynard MJ, Deng X, Wickiewicz TL, Warren RF. The popliteofibular ligament. Rediscovery of a key element in posterolateral stability. Am J Sports Med. 1996;24:311–6.
13. Muller W, Biedert R, Hefti F, Jacob RP, Munzinger U, Staubli H. OAK knee evaluation. A new way to assess knee ligament injuries. Clin Orthop Relat Res. 1998;232:37–50.
14. Noyes FR, Barber-Westin SD. Posterolateral knee reconstruction with an anatomical bone-patellar tendon-bone reconstruction of the fibular collateral ligament. Am J Sports Med. 2007;35:259–73.
15. Noyes FR, Barber SD, Simon R. High tibial osteotomy and ligament reconstruction in varus angulated, anterior cruciate ligament-deficient knees. A two- to seven-year follow-up study. Am J Sports Med. 1993;21:2–12.
16. Ross G, DeConciliis GP, Choi K, Scheller AD. Evaluation and treatment of acute posterolateral corner/anterior cruciate ligament injuries of the knee. J Bone Joint Surg Am A. 2004;86(Suppl 2):2–7.
17. Strobel MJ, Schulz MS, Petersen WJ, Eichhorn HJ. Combined anterior cruciate ligament, posterior cruciate ligament, and posterolateral corner reconstruction with autogenous hamstring grafts in chronic instabilities. Arthroscopy. 2006;22:182–92.
18. Veltri DM, Deng XH, Torzilli PA, Maynard MJ, Warren RF. The role of the popliteofibular ligament in stability of the human knee. A biomechanical study. Am J Sports Med. 1996;24:19–27.
19. Veltri DM, Deng XH, Torzilli PA, Warren RF, Maynard MJ. The role of the cruciate and posterolateral ligaments in stability of the knee. A biomechanical study. Am J Sports Med. 1995;23:436–43.
20. Lee SH, Jung YB, Jung HJ, Song KS, Ko YB. Combined reconstruction for posterolateral rotatory instability with anterior cruciate ligament injuries of the knee. Knee Surg Sports Traumatol Arthrosc. 2010;18:1219–25.

Anterior Cruciate Ligament Injury with MCL Injury

6

Abstract

The medial collateral ligament (MCL) is the most common knee ligament to be injured during knee trauma. The annual incidence of MCL injury has been reported as 0.24–7.3 per 1000 people with a male to female ratio of 2:1. It is a common injury during soccer, skiing, as a result of either a direct valgus force to players' knees or cutting maneuvers, when athletes fix one side foot and suddenly change their direction.

MCL injury usually occur as an isolated injury; however, it may present in combination with other ligament injuries. Approximately 78% of patients with grade III MCL injury had an injury combined ligament damage, of which the most common are accompanied by anterior cruciate ligament injury.

Incomplete tears (grade I, II) and isolated tears (grade III) of the MCL without valgus alignment knee can be treated conservatively, with early limited ROM (0–90 flexion) brace and quadriceps muscle strengthening exercise.

Acute repair is indicated in isolated grade III tears with moderate to severe valgus alignment knee, MCL entrapment over pes anserinus, or intra-articular entrapment or bony avulsion. The indication for primary repair is based on the resulting quality of the original MCL ligament and the time since the injury. Primary repair of the MCL is usually performed within 7–10 days after the injury.

Augmentation repair for the superficial MCL (sMCL) is a surgical technique that can be used when the original MCL ligament is not so good quality and primary repair impossible and also mid substance tear of the MCL.

Reconstruction is indicated when MCL injuries fail to heal in neutral or varus alignment. Chronic, medial-sided knee injuries with valgus malalignment should be treated with a two-stage approach. A distal femoral osteotomy should be performed first, followed by reconstruction of the MCL, posteromedial corner(PMC), posterior oblique ligament(POL).

Keywords

Medial collateral ligament • MCL reconstruction • MCL conservative treatment

6.1 Principles of Treatment of Anterior Cruciate Ligament and Posteromedial Instability

The treatment of medial collateral ligament (MCL) injuries largely depends on the severity of the injury and the needs of the patient. The MCL

Y. B. Jung et al., *Treatment of the Cruciate Ligaments Injuries*,
https://doi.org/10.1007/978-981-95-9039-1_6

is one of the four major ligaments in the knee and provides medial (inner) stability. MCL injuries are often graded on a scale of I–III, ranging from mild sprains to complete tears.

For grade I and some grade II injuries, the RICE protocol (Rest, Ice, Compression, Elevation) is often the first line of treatment. A hinged knee brace may be used to provide stability during the healing process with pain killers. Exercises may be prescribed to maintain joint mobility and muscle strength, as well as to promote healing. Patients are often advised to avoid activities that may exacerbate the injury or delay healing (Case 1, Figs. 6.9, 6.10, and 6.11).

Surgical intervention is usually reserved for grade III injuries, combined ligamentous injuries, or cases where conservative treatment has failed. Repair (Case 2, Figs. 6.12, 6.13, 6.14, 6.15, 6.16, and 6.17) or reconstruction (Case 3, Figs. 6.18, 6.19, 6.20, 6.21, 6.22, and 6.23) of the MCL may be performed using various techniques, including suturing the torn ends, grafting, and/or use of fixation devices like screws or anchors. If there is concomitant damage to other knee structures like the ACL, combined surgical procedures may be necessary.

6.2 Anatomy

The MCL consists of superficial and deep parts and superficial part. The superficial MCL(sMCL) is one of the most important structures for medial stability of the knee. It originates from 3.2 mm proximal and 4.8 mm posterior to the medial femoral epicondyle (Fig. 6.1). It has two insertions on the tibia: the proximal part attaches 12 mm distal to the articular surface, and the distal part inserts on a point 6 cm distal to the joint line. The proximal part is the primary knee stabilizer against valgus stress, while its distal part is mainly responsible for stability in external rotation to 30° and 60° of knee flexion and internal rotation.

The deep medial collateral ligament (dMCL) is the thick part of the middle third of the medial knee capsule. The dMCL presents two components—meniscofemoral and meniscotibial—and attaches the medial meniscus to the joint capsule. The structures of the medial knee posterior to the MCL known as the posteromedial corner (PMC) are another important stabilizer of the medial knee. They consist of posterior oblique ligament (POL), semimembranous insertion, oblique popliteal ligament (OPL), medial joint capsule, and posterior horn of the medial meniscus. POL is a capsular thickening of the knee joint attaching to the semimembranosus muscle. Its proximal attachment is on the distal femur near the insertion site of the medial head of the gastrocnemius muscle, and its distal attachment is on the posteromedial side of the tibia (Fig. 6.2).

During knee joint flexion, the semimembranosus muscle contracts and tightens the posteromedial knee capsule and the POL. It also pulls the medial meniscus posteriorly and prevents the anterior subluxation of the tibia. Another work of the semimembranosus muscle is internal rotation

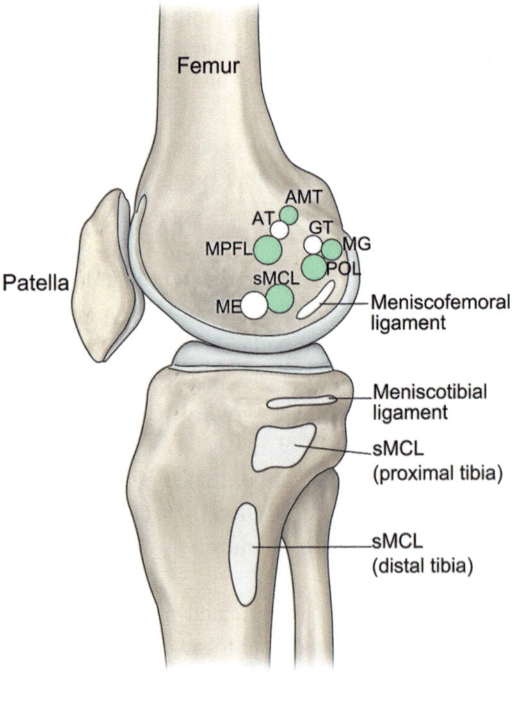

Fig. 6.1 Attachment sites of the medial knee stabilizers. Abbreviations: *AMT* Adductor Magnus tendon, *AT* adductor tubercle, *MPFL* medial patellofemoral ligament, *ME* medial epicondyle, *sMCL* superficial MCL, *POL* posterior oblique ligament, *GT* gastrocnemius tubercle, *MG* medial head of the gastrocnemius

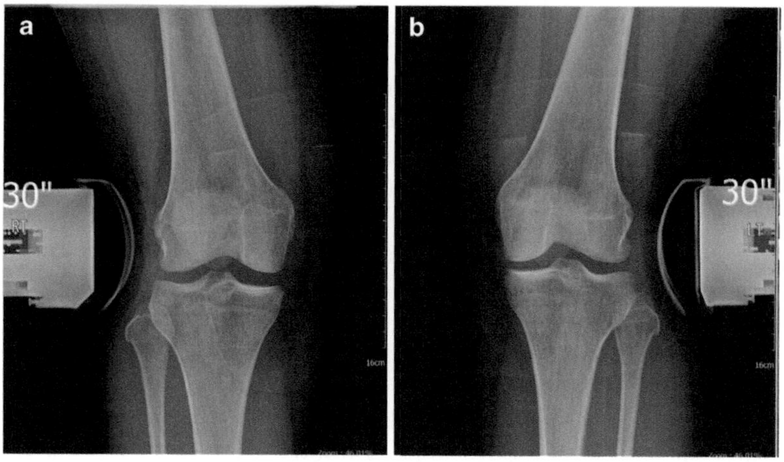

Fig. 6.2 (**a**, **b**) Valgus stress radiography, medial knee gap side-to-side difference of at least 3.2 mm suggests complete sMCL injury. In this case, the difference of medial knee joint gap between the two sides was more than 2.1 mm. Abbreviations: *sMCL* Superficial part of the medial collateral ligament

of the tibia. Therefore, PMC injuries may lead to anterior tibial subluxation by damaging the function of the semimembranosus muscle and results in external tibial rotation. The anteromedial rotatory instability (AMRI) is known as anterior subluxation of the medial tibial condyle by the flexion of the injured knee may be caused by PMC injuries.

6.3 Physical Examination

Medial laxity at 30° of knee flexion in the valgus stress test suggests MCL injury, and medial laxity at 0°, MCL with cruciate ligaments or PMC injury, may also be injured.

The physical examination should also the evaluation of the cruciate ligament (ACL and PCL), in addition to the assessment of menisci and posterolateral corner (PLC) injury. Anterior subluxation of the lateral tibial condyle at 90° of knee flexion suggests ACL injury or AMRI. However, anterior subluxation of the medial tibial condyle while the knee is 15° externally rotated and 90° flexed is specific for AMRI (Slocum test).

In the dial test, the amount of foot external rotation is evaluated in comparison with the contralateral side while the patient is in the supine or prone position and in 30 and 90° of knee flexion. A foot external rotation of at least 15° more than the other side both in 30 and 90° of knee flexion may indicate either combined PCL and PLC injury or PMC injury. If external rotation is accompanied by anterior subluxation of the medial tibial plateau, PMC injury will be the probable cause. On the contrary, posterior subluxation of the lateral tibial plateau with or without lateral laxity (posterolateral drawer test) increases the likelihood of PLC injury (and combined PCL).

6.4 Classification of Medial Collateral Ligament Injury

The American Medical Association classified the MCL injury into three grades. Grade I injuries indicate only some minimal torn fibers without any loss of ligamentous integrity (stretch injury). In grade II, there is a partial tear of the MCL. Grade III injuries show severe complete disruption of a ligament. By performing a valgus stress test in 30° of knee flexion, patients with grade III MCL injury experience valgus knee laxity. In their study, Hughston et al. subdivided grade III injuries into categories of 3–5 mm, 5–10 mm, and ≥ 10 mm based on the amount of increased medial knee space during the knee valgus stress test.

6.5 Diagnosis

Valgus stress radiographs using Telos device of the knee can be used for primary evaluation of MCL injury. Ossification of the proximal part of the MCL (Pellegrini-Stieda sign) is suggestive of chronic MCL injury. In the valgus stress radiography, the knee is flexed to 30°, medial knee gap side-to-side difference of at least 3.2 mm is suggestive of complete sMCL injury, and the gap difference is more than 9.8 mm, it indicates combined MCL/PMC injury. Side-to-side difference of less than 3.2 mm is indicated either partially injured sMCL (Fig. 6.2). However, according to the valgus stress view, the gap side-to-side difference makes it very difficult to say it's a complete MCL tear or not due to the patient's relaxation and checking if the view is in the correct position or not and also applying the Telos device correctly. Therefore, by physician's experiences by physical examine is more important to correct judgment.

Magnetic resonance imaging (MRI) help determine the presence or absence of other damage when the III valgus instability is present and to accurately identify the damage site (Fig. 6.3).

The level of agreement between MRI and clinical grading was obtained at 92% in one study.

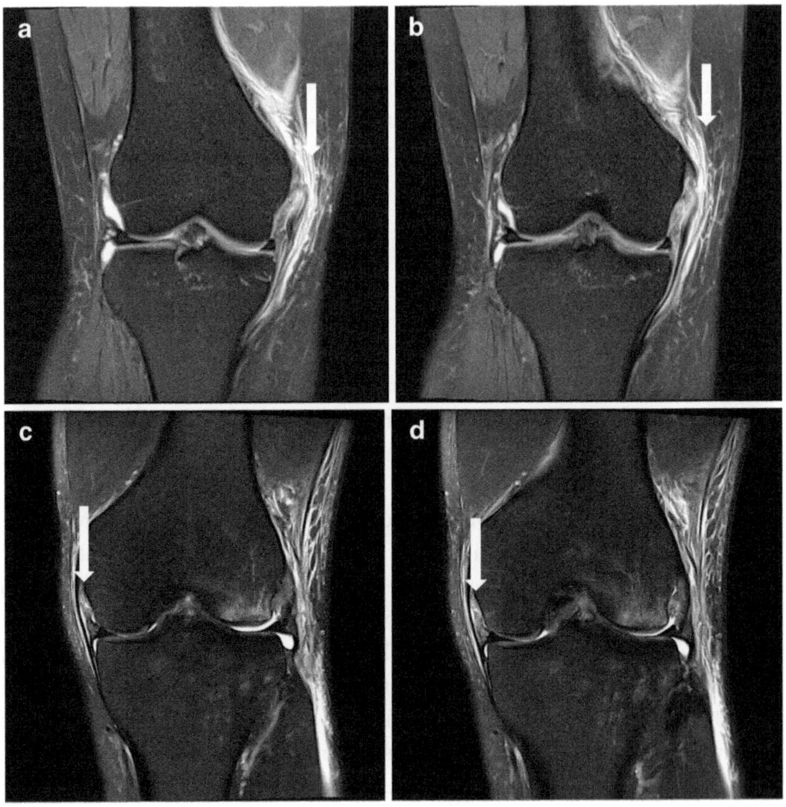

Fig. 6.3 (**a**, **b**) Magnetic resonance imaging (MRI) of a patient with MCL injury. (**c**, **d**) The injury of both superficial and deep MCL (can be detected on MRI)

6.6 Treatment

Most isolate MCL injury treatment regardless of their injury severity is conservative. However, prolong immobilization can cause degenerative changes in collagen fibers in MCL and resorption at insertion site of the ligament. Therefore, the importance of early start of range of motion (ROM) exercises is very important in conservative treatment. Grade I injury can be managed without a brace; however, a hinged knee brace is required for grade II and grade III cases. Grade II and III cases usually have to protect with a brace for at least 3 and 6 weeks (case 1, Figs. 6.9, 6.10, and 6.11). MCL brace should be fixed in full body position, and the quadriceps muscle strength that can fully extend the knee joint should be maintained.

On walking, the brace should be locked in full extension of the knee. Straight leg raising, quadriceps sets, and patella mobilization are started at the beginning of the treatment.

In avulsion of the MCL injury case, the injured MCL avulsion site not displaced, and it may be treated by conservative management. On the other hand, the pes anserinus muscle is interposed between the tibia and the injured MCL (Stener-type lesion). In case of this situation, surgical treatment is necessary.

In acute cases (≤3 weeks since injury), especially 7–10 days since injury, surgical repair is possible by direct MCL repair (Case 2, Figs. 6.12, 6.13, 6.14, 6.15, 6.16, and 6.17a, b). For subacute (3 weeks to 6 weeks from the trauma) and chronic MCL injury (more than 6 weeks), MCL reconstruction should be considered, or patients with poor ligament quality even in acute case.

6.7 Indication of Operative Management of the MCL Injury During Patients' Evaluation

1. Open MCL injury
2. Anteromedial rotatory instability (AMRI)
3. Medial laxity in valgus stress test—full extension of the knee (0 degree knee position) 6 weeks after conservative treatment or in chronic case
4. Multi-ligament injury, ACL or PCL combined injury
5. Bony avulsion with MCL which is displaced
6. Entrapment of the MCL beneath the medial meniscus
7. Stener-type lesion (tibial site rupture and entrapment pes anserinus muscle)

MLKI is an indication for surgery; however, the timing of the surgery is controversial. The delay of the surgery decreases the incidence of the adhesion or arthrofibrosis. If the inflammation or edema has subsided, delayed reconstruction of the cruciate by 3–6 weeks, ACL reconstruction will be done postsurgery and arthrofibrosis incidences will be decreased. In a systematic review, Jiang et al. demonstrated that staged management is associated with a higher excellent/good result, compared to either early or delayed operative management of MLKI. Stannard et al. showed that in MLKI, surgical repair of the PMC is associated with a higher failure rate, as compared to PMC reconstruction.

It is a well-known practice to reconstruct the ACL and manage MCL conservatively. However, in the presence of other operative indications for MCL, combined ACL-MCL injury may be done with early ACL reconstruction and MCL exploration. The timing for ACL reconstruction for cases with combined ACL-MCL injury is still open to debate. We usually treat MCL injury conservatively and postpone ACL reconstruction until we get the ROM of the knee fully recovered 3 to 6 weeks post-trauma. Dong et al. compared the outcomes of direct repair with the reconstruction of the MCL in cases with combined ACL-MCL injury. They indicated that reconstruction provides the knees with better rotational stability. However, with the introduction of internal brace augmentation techniques using high-strength sutures, more studies may be required to further determine the MCL management of choice in the MLKI cases. Moreover, a biomechanical study revealed that the moment needed to disrupt the

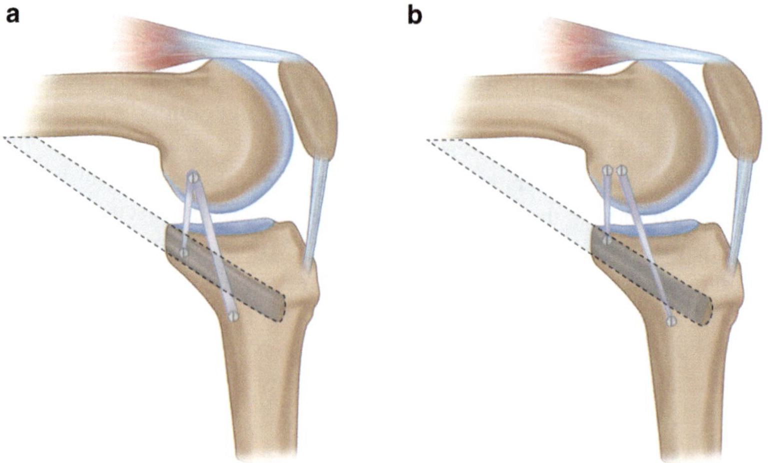

Fig. 6.4 (**a**) Schematic pictures of the triangular vector ligament reconstruction and the LaPrade anatomical ligament reconstruction. (**b**) The knee is semi-flexed, and the position of the graft relative to the MCL is shown in the pictures. The circular area in each picture shows the relative insertion site of pes anserine muscles on the tibia

internal brace was not significantly different from the force required to fail the anatomical MCL reconstruction (Gilmer BB. et al. 2016) (Fig. 6.4).

6.8 Surgical Technique

Direct repair is recommended for acute cases. The stabilizing medial knee structures are repaired from deep to superficial layers. Firstly, the medial meniscus and its attachment to the dMCL should be explored and managed. Following that, injury to the dMCL, POL, and sMCL can be addressed, respectively. Regarding the POL, its distal attachment should be repaired after the proximal counterpart. Subsequently, after drifting the POL anteriorly, the middle part of the POL's anterior border should be fixed to the sMCL by pants-over-vest sutures. This closes the gap in the medial side of the knee and tightens the PMC, stabilizing the joint further against valgus laxity. In addition, the semimembranosus muscle is evaluated. In the presence of any laxity, its capsular arm should be anteriorly advanced and fixed to the POL with pants-over-vests sutures. Historically, pants-over-vests sutures have been recommended to fix injured medial knee ligaments. However, interlocking Bunnel and Kracków sutures are also utilized for repairing MCL in the literature. Proximal or distal bony avulsions of the medial knee ligaments can be repaired by screw fixation. Nowadays, there is a growing interest to repair MCL "peel-off" injuries or small bony MCL avulsions with anchor sutures. Mid-substance tears are needed to be sutured and simultaneously augmented since they are more difficult to be repaired. Recently, the advent of ultrahigh-molecular-weight polyethylene (FiberWire®) sutures with their strength against abrasion has revolutionized the ligament repairing techniques. The use of ultrahigh-molecular-weight polyethylene/polyester suture tape (FiberTape) further enhances the strength of the ligament repairs. Ligament reconstruction is indicated whenever a chronic MCL injury or failed MCL repair is encountered or whenever the ligament quality is inappropriate. Nonetheless, similar to surgical MCL repair, it may also be associated with knee stiffness, Furthermore, any valgus malalignment of the injured knee should be addressed with osteotomy prior to the reconstruction surgery.

To date, different types of reconstruction have been proposed, which are selected by knee surgeons, depending on their experience, the presence of other ligament injuries, and the availability of surgical equipment. Isolated chronic MCL injuries unresponsive to conservative treatment can be managed with isolated MCL augmentation with semitendinosus autograft. When MLKI simultaneously affects PMC and MCL, more advanced techniques may be selected, including combined MCL reconstruction and posteromedial capsule reefing, or MCL plus POL reconstruction. Van der Wal et al. demonstrated that posteromedial capsule reefing performed simultaneously with MCL reconstruction may have a stabilizing result against valgus knee laxity, similar to the methods reconstructing both MCL and POL. LaPrade's anatomical reconstruction of sMCL and POL needs more grafts and is more technically demanding. More bone tunnels should be drilled for holding the grafts, and the MCL bone tunnels may risk the other reconstructed ligaments in cases with multi-ligament injuries. However, it will provide a better biomechanics if performed correctly. LaPrade et al. proposed to use two separate ligament grafts for the reconstruction of MCL and POL. They used two separate tunnels in the femur and two tibial tunnels to fix the grafts at the anatomical attachment points of MCL and POL. They also reported that the use of this technique gives the best biomechanical property to the knee joint. Moreover, they found that 100% of patients had less than 3 mm medial knee gap on valgus stress radiographs during a follow-up period of 18 months. Hongtao Xu proposed a method with one femoral tunnel and one tibial tunnel to reconstruct MCL and POL. In this method called triangular vector ligament reconstruction, the attachment sites of MCL and POL on the femur and tibia are marked. Thereafter, two pins are positioned on the knee joint between the origin and insertion site of each of the two ligaments (POL and MCL) to simulate the relative path of each ligament. The intersection of the two pins on the femur is marked as the best place to position the femoral tunnel. The insertion sites of the two ligaments on the tibia are used as the endpoints of the tibial tunnels. After drilling the femoral tunnel mediolaterally and the tibial tunnel posteroanteriorly, an allograft is inserted through the tibial tunnel. Finally, the endpoints of the graft are fixed at the femoral tunnel. Hongtao found that the medial knee gap on the valgus stress radiographs (with 30° of knee flexion) decreases from 10.32 to 3.13 mm using this method.

6.9 My Preferred Technique

For each sMCL reconstruction, an Achilles allograft was used. The medial epicondyle was identified through a longitudinal incision, which was distal and anterior to the adductor tubercle. Then, the attachment site of the sMCL was identified, which was slightly proximal and anterior to this location. At this point, an eyelet passing pin was drilled transversely across the femur. Another longitudinal incision was made medially to the tibial tubercle. The distal tibial attachment of the sMCL was identified deep within the pes anserine bursa. A Kirschner wire was drilled through the center of the distal attachment site. An isometry test was performed with a suture looped over the passing pin at the femoral site and the Kirschner wire at the tibial site (Fig. 6.5).

A bone tunnel was drilled at the femoral attachment according to the measured diameter of the bone plug of the Achilles allograft (Fig. 6.6).

The location of the central arm of the POL is in the posteromedial tibia epiphysis, immediately anterior to the insertion of the direct arm of the semimembranosus tendon. A pin is once again employed in an oblique direction to Gerdy's tubercle. The tunnel is completed in this position at a depth of 25 mm. Then, the allograft was passed to the POL tibial attachment first in a 90-degree flexion position and was fixed with a bio-screw. Then, the bone plug was fixed with a bio-screw on the femoral side at full extension position. Finally, the tibial tunnel for sMCL was fixed with a bio-screw in the 30-degree flexion position (Fig. 6.7).

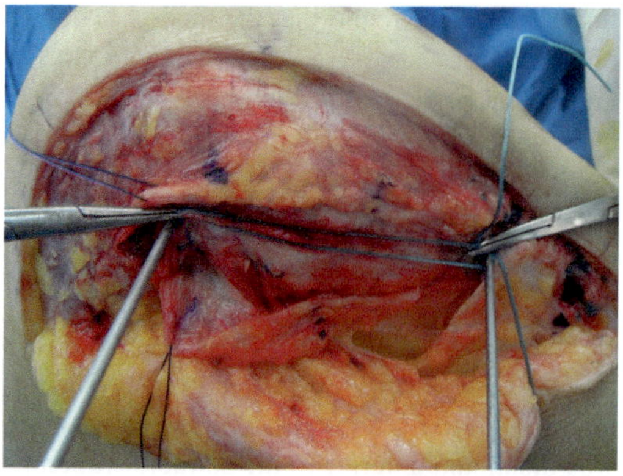

Fig. 6.5 The isometry for sMCL was checked

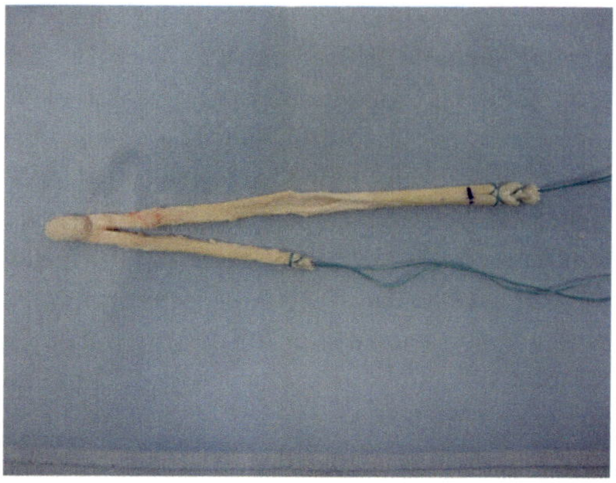

Fig. 6.6 Bifurcated Achilles tendon was prepared

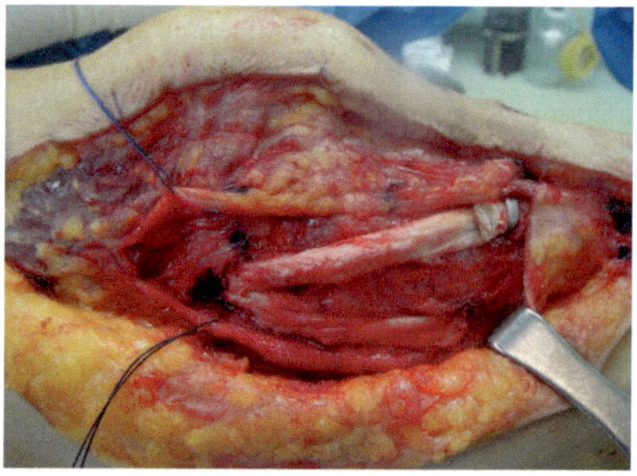

Fig. 6.7 sMCL and POL was reconstructed

6.10 Postoperative Rehabilitation

The exact postoperative protocol is still a topic of debate. It is a common practice to give the patient a hinged knee brace postoperatively for at least 4–6 weeks. Jacobson recommended that the brace be set at 45° of flexion in isolated medial knee repair and increment 15° of passive knee extension every 2 weeks. The weight-bearing would be started when a 15 degree of flexion is reached. In the presence of ACL injury, however, he was a proponent of keeping the brace at full extension and following an ACL rehabilitation protocol. Nevertheless, delayed initiation of knee motion, as proposed in this approach, makes the patients more prone to arthrofibrosis. According to LaPrade et al., postoperatively, patients with MCL injury should be encouraged to start knee ROM within the safe zone determined during the operation for the first 2 weeks, and since then, they can gradually increase their ROM to the normal limits. Moreover, patients are recommended to exercise straight leg raise in braces until they can do this without knee extension lag. After 6 weeks, MCL-injured individuals are recommended to start weight-bearing as tolerated. Strengthening exercises can be initiated once their gait is normalized, commonly after 4–5 months. It may be possible to begin weight-bearing earlier by augmenting MCL surgical repair with an internal bracing technique using high-strength sutures. Golden et al. proposed to initiate ROM within 0–90° of flexion and partial weight-bearing in the first 2 weeks postoperatively. After 2 weeks, the ROM could be increased to 120-degree flexion with a full weight-bearing protocol. The majority of patients with MCL injury can be treated conservatively by hinged knee brace and early ROM. Nonetheless, understanding the surgical indications of the MCL injury, including Stener-type lesion, AMRI,

MLKI, and chronic MCL injuries unresponsive to conservative treatment, may help the orthopedic surgeon to decide if the patient benefits from the surgical intervention. Whether operative or conservative therapy is selected, the early initiation of ROM would be a key part of the MCL management in order to prevent arthrofibrosis.

(a) Rehabilitation Phase I (0–2 weeks)

Hinged knee brace.

0–90° of passive or passive-assisted knee flexion.

No weight-bearing.

Isometrics quadriceps sets and straight leg raises.

(b) Phase II (2–6 weeks)

ROM may progress as tolerated, with the goal of restoring full ROM.

Closed-chain kinetic exercise.

Weight-bearing must not be allowed. This fact does not depend on the procedure (repair vs. repair/reconstruction).

(c) Phase III (6–12 weeks)

Weight-bearing as tolerated.

Walking, elliptical training, cycling encouraged.

(d) Phase IV (> 12 weeks)

Discontinue brace except for activities (lower-profile hinged brace used).

Light jogging, gradual return to sport-specific drills.

Return to play when greater than 80% quadriceps strength returns and adequate performance on functional tests.

6.11 Complications

Surgical treatment of medial knee lesions can injure the saphenous nerve. The saphenous nerve divides into the infrapatellar branch and sartorial branch. The infrapatellar branch travels anteriorly and travels inferior to the patella and sartorial terminal to innervate the anteromedial aspect of the knee.

The sartorial branch has a vertical course posterior to the medial knee structure and provides sensation to the medial part of the leg.

The distance of the sartorial branch of the saphenous nerve from the adductor tubercle was 5.0 ± 1.1 cm, 6.1 ± 1.0 cm from the medial epicondyle, and 4.8 ± 0.9 cm from the anterior border of the sMCL to 2 cm distal from the joint line.

Postoperative stiffness is common in medial knee surgeries. Performing anatomical reconstruction techniques that allow early postoperative knee motion is important. The stiffness can be associated with the timing of repairs and with non-anatomical repairs. Residual laxity is another common complication and can be caused by failure to recognize all components of the injury, especially the meniscus and posteromedial structures.

Incomplete tears (grade I, II) and isolated tears (grade III) of the MCL without valgus instability can be treated nonsurgically with early functional rehabilitation. Failure of nonsurgical treatment can lead to debilitating, persistent medial instability, secondary ACL dysfunction, weakness, and osteoarthritis. Acute repair is indicated in isolated grade III tears with severe instability, MCL entrapment over the pes anserinus, and intra-articular or bony avulsion. The indication for primary repair is based on the resulting quality of the native ligament and the length of time since the injury. Primary repair of the MCL is usually performed within 7–10 days after the injury. Augmentation repair for the sMCL can be used when the resulting quality of the native ligament makes the primary repair impossible. Reconstruction is indicated when MCL injuries fail to heal in neutral or varus alignment. Reconstruction might be advisable for correcting chronic instability. Chronic, medial-sided knee injuries with valgus malalignment should be treated using a two-stage approach. A distal femoral osteotomy should be performed first, followed by reconstruction of the medial knee structures.

6.12 Cases of MCL Injury

Case 1—MCL Conservative Treatment Case

A 25-year-old male patient with no previous history of knee visited the outpatient clinic complaining of left knee pain. The symptoms began to occur at his knee bent left and right while doing jiujitsu 4 days ago. There were no specific findings on the radiograph taken immediately after the injury and MCL tenderness with valgus stress test grade 1 were checked on physical examination (Fig. 6.8).

The MRI taken at the time of the injury showed that the MCL was thinned overall due to an acute tear, and the T2 imaging test showed a high signal, showing an acute complete rupture of proximal MCL (Figs. 6.9 and 6.10a, b). There were accompanied MMPH horizontal tear involving inferior surface.

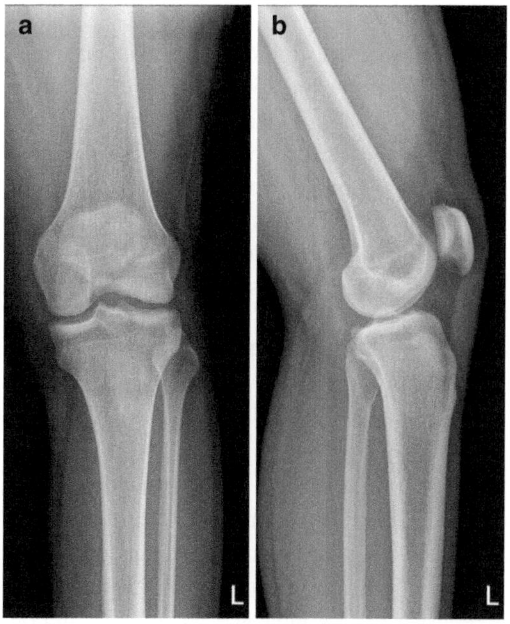

Fig. 6.8 (**a**, **b**) Preoperative x-ray were shown

During the patient's outpatient follow-up, he was felt that the pain and instability gradually improved over time. The patient is in a state where he does not feel any discomfort or valgus laxity in everyday life.

Case 2—MCL Repair Case

A 64-year-old man, 1 month ago, landed during a jump while playing tennis, causing flexion and internal rotation of his left knee. Afterwards, discomfort and instability in his left knee persisted and was referred to our outpatient clinic via another hospital. He had a history of conservative treatment for right knee ACL rupture 20 years ago. There were no specific findings on the plain radiograph taken immediately after the injury (Fig. 6.11a, b), and Lachman test grade 2 and valgus stress test grade 2 were checked on physical examination (Figs. 6.12, 6.13, 6.14 and 6.15).

In the follow-up valgus stress x-ray after surgery, SSD was almost zero (Fig. 6.16).

There was no discomfort in the patient's left knee during outpatient follow-up after surgery, and laxity was not confirmed in the ADT and valgus stress tests on physical examination.

Case 3—MCL Reconstruction Case

A 61-year-old man, who underwent multiple surgical treatments for Fx. patella, Lt. &Fx. shaft, femur, Lt. after motorcycle TA, visited our outpatient department 2 years after the injury, complaining of pain in the medial part of his right knee and a feeling of instability in his knee during exercise (Fig. 6.17).

Fig. 6.9 (**a**, **b**) The patient's pain was not severe, and there were no instability findings complaining in daily life, so it was decided to perform conservative treatment first, and a long leg cast was applied for 2 weeks. Afterwards, MCL brace was applied for 3 weeks

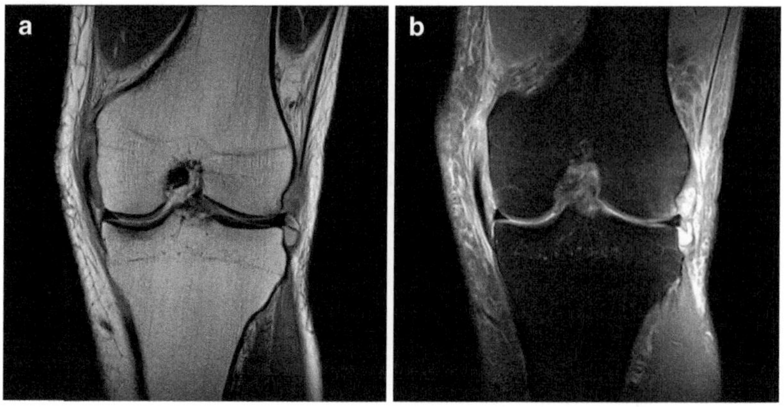

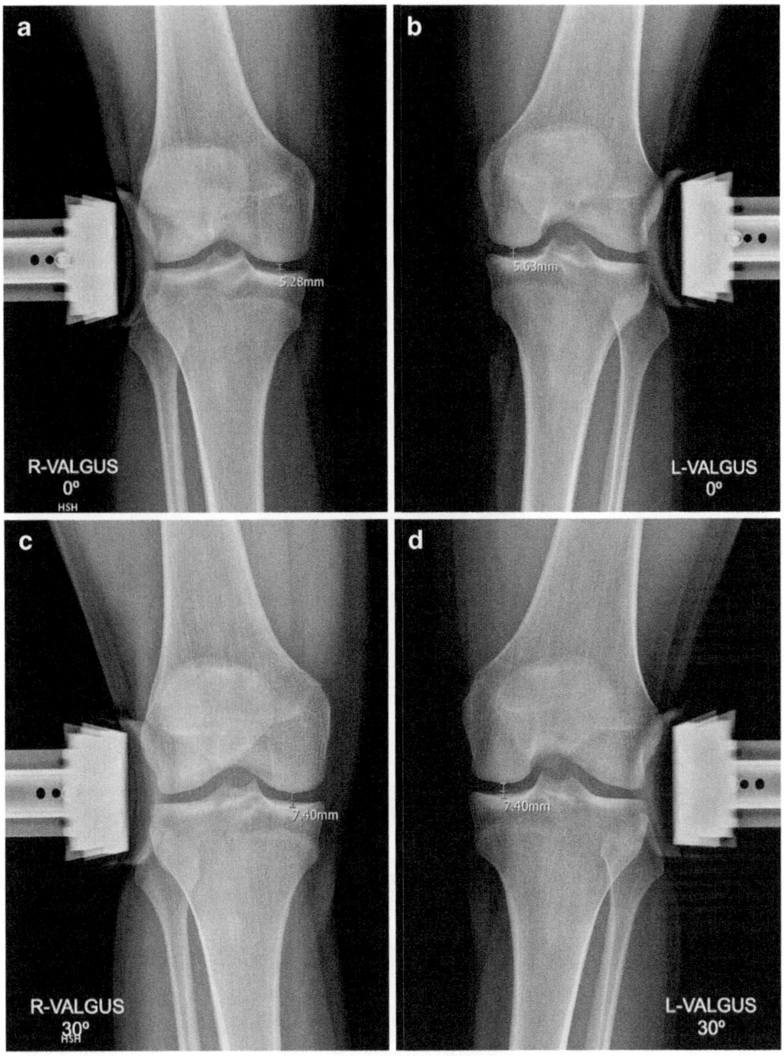

Fig. 6.10 (**a**, **b**) 0°, (**c**, **d**) 30° flexion. In the valgus stress radiographic examination taken at 3 months after injury, a no SSD (side to side difference), no valgus laxity was checked compared to the unaffected side

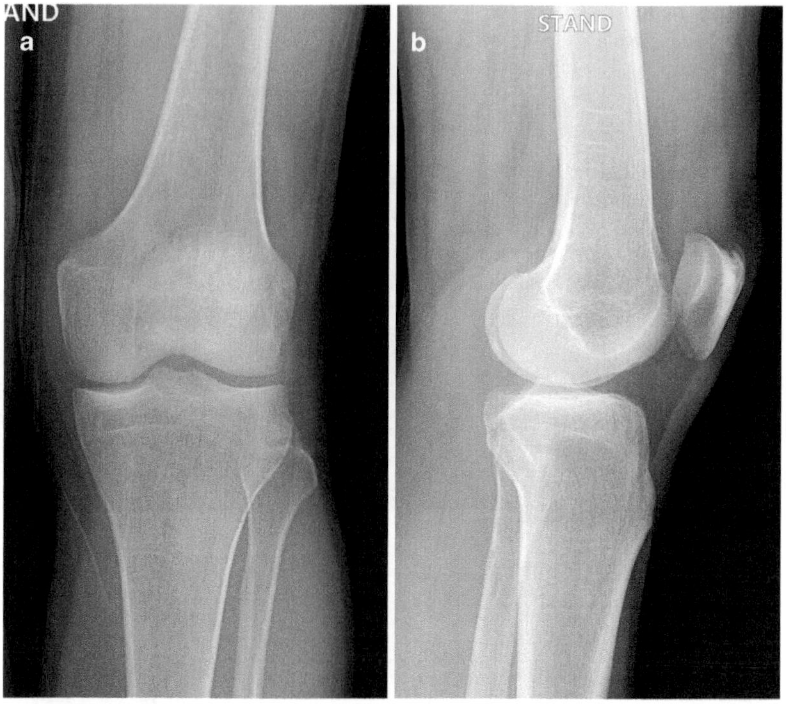

Fig. 6.11 (**a**, **b**) There were no specific findings on the plain radiograph taken immediately after the injury (**a**, **b**), and Lachman test grade 2 and valgus stress test grade 2 were checked on physical examination

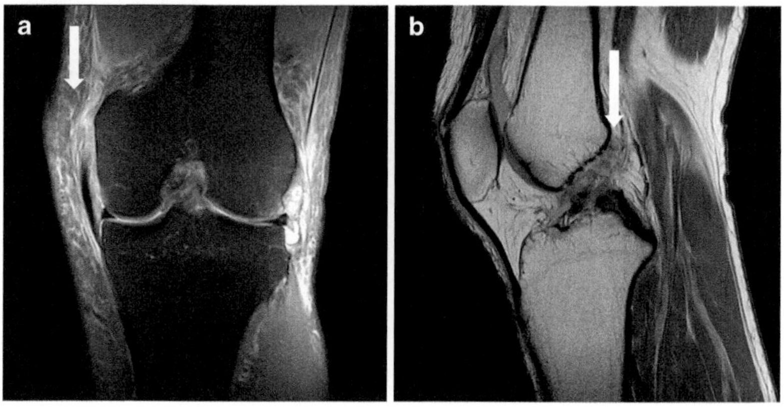

Fig. 6.12 (**a**, **b**) A complete rupture of the ACL was accompanied by a complete rupture of the femur side of the MCL on MRI

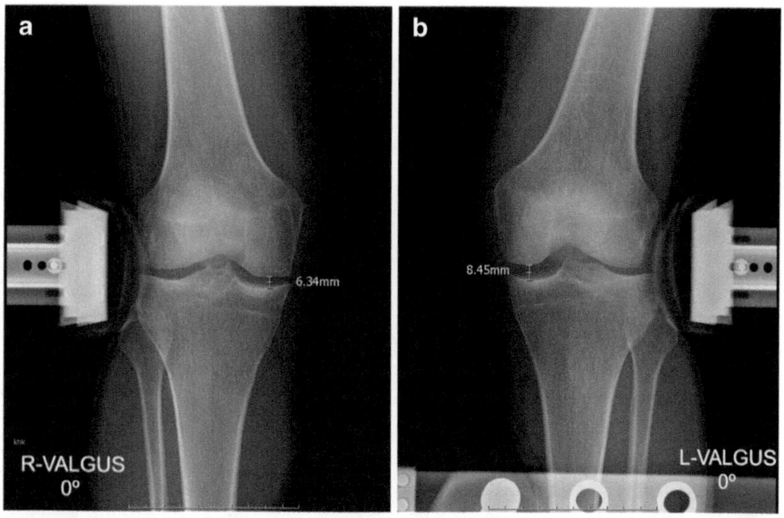

Fig. 6.13 (**a**, **b**) In the 0′ valgus stress radiographic examination, a 2.1 mm SSD (side to side difference) was checked compared to the unaffected side

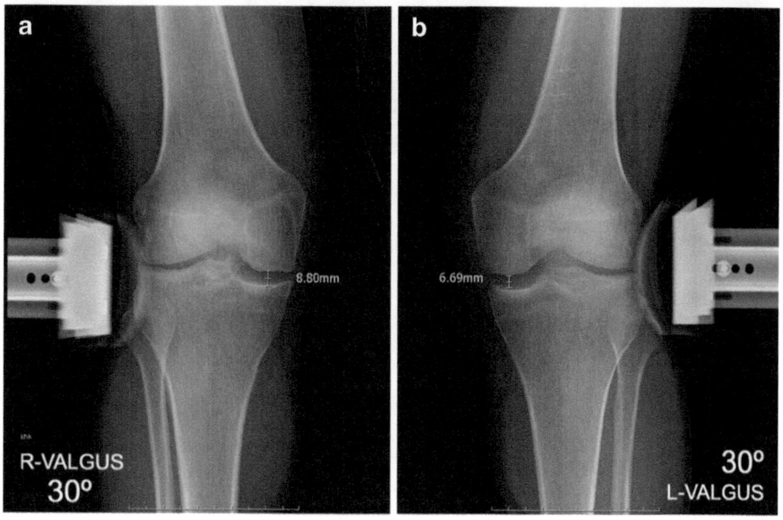

Fig. 6.14 (**a**, **b**) In the 30′ valgus stress radiographic examination, a 2.1 mm SSD as checked compared to the unaffected side

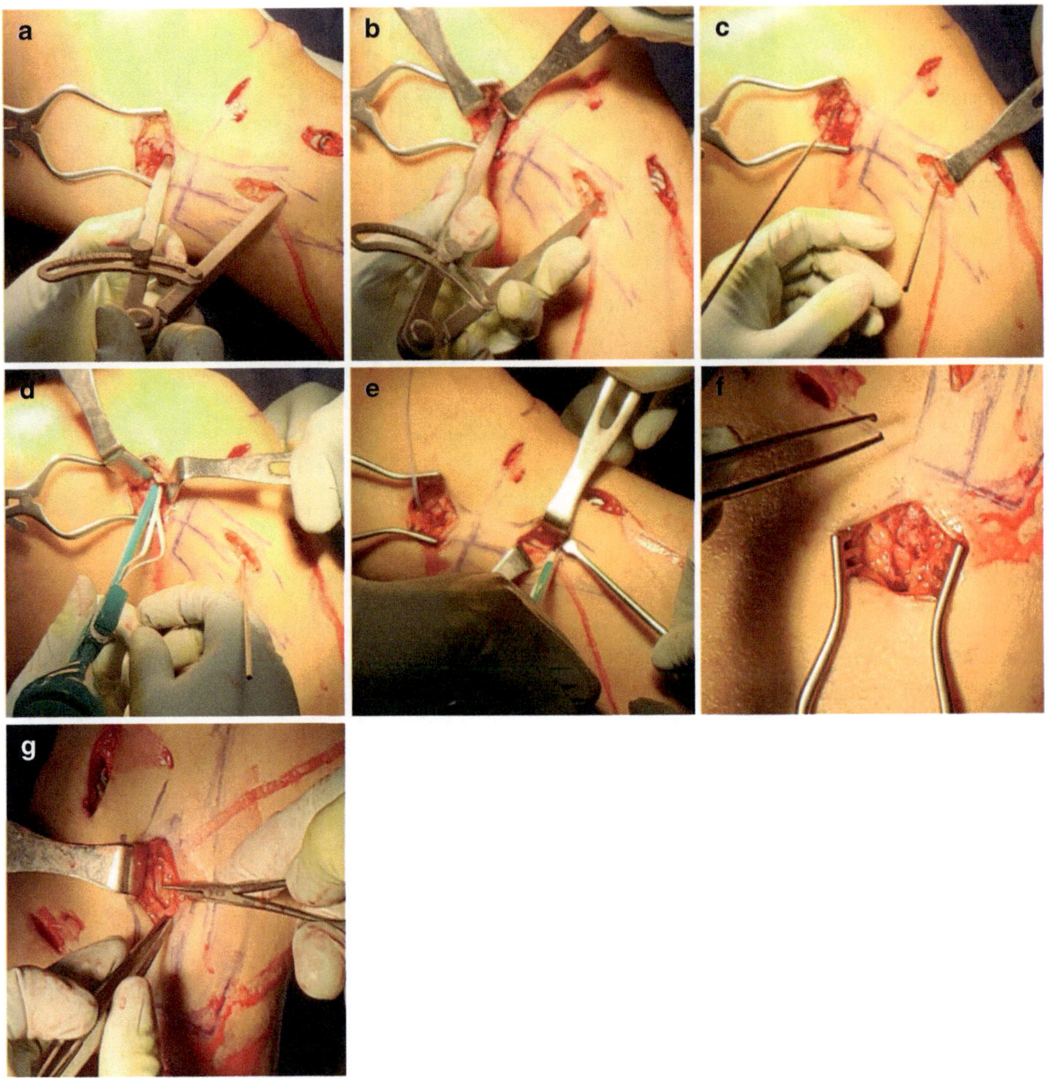

Fig. 6.15 (**a**, **b**) MCL repair was performed using an anchor with fiber tape for acute MCL injury findings along with ACL reconstruction in an unstable pattern during valgus stress. (**c**) K-wires were inserted to the isometric points. (**d**, **e**) MCL augmentation was performed using a Swivelock anchor. (**f**, **g**) Finally, MCL repair was performed using the anchors. The repaired ligament was shown with fiber tape augmentation. An isometric point was found using a compass

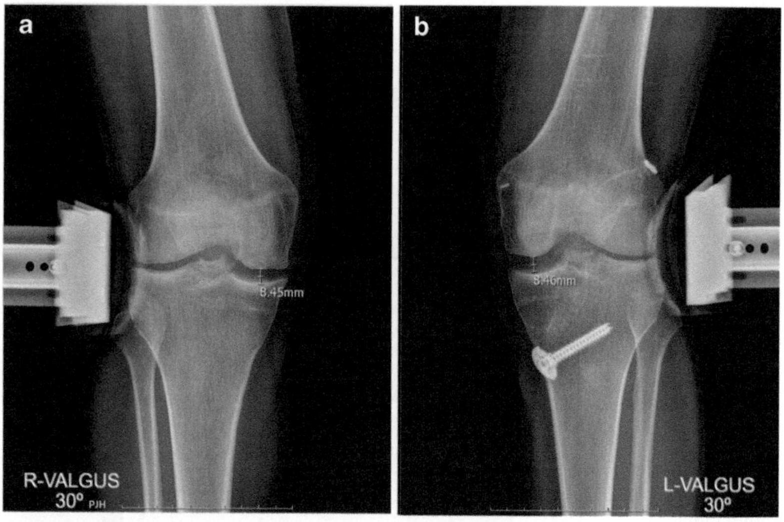

Fig. 6.16 (**a**, **b**) No laxity on valgus test was found

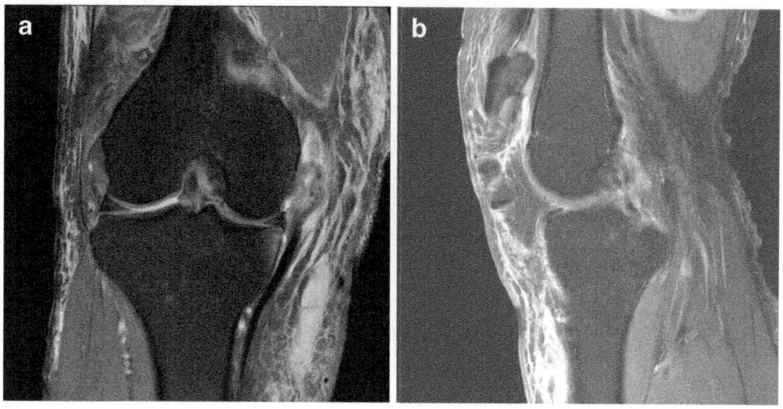

Fig. 6.17 (**a**) The findings of acute MCL complete rupture and (**b**) PCL complete rupture are confirmed on MRI taken at the time of injury

Chronic MCL and PCL rupture findings are consistently confirmed on f/u MRI taken 2 years after treatment for fracture injuries (Fig. 6.18a, b).

On physical examination, valgus stress test grade 2/1, PDT grade 3/3, and PLRI grade 2/2 were confirmed (Figs. 6.19 and 6.20).

It was checked that medial instability and discomfort persisted even after 2 years of conservative treatment, and it was difficult to expect improvement with primary sutures due to chronic rupture findings. Therefore, anatomical reconstruction of MCL was performed using an Achilles allograft because there was persistent valgus instability despite conservative treatment along with PCL reconstruction (Fig. 6.21a, b).

A tunnel was made on the femur lateral side along the guide pin, reamed, and the allogeneic tendon was inserted and fixed with a bio-screw. Afterwards, the graft tendon was moved to the tibia to find an isometric point, and after confirming that there was no change in ligament length during ROM, it was fixed.

After surgery, the CT showed the properly positioned tunnel and bioabsorbable screw in the femur and tibia. The posterior cruciate ligament and medial collateral ligament on the femoral side were well maintained without overlapping (Fig. 6.22a–f and 6.23).

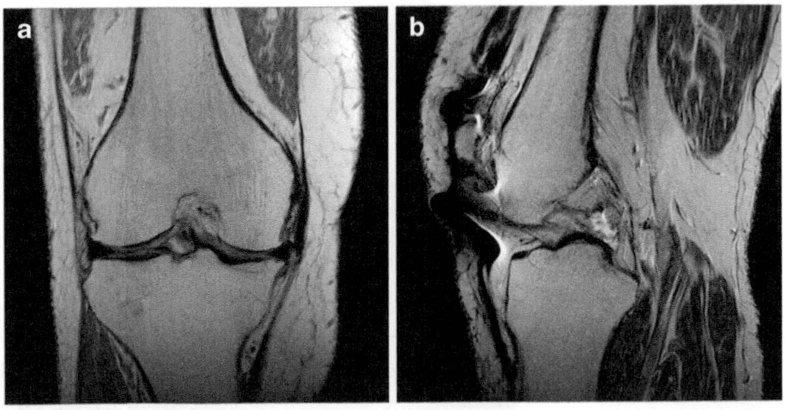

Fig. 6.18 (**a**, **b**) Chronic MCL and PCL injury (no ligament) were found

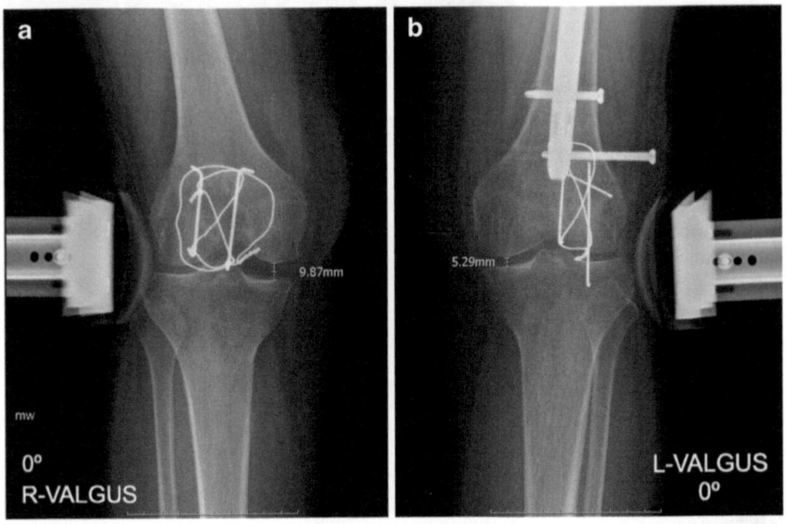

Fig. 6.19 (**a**, **b**) In the 0′ valgus stress radiographic examination, a 4.6 mm SSD (side to side difference) was checked compared to the unaffected side

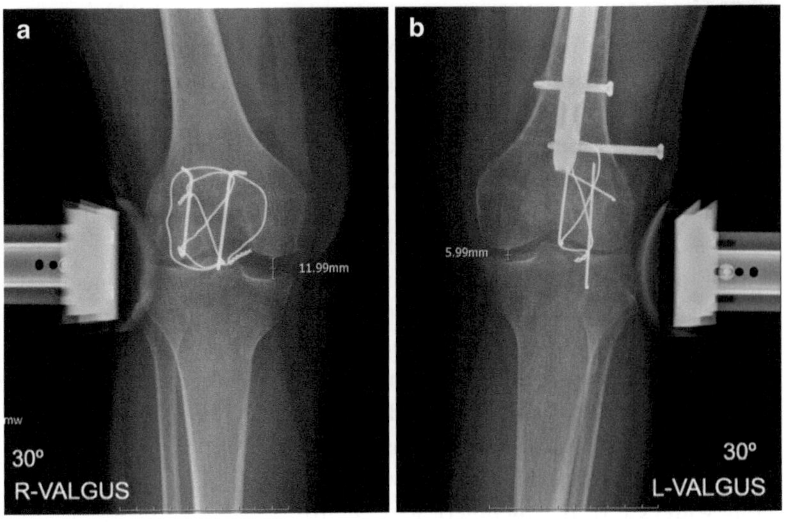

Fig. 6.20 (**a**, **b**) In the 30′ valgus stress radiographic examination, a 6 mm SSD was confirmed compared to the unaffected side

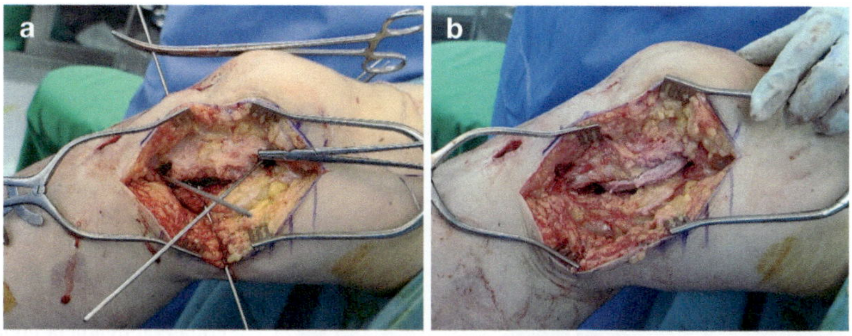

Fig. 6.21 (**a, b**) Anatomical reconstruction of MCL was performed using an Achilles allograft because there was persistent valgus instability despite conservative treatment along with PCL reconstruction

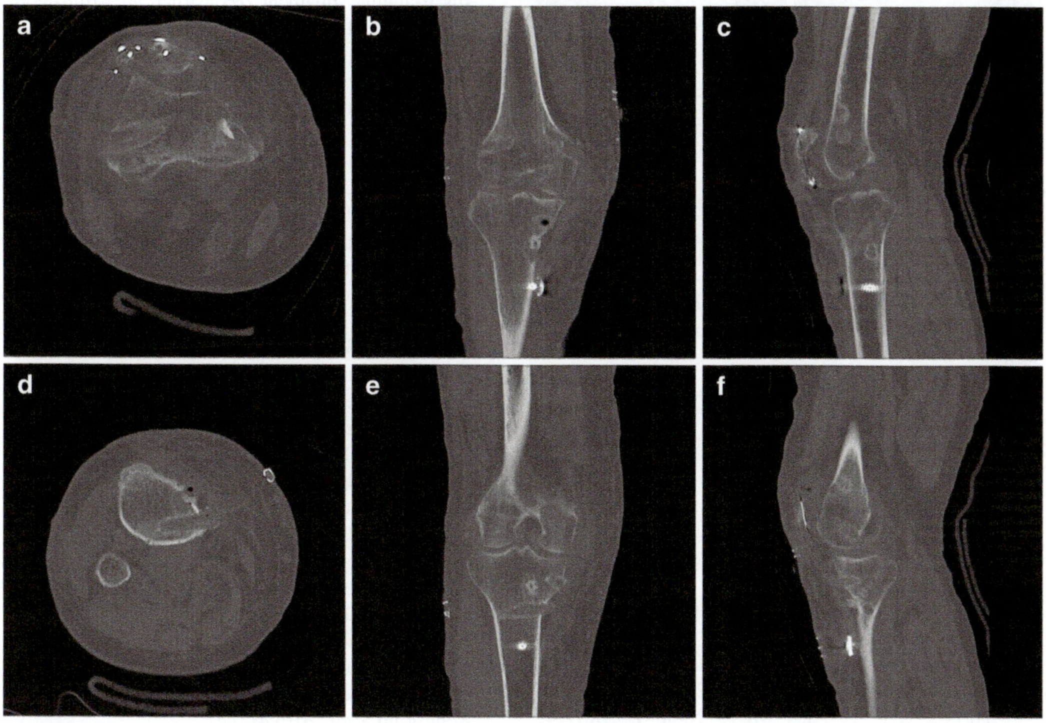

Fig. 6.22 Postoperative CT images. (**a**) Reconstructed PCL and MCL femoral tunnel were shown on axial image. (**b**) No collision of femoral tunnels. (**c**) Well-reconstructed PCL was found on sagittal image. (**d**) MCL tunnels were shown. No overlapping was found. (**e**) The tibial tunnels of sMCL and POL were shown. No overlapping was found. (**f**) No collision were found among the tunnels. During outpatient follow-up after surgery, laxity was not seen in the patient's right knee valgus stress test and posterior draw test, and medial discomfort improved

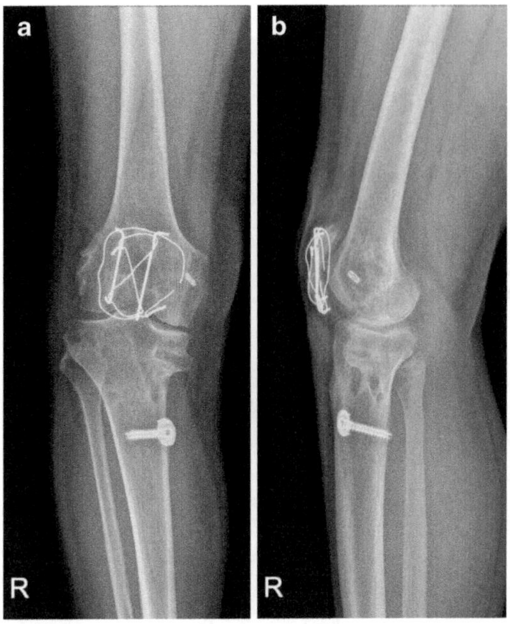

Fig. 6.23 (**a**, **b**) The x-ray taken during outpatient follow-up showed no unusual findings and was maintained well

References

1. Memarzadeh A, Melton J. Medial collateral ligament of the knee: anatomy, management and surgical techniques for reconstruction. Orthop Trauma. 2019;33(2):91–9.
2. DeLong J, Waterman B. Surgical techniques for the reconstruction of medial collateral ligament and posteromedial corner injuries of the knee: a systematic review. Arthroscopy. 2015;31(11):2258–72.
3. Andrews Kyle L, Alex MKL, Nabil E. Review: medial collateral ligament injuries. J Orthop. 2017;14(4):550–4.
4. Robinson J, Bull A, Thomas R, Amis A. The role of the medial collateral ligament and posteromedial capsule in controlling knee laxity. Am J Sports Med. 2006;34(11):1815–23.
5. Phisitkul P, James S, Wolf B, Amendola A. MCL injuries of the knee: current concepts review. Iowa Orthop J. 2006;26:77–90.
6. LaPrade R, Engebretsen A, Ly T, Johansen S, Wentorf F, Engebretsen L. The anatomy of the medial part of the knee. J Bone Joint Surg Am. 2007;89(9):2000–10.
7. Wijdicks C, Ewart D, Nuckley D, Johansen S, Engebretsen L, LaPrade R. Structural properties of the primary medial knee ligaments. Am J Sports Med. 2010;38(8):1638–46.
8. Griffith C, LaPrade R, Johansen S, Armitage B, Wijdicks C, Engebretsen L. Medial knee injury: part 1, static function of the individual components of the main medial knee structures. Am J Sports Med. 2009;37(9):1762–70.
9. Jacobson K, Chi F. Evaluation and treatment of medial collateral ligament and medial-sided injuries of the knee. Sports Med Arthrosc Rev. 2006;14(2):58–66.
10. Chen L, Kim P, Ahmad C, Levine W. Medial collateral ligament injuries of the knee: current treatment concepts. Curr Rev Musculoskelet Med. 2008;1(2):108–13.
11. Dong J, Wang X, Men X, Zhu J, Walker G, Zheng X, et al. Surgical treatment of acute grade III medial collateral ligament injury combined with anterior cruciate ligament injury: anatomic ligament repair versus triangular ligament reconstruction. Arthroscopy. 2015;31(6):1108–16.
12. Serra Cruz R, Olivetto J, Dean C, Chahla J, LaPrade R. Superficial medial collateral ligament of the knee: anatomic augmentation with semitendinosus and Gracilis tendon autografts. Arthrosc Tech. 2016;5(2):e347–e52.
13. Lundblad M, Hägglund M, Thomeé C, Hamrin Senorski E, Ekstrand J, Karlsson J, et al. Medial collateral ligament injuries of the knee in male professional football players: a prospective three-season study of 130 cases from the UEFA elite club injury study. Knee Surg Sports Traumatol Arthrosc. 2019;27(11):3692–8.
14. Edson C. Conservative and postoperative rehabilitation of isolated and combined injuries of the medial collateral ligament. Sports Med Arthrosc Rev. 2006;14(2):105–10.
15. Tandogan R, Kayaalp A. Surgical treatment of medial knee ligament injuries: current indications and techniques. EFORT Open Rev. 2016;1(2):27–33.
16. Encinas-Ullán CA, Rodríguez-Merchán E. Isolated medial collateral ligament tears: an update on management. EFORT Open Rev. 2018;3(7):398–407.
17. Burrus MT, Werner B, Griffin J, Gwathmey F, Miller M. Diagnostic and management strategies for multiligament knee injuries a critical analysis review. J Bone Joint Surg. 2016;4(2):e1.
18. Elkin J, Zamora E, Gallo R. Combined anterior cruciate ligament and medial collateral ligament knee injuries: anatomy, diagnosis, management recommendations, and return to sport. Curr Rev Musculoskelet Med. 2019;12(2):239–44.
19. Grant J, Tannenbaum E, Miller B, Bedi A. Treatment of combined complete tears of the anterior cruciate and medial collateral ligaments. Arthroscopy. 2012;28(1):110–22.
20. Lubowitz J, Mackay G, Gilmer B. Knee medial collateral ligament and posteromedial corner anatomic repair with internal bracing. Arthrosc Tech. 2014;3(4):e505–8.
21. Hughston JC. The importance of the posterior oblique ligament in repairs of acute tears of the medial ligaments in knees with and without an associated rupture of the anterior cruciate ligament. Results of long-term follow-up. J Bone Joint Surg Am. 1994;76(9):1328–44.

22. Van der List J, Difelice G. Primary repair of the medial collateral ligament with internal bracing. Arthrosc Tech. 2017;6(4):e933–e7.
23. Golden T, Friedman A, Jazayeri R, Sanderson B, Levy E. Primary repair of the medial collateral ligament with a double row suture technique and suture tape augmentation for acute tibial-sided injuries. Arthrosc Tech. 2019;8(4):e395–e8.
24. Trofa D, Sonnenfeld J, Song D, Lynch TS. Distal knee medial collateral ligament repair with suture augmentation. Arthrosc Tech. 2018;7(9):e921–6.
25. Van der Wal WA, Van Gennip S, Heesterbeek PJ, Busch VJ, Wymenga AB. Anatomical superficial medial collateral ligament reconstruction with posteromedial capsule reefing successfully restores valgus knee laxity. Acta Orthop Belg. 2020;86(1):69–76.
26. Joshi A, Nagmani S, Thapa S, Pradhan I. Weave technique for reconstruction of medial collateral ligament and posterior oblique ligament: an anatomic approach using semitendinosus tendon. Arthrosc Tech. 2019;8(11):e1417–e23.
27. LaPrade R, Wijdicks C. Surgical technique: development of an anatomic medial knee reconstruction. Clin Orthop Relat Res. 2011;470(3):806–14.
28. Xu H, Kang K, Zhang J, Xin D, Liu W, Jin G, et al. An anatomical-like triangular-vector ligament reconstruction for the medial collateral ligament and the posterior oblique ligament injury with single femoral tunnel: a retrospective study. J Orthop Surg Res. 2017;12(6)
29. Vosoughi F, Rezaei Dogahe R, Nuri A, Avati Firoozabadi M, Mortazavi J. Medial collateral ligament injury of the knee: a review on current concept and management. Arch Bone Jt Surg. 2021;9(3):255–62.

7 Anterior Cruciate Ligament Reconstruction Revision

Abstract

Preoperative Evaluation for ACL Revision

The surgeon should have an understanding of the etiology of ACL reconstruction failure. In order to have accurate information, the medical history, current symptoms, type of graft, method of fixation, surgical approach, previous surgical notes, etc., should be obtained. The surgeon should also be aware of the patient's activity level, functional goals, and expectations. Finally, to achieve a successful revision, the surgeon should know the etiology of the reconstruction failure.

The physical examination should begin by inspecting the affected knee to look for effusion, signs of infection, and previous surgical incisions. Stance and gait should be assessed to identify any possible malalignment of the limb. The varus or valgus thrust gait should be further assessed. Specific maneuvers should be performed to evaluate the posterolateral or posteromedial corners. The valgus and varus stress tests at 0* and 30*, the position of the knee, and the range of motion should be compared to the normal side. The major cause of ACL reconstruction failure is technical error. Tunnel malposition, hardware malposition or failure, and unrecognized limb malalignment are the most common errors. A malpositioned graft will have a non-physiologic load, and if it is loaded beyond its yield point, the graft will be a failure. The most common type of tunnel malposition is an anterior (anatomically distal) femoral tunnel. This position results in reduced knee flexion due to increased graft tension, or if physiologic knee flexion is achieved, graft attenuation and/or failure. Vertical placement of the femoral tunnel will provide adequate anterior-posterior restraint but will compromise the rotational stability of the knee, e.g., negative Lachman test but positive pivot shift test.

Malpositioning of the tibial tunnel also affects the graft. If the tibial tunnel is placed too anteriorly, the graft will hit the notch when the knee is extended. Posterior placement causes graft laxity in flexion and PCL impingement.

Graft fixation is critical to maintain proper graft placement and tension, especially at approximately 2 weeks postoperatively when the graft is at its weakest.

The risk of ACL reconstruction failure has been shown to be influenced by unrecognized bony malalignment and missed comorbidities, such as MCL laxity, LCL laxity, or neglected posteromedial, posterolateral rotatory insufficiency. The risk of graft failure may also be increased by untreated injuries to the posterolateral or posteromedial structures and the medial meniscus at the time of initial ACL reconstruction.

Y. B. Jung et al., *Treatment of the Cruciate Ligaments Injuries*,
https://doi.org/10.1007/978-981-95-9039-1_7

Posteroanterior tibia slope and varus malalignment place increased stress on the graft, and a posteroanterior tibia slope of 12* or more has been shown to be the strongest predictor of recurrent ACL injury (Salmon et al). Preoperative evaluation for ACL revision.

Keywords

Etiology of the failure • Neglected posteromedial and posterolateral instability • Varus or valgus thrust gait • Malalignment • Posterior tibial slope

7.1 Principles of Treatment of Anterior Cruciate Ligament Revision

According to the reference, anterior cruciate ligament (ACL) reconstruction is performed at a rate of 74.6 per 100,000 in the United States, and 75–97% of patients have a satisfactory outcome. However, patients younger than 20 years of age have a higher rate of graft failure.

7.2 Etiology of Graft Failure

The key to successful ACL revision surgery is to identify the cause of graft failure. The Multicenter ACL Revision Study Group detailed the causes of ACL graft failure. They showed that multiple factors were responsible for the majority of ACL re-tears (37%). A single cause of revision was responsible for the majority of traumatic re-injuries (32%), technical errors (24%), and biological factors (7%) of patients. Autografting has been shown to have good results.

However, the graft used in previous autograft harvesting procedures determines the available autograft donor sites for revision ACL reconstruction. In the young and active population, allografts are associated with a significantly higher risk of revision surgery, according to the literature.

Traumatic ACL graft failures can be divided into those that occur before graft incorporation and those that occur after graft incorporation.

Early physical therapy is recommended for the initiation of range of motion and gentle muscle strengthening. However, a new graft may be compromised by aggressive early strengthening (2 weeks postoperatively). This is because an animal study showed that the ACL graft lost 30% of the strength of the native ACL during the first year after surgery. At any time during rehabilitation, acute trauma to the surgical knee may occur. However, high-level sports with increased cutting movements have been shown to cause microtrauma to the graft. This can eventually lead to graft attenuation and failure.

Risk factors for graft attenuation or re-rupture after return to full activity include

1. Young age < 25 years.
2. Return to contact sports such as spinning and jumping activities.
3. Decreased quadriceps/hamstring strength.
4. Poor performance on postoperative single-leg hop/jump tests has also been shown to correlate with a higher risk of reinjury.

7.3 Preoperative Evaluation for ACL Revision Surgery

The surgeon should have an understanding of the etiology of ACL reconstruction failure. The patient's medical history, current symptoms, graft type, fixation method, surgical approach, and previous surgical notes, as well as the patient's activity level, desired functional abilities, and patient expectations, should be obtained to have accurate information. Finally, in order to perform a successful revision, the surgeon should be aware of the etiology of the reconstruction failure.

The physical examination should begin with an inspection of the affected knee. Look for effusion, signs of infection (Figs. 7.1, 7.2, and 7.3a, b), and previous surgical incisions. Stance and gait should be assessed to identify any possible malalignment of the limb.

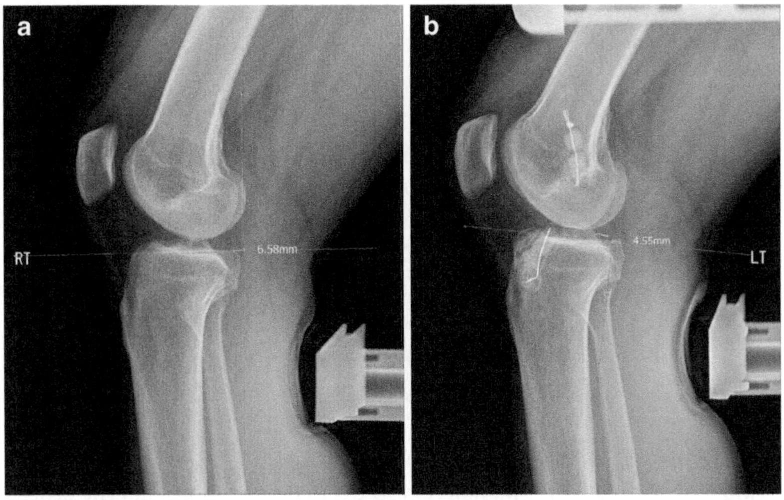

Fig. 7.1 (**a**, **b**) More than 2–3 mm difference was checked compared to the unaffected side in the pull stress test imaging. For the physical exam, the Lachman test was positive, and a definite positive pivot shift test was observed

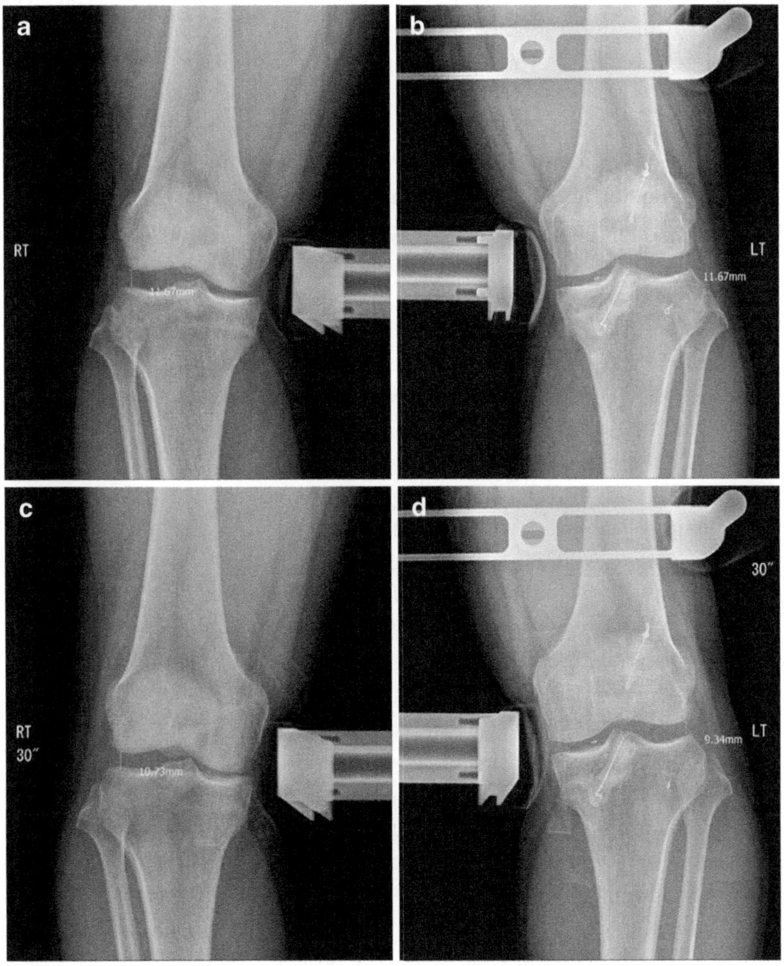

Fig. 7.2 (**a**, **b**) 0° and (**c**, **d**) 30° flexion view and varus view, respectively; a 1–2 mm difference was shown

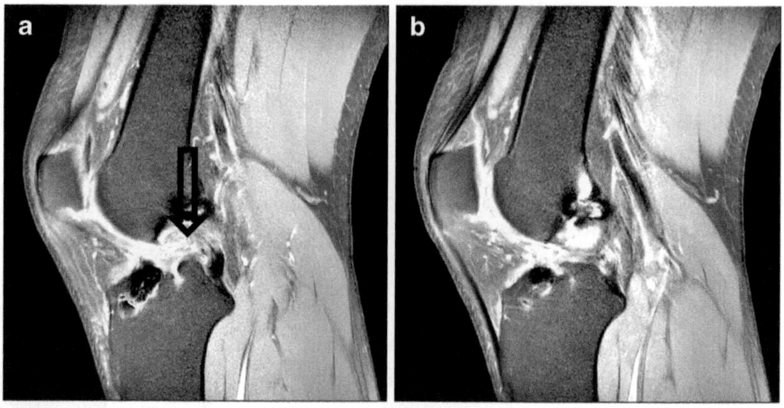

Fig. 7.3 (**a**, **b**) ACL is absent on MRI due to infection

Varus or valgus thrust gait should be further evaluated with specific maneuvers to evaluate the posterolateral or posteromedial corners. Valgus and varus stress testing at 0* and 30*, knee position, and range of motion should be compared with the normal side (Figs. 7.2 and 7.4c–f).

Technical errors are the second most common cause of failure in ACL reconstruction. The most common errors are improper tunnel placement, incorrect hardware placement or hardware failure, and unrecognized limb malalignment. A malpositioned graft will receive non-physiologic loads, and if stressed beyond its yield point, the graft will fail. The most common type of tunnel malposition is an anterior (anatomically distal) femoral tunnel. This position results in decreased knee flexion due to increased graft tension, or if physiologic knee flexion is achieved, the graft will be attenuated and/or fail. Vertical femoral tunnel placement (Figs. 7.2a–d and 7.25c, d) provides adequate anterior-posterior restraint but compromises rotational stability of the knee, resulting in a negative Lachman test but a positive pivot shift test. Malpositioning of the tibial tunnel also affects the graft. Placement of the tibial tunnel that is too anterior will result in impingement of the graft on the notch during extension. Posterior placement will result in graft laxity in flexion and impingement on the posterior cruciate ligament.

Graft fixation is critical to maintain proper graft placement and tension. This is especially true at approximately 2 weeks postoperatively when the graft is at its weakest.

Bone-tendon-bone grafts may fail at the bone-to-bone interface or with pullout failure of the interference screw fixation. Soft tissue graft fixation failure typically occurs due to improper placement of the endoscopic fastener or tension failure of the suspended fixation.

The risk of ACL graft rupture has been shown to be influenced by unrecognized bony malalignment and missed comorbidities, such as MCL laxity, LCL laxity (Fig. 7.4c–f), or neglected posteromedial PLRI (posterolateral rotatory instability) (Figs. 7.7, 7.8, 7.21, 7.22, 7.23, 7.24, 7.25, 7.26, and 7.27). Posterior tibial slope and varus malalignment place increased stress on the graft, and a posterior tibial slope greater than 12* has been shown to be the strongest predictor of ACL injury recurrence (by Salmon et al.).

Varus or valgus thrust gait should be further evaluated with specific maneuvers to evaluate the posterolateral or posteromedial corners. Valgus and varus stress testing at 0* and 30* knee position and range of motion should be compared with the normal side.

Technical errors are the second most common cause of ACL reconstruction failure. The most common errors are inappropriate tunnel placement, incorrect hardware placement or hardware failure, and unrecognized limb malalignment. A malpositioned graft will sustain non-physiologic loads, and if stressed beyond its yield point, the graft will fail. The most common tunnel malposition is an anterior (anatomically distal) femoral tunnel. This position results in decreased knee flexion due to increased graft tension, or if physiologic knee flexion is achieved, the graft will be attenuated and/or fail.

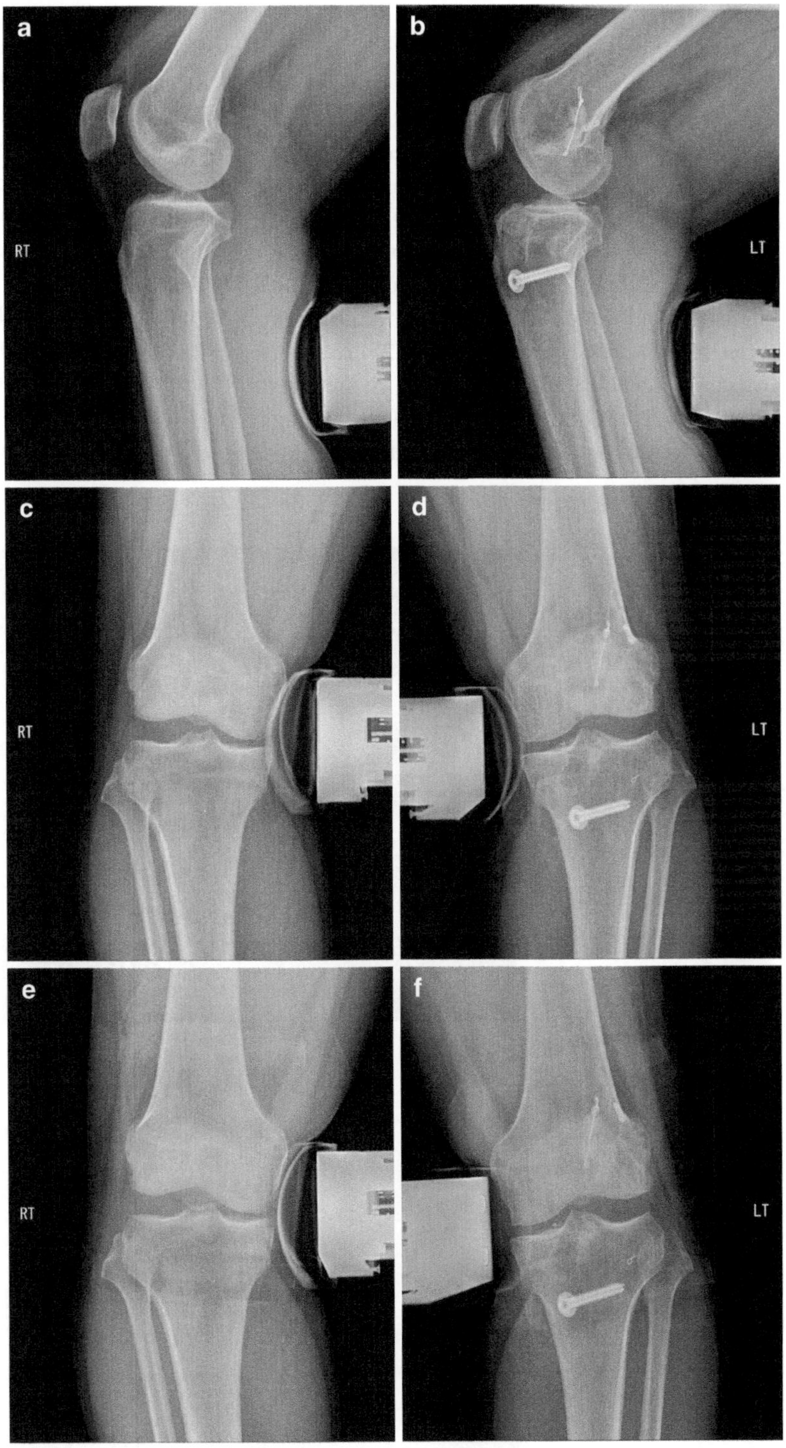

Fig. 7.4 Seven months after ACL revision. (**a**, **b**) Pull view, (**c**, **d**) 0°, (**e**, **f**) 30° varus stress view of both knees. There was not much instability in the pull and varus stress view

7.4 Imaging Techniques

Determine whether, in one in all patients who present with recurrent instability of the knee, an initial radiograph of the affected knee should be obtained. For tibial and femoral tunnel placement, anterior, posterior, and lateral views can be obtained. The ACL tunnel will be placed in an accurate location with no need for redirection, in an inaccurate location with a need for redirection through native bone (Figs. 7.4 and 7.25) or in an inaccurate location with a need for redirection through a preexisting tunnel. Weight-bearing knee radiographs and standing alignment radiographs should also be obtained. These images are evaluated for degenerative changes or malalignment of the limb, including varus, valgus, and excessive posterior tibial slope (Figs. 7.5, 7.6, and 7.7). The tibial slope can be measured on lateral radiographs of the knee. MRI can be used primarily for evaluation of graft status and associated injuries such as chondral damage; meniscal, coronal, and sagittal planes should be measured at the widest visualized diameter (Figs. 7.8, 7.9, and 7.10). Measurements >15 mm are consistent with significant tunnel osteolysis. The literature supports performing bone grafting prior to revision ACL reconstruction.

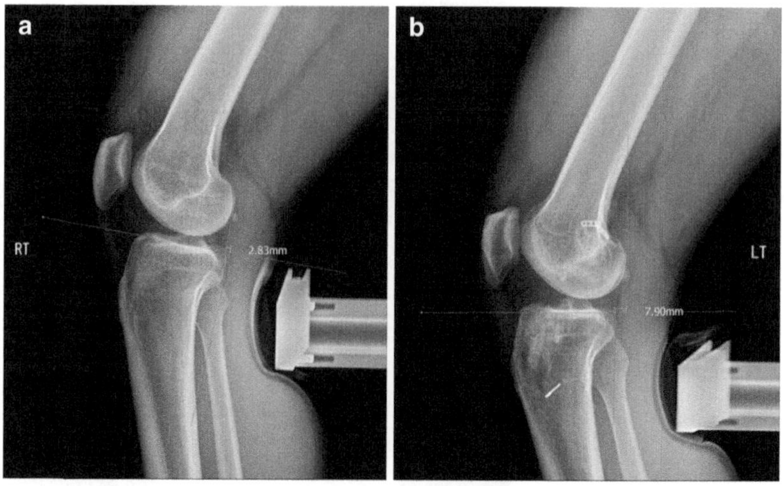

Fig. 7.5 (**a**, **b**) A side-to-side difference of 5.1 mm compared to the unaffected side was verified in the pull stress test image

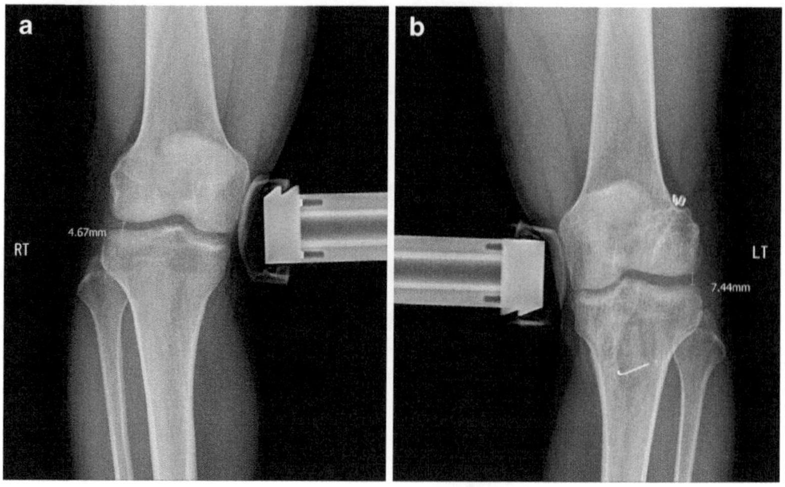

Fig. 7.6 (**a**, **b**) Varus stress view; left knee lateral joint space is wider than the right knee

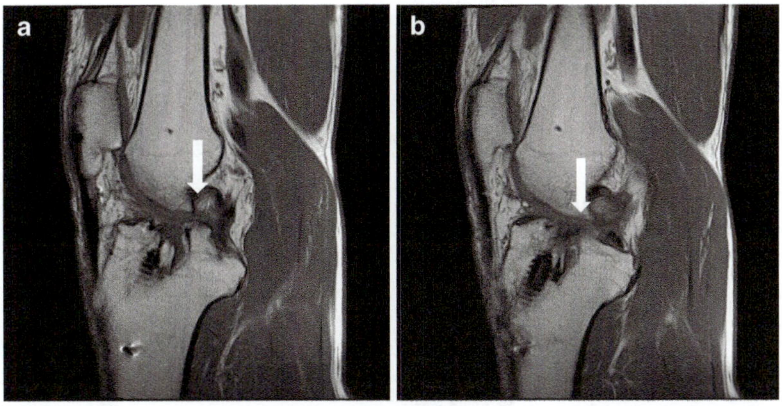

Fig. 7.7 (**a**, **b**) The ACL graft was partially ruptured and had melted away on the femoral side

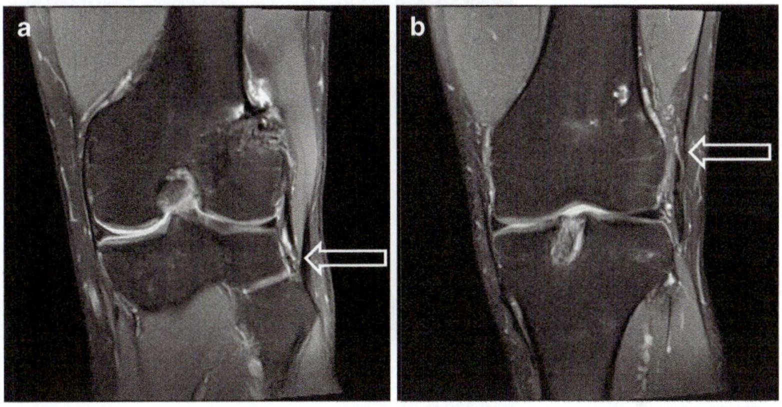

Fig. 7.8 (**a**, **b**) Absent ACL graft was shown. (**a**, **b**) LCL injury was observed on MRI

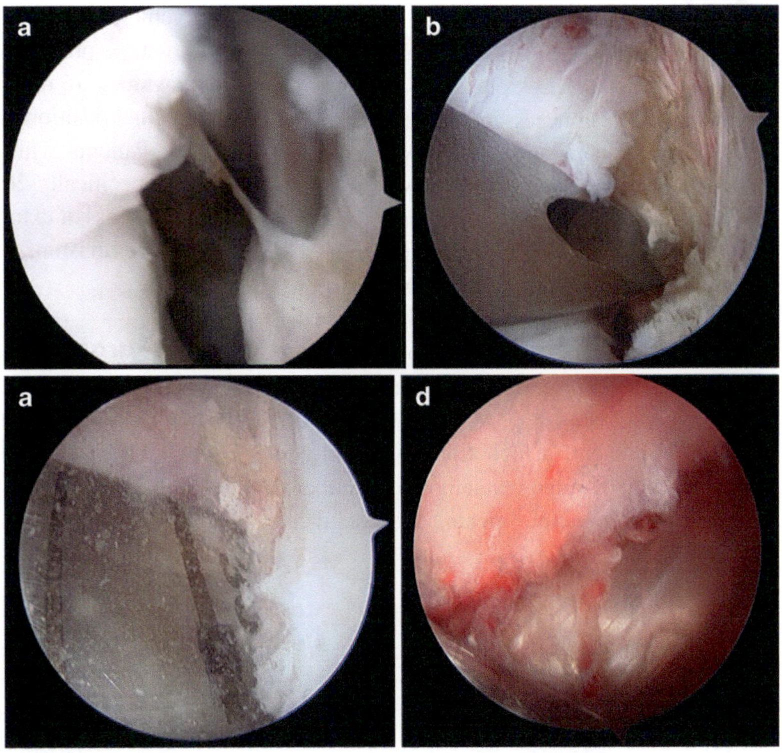

Fig. 7.9 (**a**) Lateral femoral condyle articular upper margin, (**b**) 7 mm offset guide applied just above the lateral femoral condyle articular upper margin, (**c**, **d**) ACL revision surgery using the rectangular dilator was shown. Using the rectangular dilator, the tunnels could be impacted and a more anatomical shape of the graft

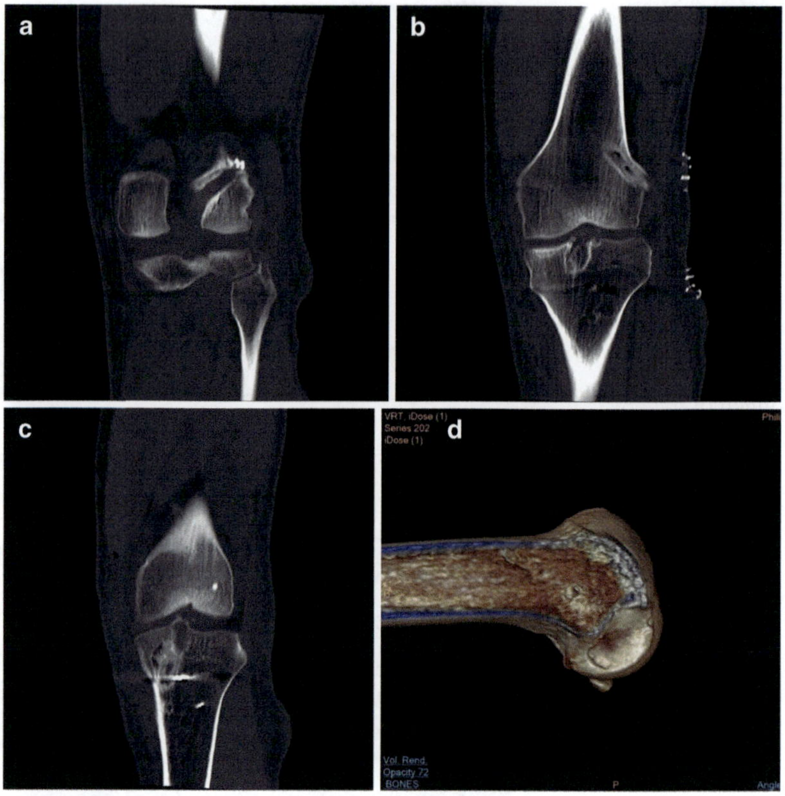

Fig. 7.10 (**a**) A femoral tunnel formed at the anatomical location of the femoral side of the ACL was checked. (**b**) Femoral tunnel for the PLCS (**b**, **c**) Tibial tunnel for the ACL. (**d**) Femoral tunnel just below the posterior femoral cortical line on the 3D CT image taken after ACL revision using a rounded rectangular dilator with PLCS through the fibular head tunnel to the lateral epicondyle area

7.5 Preoperative Considerations

In the planning of revision ACL reconstruction, the surgeon should check one-stage or two-stage procedure will be necessary. As noted above, patients with limb malalignment may need to correct this to prevent recurrent graft laxity or injury. Procedures to correct limb malalignment are typically performed at the same time as revision ACL reconstruction. However, they may be performed in a staged fashion. An anterior closing wedge tibial osteotomy for excessive posterior tibial slope has been performed to reduce anterior tibial translation and force on the ACL. In patients with varus malalignment, a high tibial osteotomy is recommended. In valgus malalignment, either a varus-producing lateral opening wedge distal femoral osteotomy or a medial closing-wedge distal femoral osteotomy can be performed.

Two-stage procedures are performed when a tunnel width > 15 mm is present or when the previous tunnel position interferes with placing new tunnels. Patients with decreased knee range of motion, specifically 20* loss of terminal flexion or > 5–10* loss of extension, should also undergo a two-stage revision.

7.6 Surgical Technique

As a routine arthroscopic evaluation, diagnostic examination, chondral lesion, meniscal tear, intercondylar notch narrowing, ACL graft remnant, etc.

7.7 Single-Stage Revision

If the tunnel widening is <15 mm and the previous tunnels are either in the appropriate positions or are out of the range of the planned tunnels, then a single-stage revision can be performed. Tunnel overlap is not a contraindication to single-stage revision. However, it does require additional techniques to ensure proper graft fixation. Techniques to manage tunnel overlap include the following: Filling the tunnel (either with bone graft or with bone-attached allograft to fill as much of the bone defect as possible). When graft fixation is questionable, a two-stage procedure needs to be considered. If the previous tunnels are used, the surgeon should ream the tunnel to the desired diameter for the new graft or when a circumferential bone margin has been achieved.

7.8 Two-Stage Revision

All hardware should be removed from the tunnel and the immediate area. Bone grafting of the tunnels can be accomplished in a variety of ways, including allograft (shavings or dowels) and autograft. The insertion of dowels must be performed with caution, as a fracture of the dowel is possible and may result in inadequate fixation and bone incorporation. After the initial procedure, the second stage can be performed in 4–6 months. Incorporation of the bone graft is confirmed by plain radiography or CT scan.

7.9 Graft and Fixation Choices

There is controversy regarding the use of autograft versus allograft in revision reconstruction. Some large systematic reviews suggest that the use of autograft is associated with a decreased risk of failure and improved overall clinical outcomes. However, others have found that this difference may be minimal or clinically insignificant. To reduce the risk of graft failure in primary ACL reconstruction, grafts should be at least 8 mm in diameter. In revision ACL reconstruction, loss of graft fixation is a common cause of early failure. If adequate bone stock is available, interference screw fixation should be considered. Suspensory fixation is another option to consider.

If there is concern for fixation integrity, supplemental extra-cortical graft fixation should be used. A suture anchor, staples, a screw, and a washer are options for supplemental fixation.

7.10 Extra-Articular Complementation

The anterolateral complex (ALC) of the knee is an important contributor to rotational stability. It may be injured or deficient in patients with ACL tears. Several biomechanical studies have shown that ACL reconstruction alone does not restore normal knee kinematics in the setting of ACL and ALC injuries. The addition of ALC augmentation reduces anterolateral rotational instability. Therefore, reconstruction of the AL complex, either by lateral extra-articular tenodesis (LET) or anterolateral ligament reconstruction, in the setting of ALC injury has been suggested in both primary and revision ACL reconstruction. However, there is ongoing research and debate regarding the exact indications and clinical significance of ALC augmentation. Recently, Getgood et al. prospectively evaluated the outcomes of adding LET (lateral extra-articular tenodesis) to primary ACL reconstruction and found that LET may reduce the risk of ACL reconstruction failure in young (<25 years), active, ligamentous lax patients in the setting of primary ACL reconstruction with hamstring autograft.

7.11 Revision ACL Results

Recent studies have shown that the objective results of revision ACL reconstruction are less favorable than those of primary ACL reconstruction. Revision ACL reconstructions had lower Lysholm and International Knee Documentation Committee (IKDC) scores in the most recent meta-analysis comparing revision and primary ACL reconstructions. Revisions also showed lower rotational stability. However, AP stability was similar. However, it is interesting to note that several large studies have reported the proportion of repeat revision ACL reconstructions to be 2.0–5.4%. This is comparable to that reported for revision of primary ACL reconstructions (1.7–7.7%). These findings are not consistent with other reports of worse patient-reported and objective outcomes in revision ACL surgery.

Using several objective criteria, including KT-2000 measurements and pivot shift grades, a recent systematic review by Wright et al. reported a failure rate of 13.7% for revision ACL reconstruction. However, using other failure criteria, such as swelling, pain, or knee stiffness, failure rates as high as 25% have been reported. Studies have shown an increased incidence of meniscal pathology in revision ACL surgery, which can lead to a higher degree of osteoarthritis in the knee. In fact, it has been estimated that up to 60% of patients who undergo a revision ACL reconstruction will develop osteoarthritis of the knee joint within approximately 6 years.

In the most recent meta-analysis comparing revision procedures, the lateral augmentation procedures may be considered in any of the following situations: Young patients, multiple revision situations, patients with preoperative grade 2–3 pivot shifts (clunk or locking), patient intent to return to high-risk cutting sports, increased posterior tibial slope not meeting criteria for slope correction osteotomy, and persistent rotational instability after ACL reconstruction. Alternatively, the anterolateral ligament complex can be reconstructed with an allograft tendon. A major concern with ALC augmentation is the potential for overstraining the knee, reducing physiologic rotational motion, and thereby altering normal knee biomechanics.

Nonetheless, over-constraint has been demonstrated in biomechanical studies. Despite early data suggesting that the addition of ALC augmentation to ACL reconstruction results in an increased risk of knee osteoarthritis, this has not been found in more recent, highly powered studies with long-term follow-up.

Authors' preferred control under anesthesia, anterolateral rotatory instability or posterolateral rotatory instability (PLRI), and also lateral laxity or not by the varus stress test at 0 and 30° of flexion of the knee. For PLRI grade 1–2, we should perform the posterolateral corner sling through the fibular head tunnel as the modified Larson technique. For anterolateral rotatory instability, we should do ALC augmentation. In my opinion, PLCS through the fibular head tunnel to the lateral femoral epicondyle, which will cover all lateral rotatory instability, even if anterolateral rotatory instability (Figs. 7.21, 7.22, 7.23, 7.24, 7.25, 7.26, and 7.27). However, be careful not to over-constrain the lateral side of the knee.

7.12 Authors Prefer ACL Revision Technique

In the author's experience, almost all revision anterior cruciate ligament reconstruction is a single stage, even if it is a fourth operation, a tunnel in the femur: (1) when the tunnel is in the correct position, (2) when the tunnel is completely out of position, and (3) when the tunnel is overlapped and is technically problematic. In the case of the transtibial tunnel technique, outside-in technique, in previous ACL reconstruction, using the accessory lower anteromedial portal (AMP) technique makes it easier to solve the problems during revision ACL reconstruction, as the tunnel direction is different (Figs. 7.9, 7.10, 7.11, and 7.12). The creation of the femoral tunnel started at 90 degrees of knee flexion to ensure proximity to the anatomical position. The guide pin was first placed and then completed at nearly 120* knee flexion through the low AM portal, with gradual flexion from the 90-knee position under arthroscopic visualization. At the first marking point (guide pin starting point with awl or electrocautery) and then arthroscope, change through the lower AM portal to confirm the correct position or not, to see the intercondylar ridge and posterior femoral cortical line, which is a linear ACL femoral origin arising in continuity with the pos-

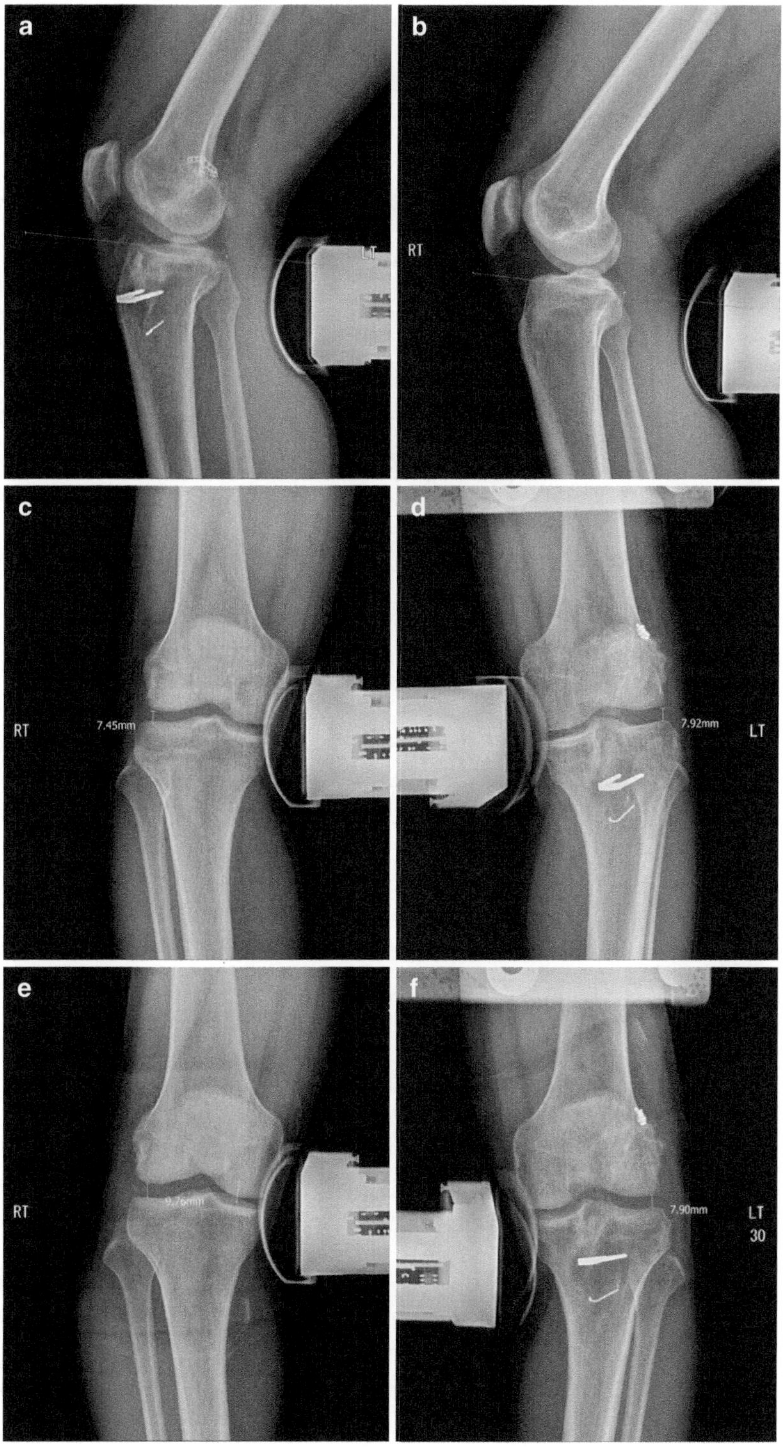

Fig. 7.11 Six months after ACL revision. (**a**, **b**) Pull view, (**c**, **d**) 0°, varus (**e**, **f**) 30° stress view of both knees. There is no instability in the pull and varus stress view

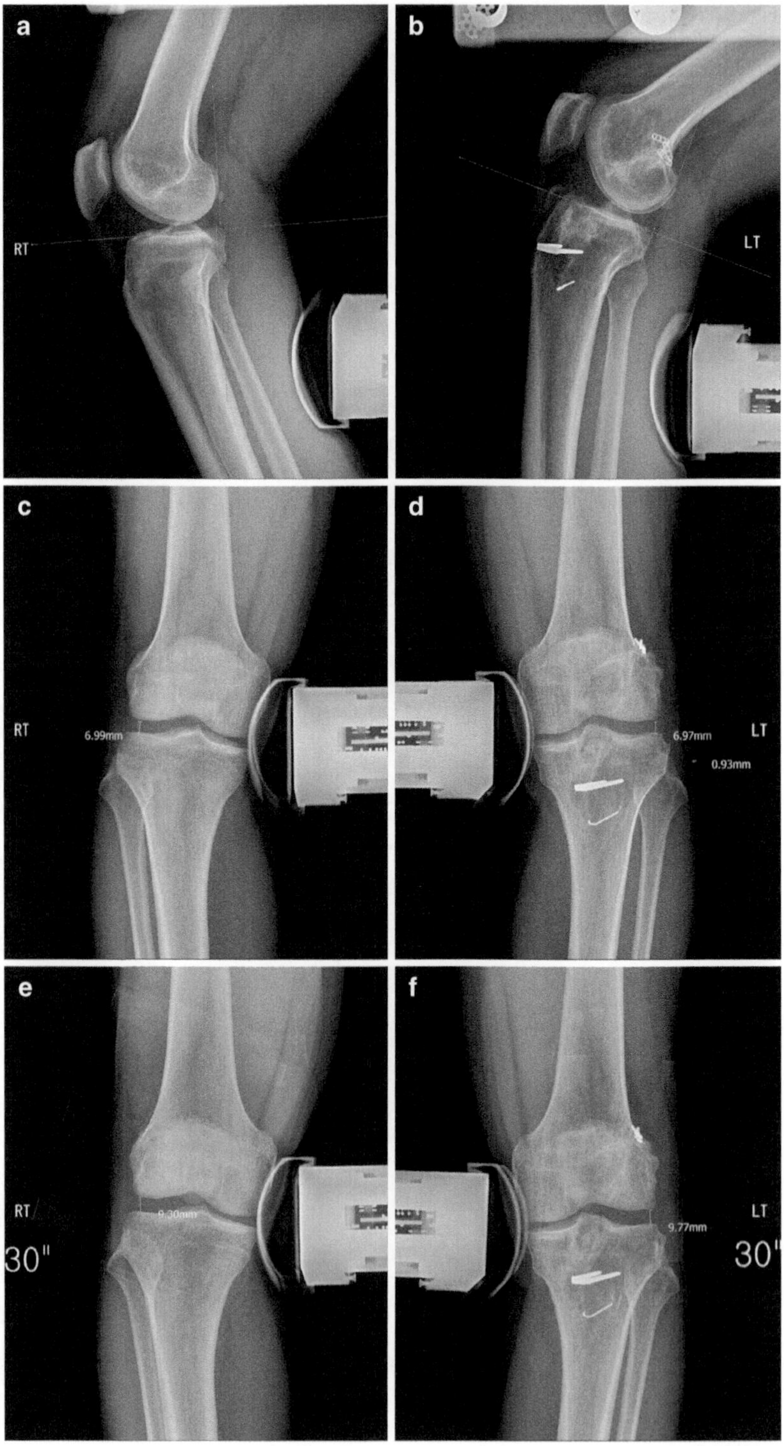

Fig. 7.12 Twelve months after ACL revision. (**a**, **b**) Pull view, (**c**, **d**) 0° varus stress view (**e**, **f**) 30° flexion, varus stress view of both knees. There is no instability in pull and varus stress view

terior femoral cortex (Smigielsky et al. 2015, KSSTA). Then, reaming with a covered clear plastic tube overlapped the 4.5mm diameter reamer to allow the tunnel to be easily removed of bone debris during reaming. Then, using a rounded rectangular dilator, make a rounded rectangular tunnel (Fig. 7.9); the direction of the tunnel is different, so the overlapping part of the tunnel is relatively easy to solve. If a part of the tunnel overlaps at the entrance of the tunnel, it can be solved by hitting with a bone plug. We can use a thicker one (use allograft + autograft, mixed graft if possible). If the femoral tunnel is also widened and bone grafting is required, a method of filling the tunnel with an allograft attached to a bone block in the femoral tunnel area, and, in some cases, an outside-in technique may also be a solution. When creating a tibial tunnel, if the tunnel is overlapped and widened, using a bone block attached Achilles allograft and autogenous ST mixed graft is filled as much as possible with bone block and tendon. Fixation with the intrafix technique (sheath with non-absorbable screw fixation, Depuy Co.) and back-up fixation. When the tibial tunnel, the revision tunnel is closed past tunnel then the starting point of the tibial tunnel further down, that is, the 55–65 degree angle guide use, so that part of the tunnel is a new tunnel bone (Fig. 7.10c). In addition, the use of a rounded, rectangular (Fig. 7.18b), or oval shape dilator has the advantage of less bone loss and somewhat easier one-stage revision because usually the tunnel is not reamed, only dilated with the dilator, thus preserving more bone compared to using the round reamer. Recently, I have had several cases of ACL revision, even though anterolateral ligament reconstruction (ALL) was performed with ACL reconstruction. Because there were neglected PLRI, in my experiences, when PLRI or LCL laxity cases, ALL reconstruction was not enough to protect posterolateral rotatory instability. When we additionally do ALL reconstruction will be done at anterolateral rotatory instability with ACL injured case. Otherwise such as ACL combined LCL injury or PLRI cases, we should PLCS through fibular head tunnel to lateral epicondylar area. When grade III PLRI case, we should do anatomical reconstruction of posterolateral structures. Even more reinforcement LCL as possible as we can do. Fortunately, grade III PLRI case was very rare in my experience.

7.13 Tension

The appropriate amount of tension to apply during graft fixation remains controversial. However, excessive or inappropriate tension can lead to ACL reconstruction failure. It is generally accepted that 20–40 N is appropriate for physiological tension and relaxation of the graft and biomechanical tension. The author usually performs cyclic loading of about 20 times flexion-extension (0–90*) ROM. The graft is fixed to the knee joint at about 0–5° of extension with 12–15 lbs. of tension.

Finally, the surgeon should be aware of the etiology of reconstruction failure in order to achieve a successful revision of ACL reconstruction. In my experience, the most common cause of failure is a neglected PLRI with too vertical a femoral tunnel or anterior placement of the femur. Correct surgical technique is also very important. Graft fixation is critical to maintain proper graft placement and tension. Rehabilitation is also important pre- and postoperatively, especially during the first 2 weeks postoperatively when the graft is at its weakest.

7.14 Cases of ACL Reconstruction Revision

Case 1: ACL Revision

A 33-year-old male patient with previous history of ACL reconstruction and ACL graft removal (due to septic knee) presented to the outpatient department complaining of pain in his left knee. He had no clear history of trauma, but the pain developed after hiking. Anterior drawing test grade 1, Lachman test grade 1, PLRI grade 2, and varus stress grade 1 were checked on physical examination.

KT-2000 arthrometer maximum manual test (MMT): 8 mm right and 14 mm left were checked.

KT-2000 arthrometer maximum manual test (MMT): 9 mm right and 10 mm left were checked on physical examination.

Case 2: ACL Revision Combined with PLRI

A 29-year-old male patient with a history of six times previous ACL revisions (5 allograft, 1 autograft) presented to the outpatient clinic complaining of pain and instability in his left knee. Physical examination revealed Lachman test grade 2, pivot shift grade 1, PLRI grade 2, and varus stress grade 1.

KT-2000 arthrometer maximum manual test (MMT): 7 mm right and 15–16 mm left were checked.

Therefore, ACL seventh revision and PLCS were done.

KT-2000 arthrometer maximum manual test (MMT): 8 mm right and 9 mm left were checked on physical examination.

Case 3: ACL Revision

ACL revision, knee, Lt.

A 21-year-old female patient with a history of left knee PCL reconstruction 10 years ago and ACL reconstruction 6 years ago presented to the outpatient clinic complaining of left knee pain. She injured her knee 2 weeks ago. Physical examination showed Lachman test grade 1–2 and pivot shift test grade 1 (Figs. 7.13, 7.14, 7.15, 7.16, 7.17, 7.18, and 7.19).

Therefore, PCL reconstruction and PCLS were performed

Her knee was very stable, and she returned to her job as a physical education teacher (Fig. 7.20).

Case 4: ACL Revision

A 27-year-old male patient with a history of right knee ACL reconstruction 2 years ago presented to the outpatient clinic complaining of right knee pain after a slip-down injury. He injured his knee 3 months ago. Physical examination showed Lachman test grade 2, pivot-shift test grade 2, PLRI grade 2, and positive varus stress test (Figs. 7.21 and 7.22).

So, ACL revision and PLCS were performed (Figs. 7.23 and 7.24).

Case 5

A 40-year-old male has some instability and discomfort to his knee for 3 years. He had two times ACL reconstruction at other university hospital (Fig. 7.25).

By KT 1000 arthrometer examination; maximal manual test; Rt 7–8 mm, Lt 12–13 mm (Figs. 7.26 and 7.27).

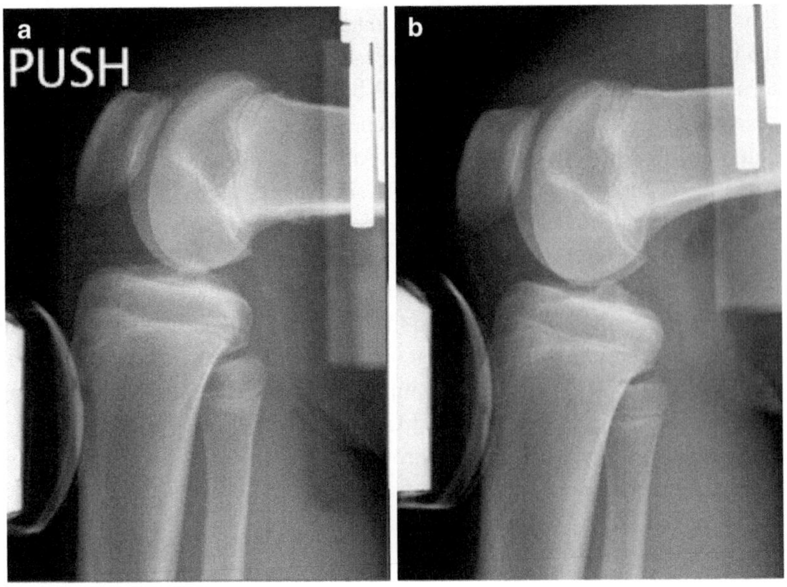

Fig. 7.13 (**a**, **b**) These are the push stress view plain radiograph at initial. Severe posterior instability at the left knee is identified

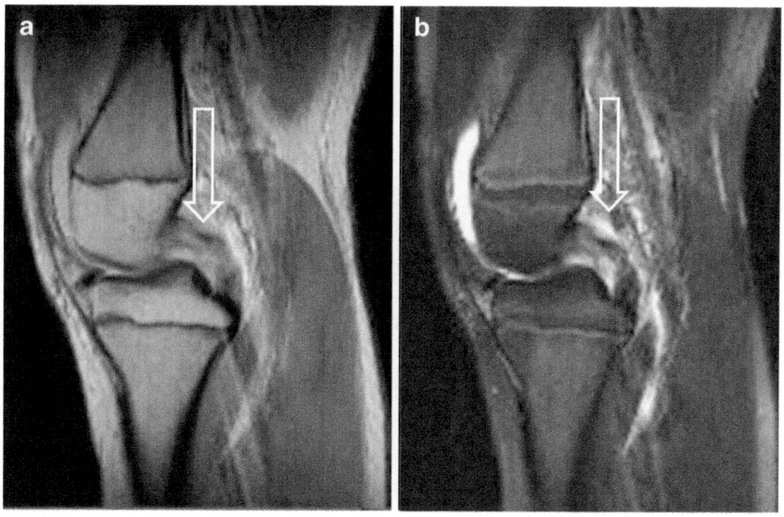

Fig. 7.14 (**a**, **b**) Rupture of the PCL is identified in the sagittal view of the MRI

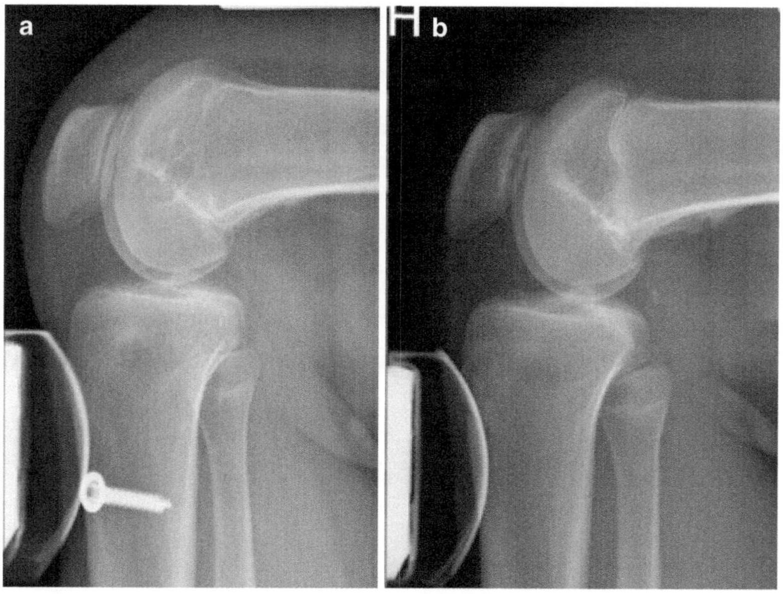

Fig. 7.15 (**a**, **b**) These are the push stress views 1 year after PCL with PLCS reconstruction. We can see that posterior instability is reduced compared to the initial push stress view X-ray

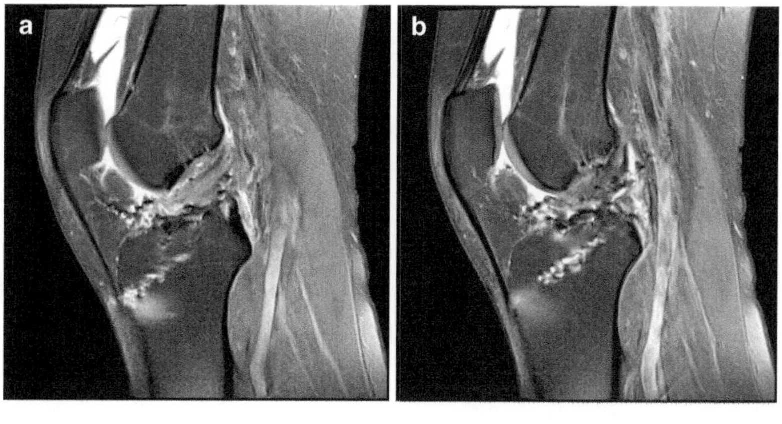

Fig. 7.16 (**a**, **b**) This is the MRI taken 1 year after ACL reconstruction. The ACL graft was completely ruptured of ACL graft

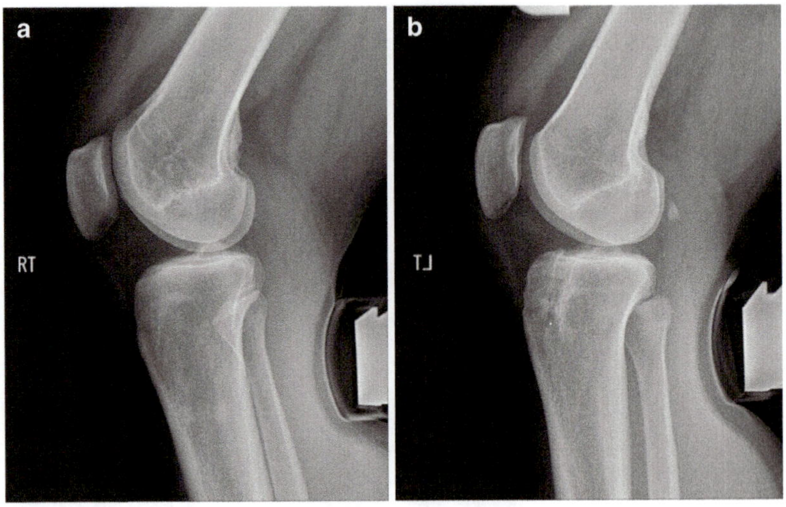

Fig. 7.17 (**a**, **b**) In the pull stress x-ray, a 3–4 mm side-to-side difference was checked compared to the unaffected side

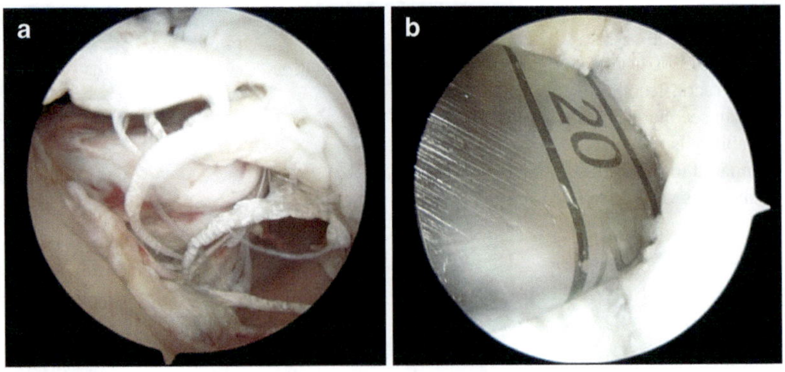

Fig. 7.18 (**a**, **b**) In arthroscopy, the previous ACL graft was ruptured completely, and ACL revision with a rectangular dilator was done

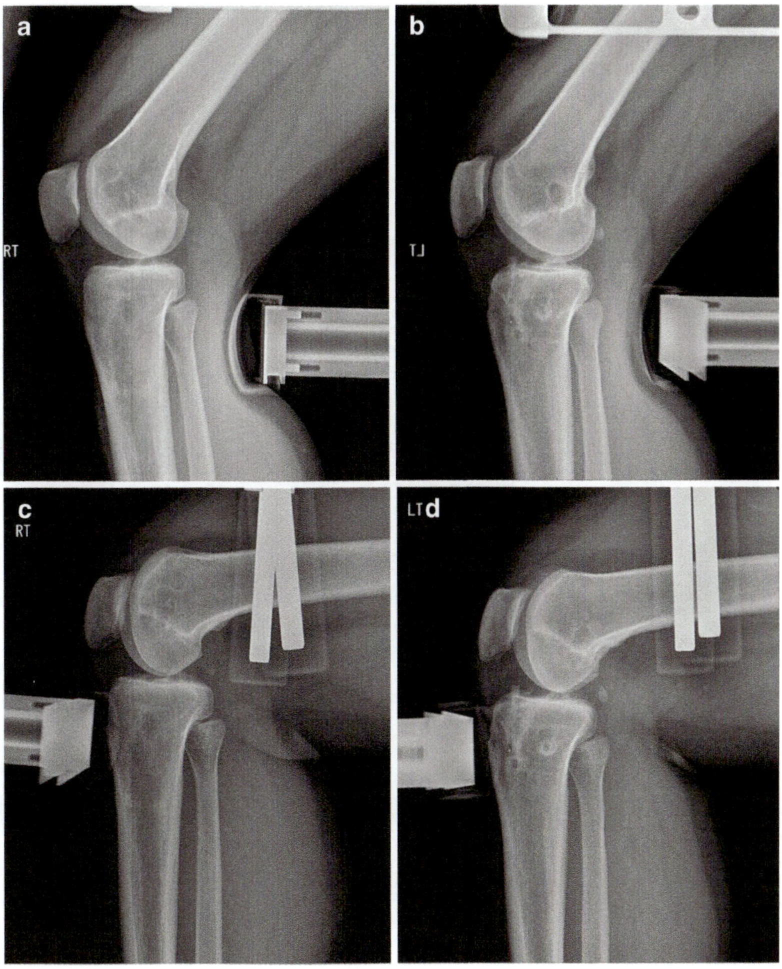

Fig. 7.19 (**a**, **b**) After the surgery, postoperative 1 year and 4 months later, there is no significant side-to-side difference on pull and (**c**, **d**) push stress view

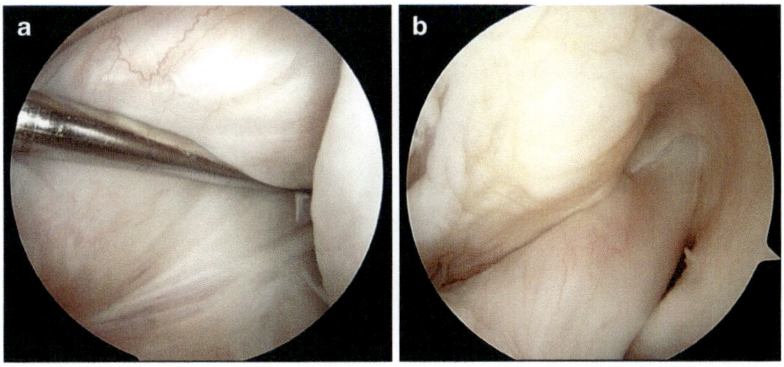

Fig. 7.20 (**a**, **b**) A second look arthroscopic exam was performed postoperative 1 year and 4 months later. Well-synovialized graft was found without any degeneration

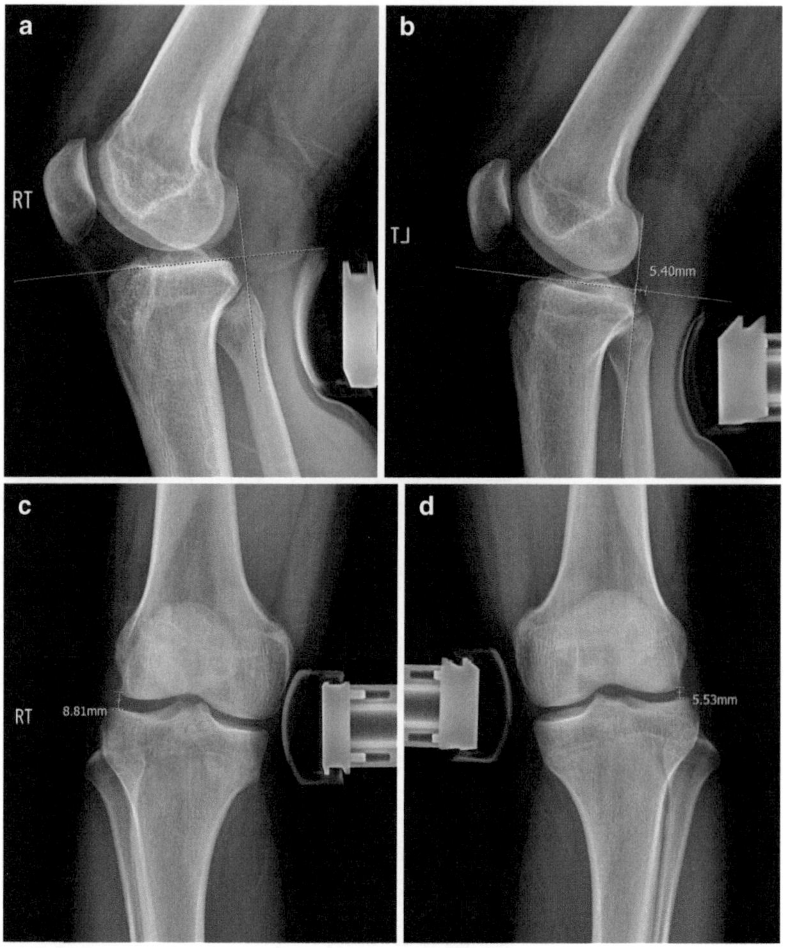

Fig. 7.21 (**a**, **b**) A 5.4 mm side-to-side difference was observed at the pull stress view. (**c**, **d**) A wider lateral joint space was also observed compared to the unaffected side of the knee

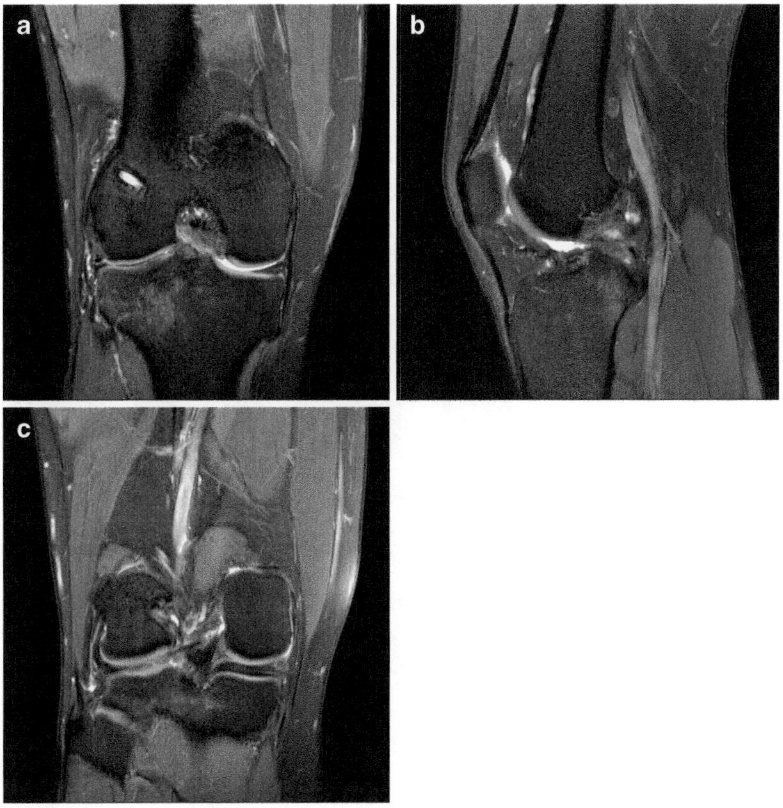

Fig. 7.22 (**a**, **c**) The previous ACL graft and fibular collateral ligament rupture were seen on the MRI image. (**b**) The ACL graft was torn and distorted in shape

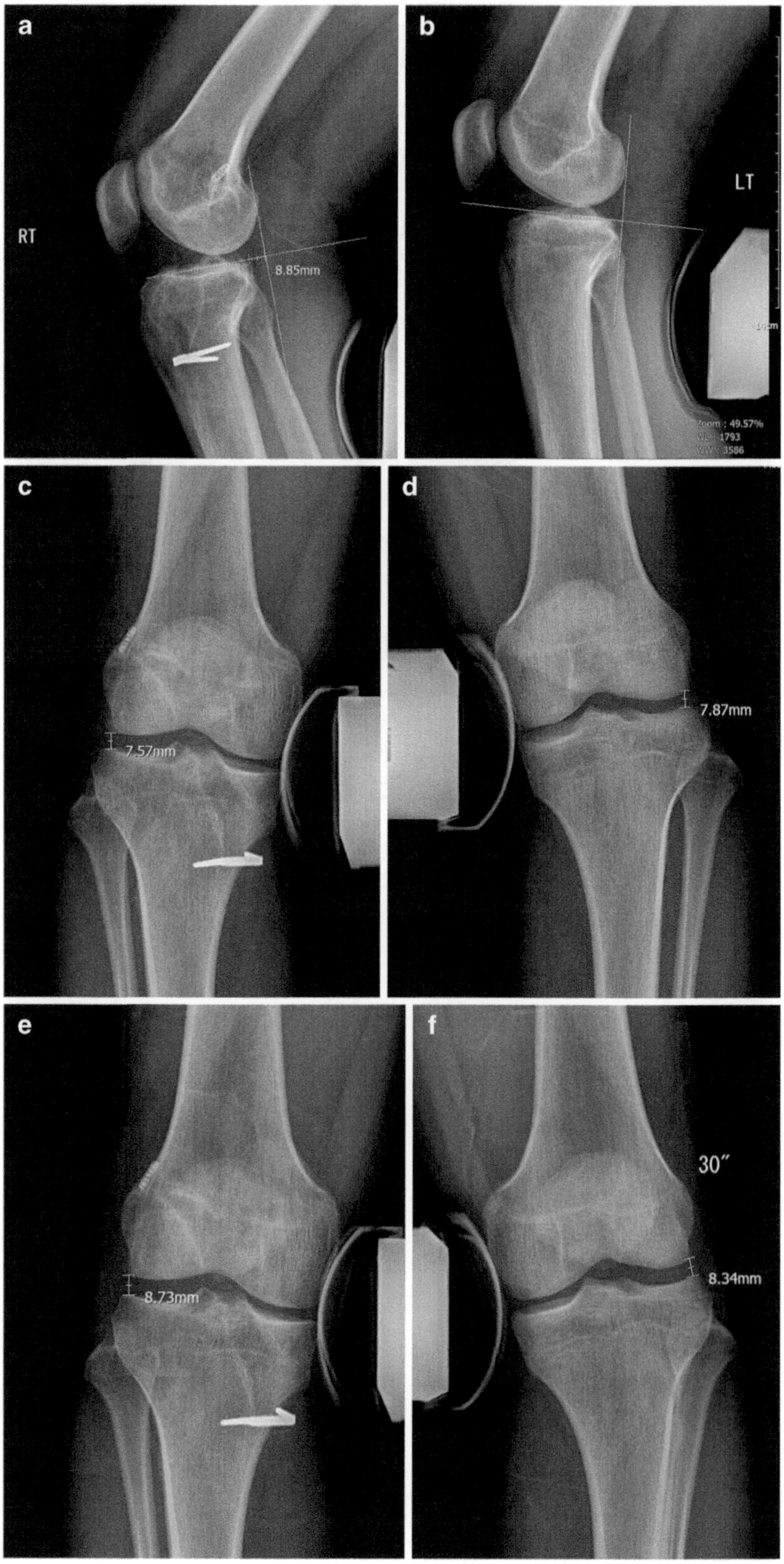

Fig. 7.23 After surgery, at 2 years and 2 months postoperatively, (**a**, **b**) there was no significant difference in the side-to-side view of the pull and (**c**, **d**) 0° varus stress, and (**e**, **f**) 30° varus stress

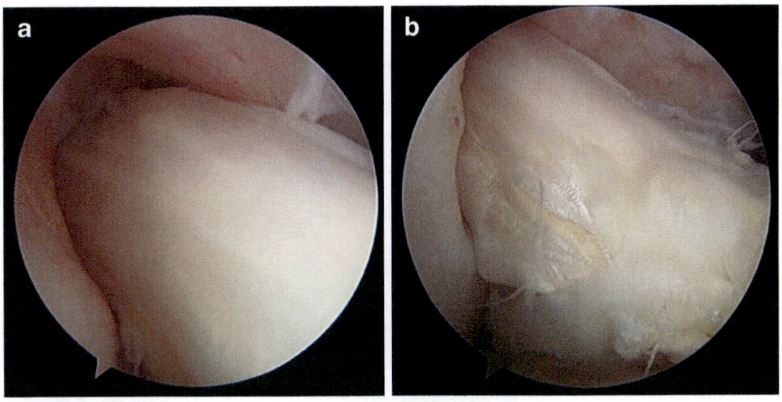

Fig. 7.24 (**a**, **b**) These were the second-look arthroscopic findings, postoperative 2 years and 3 months after ACL revision, showing a well-synovialized ACL graft

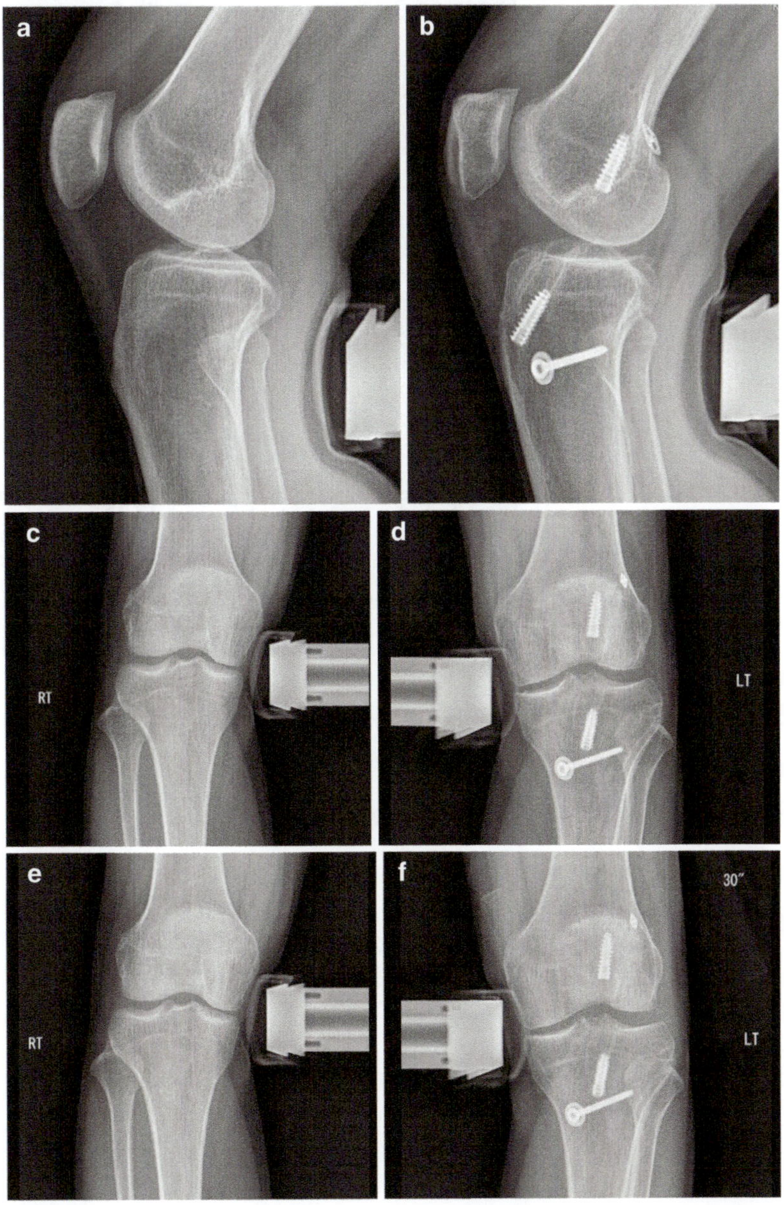

Fig. 7.25 (**a**, **b**) ACL reconstruction 2 times; third revision preop; side-to-side differences; 4–5 mm. (**c**, **d**) varus stress view 0*, (**e**, **f**) varus stress view 30* flexions third revision preop

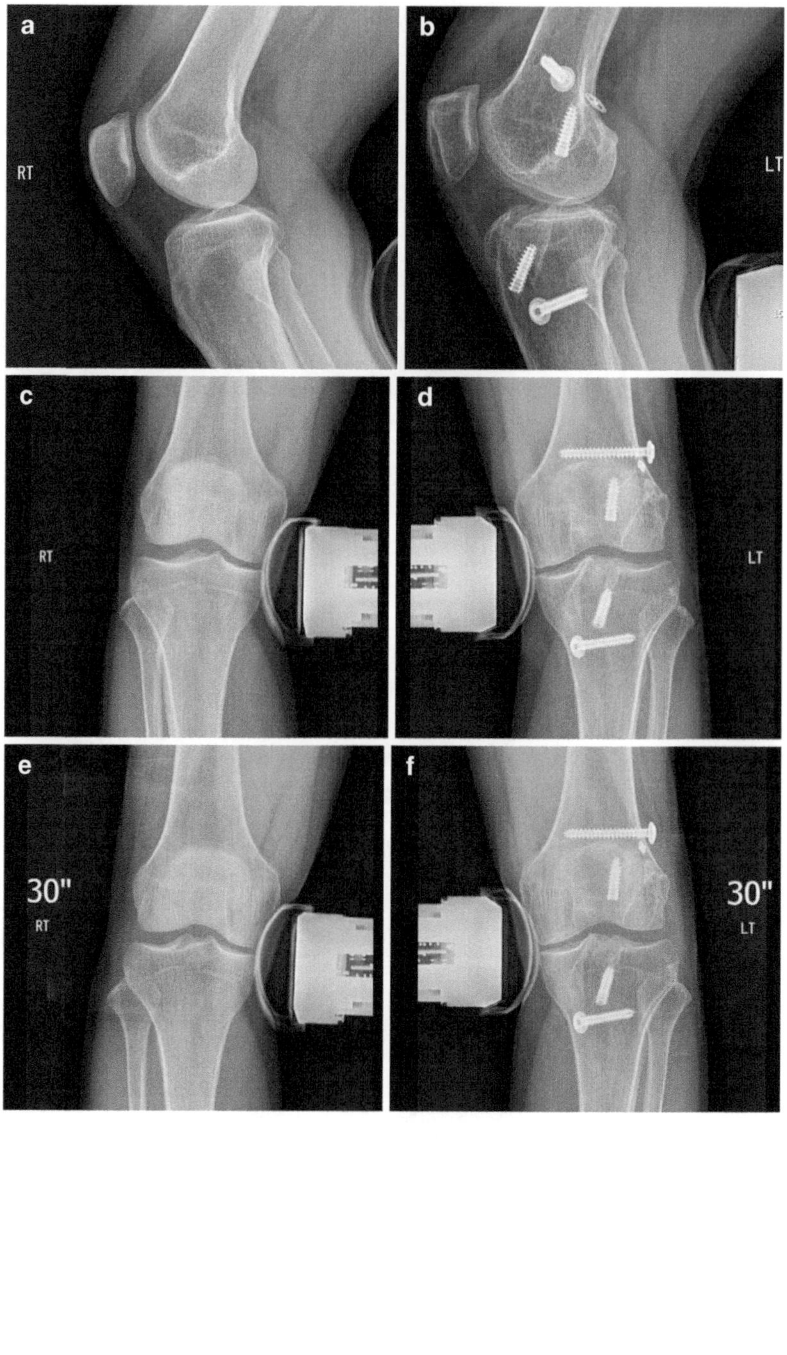

Fig. 7.26 (**a**, **b**) Pull view 2 years after the third revision of the ACL with PLCS. (**c**, **d**) Varus stress 0*, (**e**, **f**) varus stress 30* flexion 2 years after third revision of the ACL with PLCS

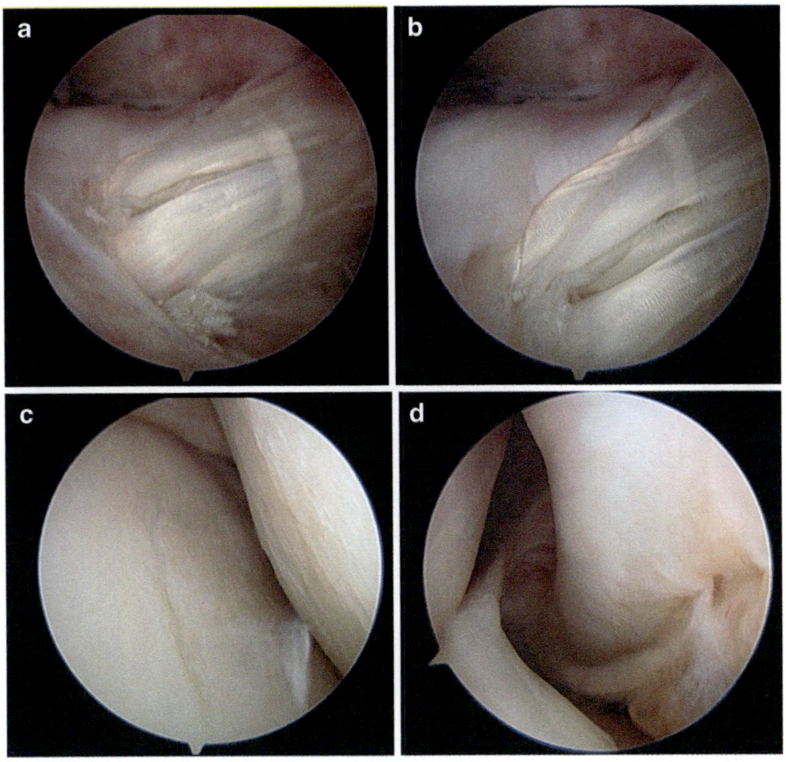

Fig. 7.27 (**a**, **b**) A second look 2 years after the third revision of the ACL with PLCS. The ACL graft looks good, and synovialization was not bad. (**c**) However, there was mild degenerative change of the medial femoral condyle cartilage (**d**) and the popliteal tendon and lateral meniscus look good

Further Reading

1. Christensen JJ, Krych AJ, Engasser WM, Vanhees MK, Collins MS, Dahm DL. Lateral tibial posterior slope is increased in patients with early graft failure after anterior cruciate ligament reconstruction. Am J Sports Med. 2015;43(10):2510–4.
2. Burnham JM, Herbst E, Pauyo T, et al. Technical considerations in revision anterior cruciate ligament (ACL) reconstruction for operative techniques in orthopaedics. Oper Tech Orthop. 2017;27(1):63–9.
3. Engler ID, Salzler MJ, Wall AJ, Johnson WR, Makani A, Shields MV, Gill TJ. Patient-reported outcomes after multiple-revision ACL reconstruction: good but not great. Arthrosc Sports Med Rehabil. 2020;2:e539–46.
4. Kanakamedala AC, Edgar CM, Fanelli GC, Musahl V, Alaia MJ. Surgical considerations in revision anterior cruciate ligament reconstruction. Instr Course Lect. 2022;71:475–87.
5. Gifstad T, Drogset JO, Viset A, Grøntvedt T, Hortemo GS. Inferior results after revision ACL reconstructions: a comparison with primary ACL reconstructions. Knee Surg Sports Traumatol Arthrosc. 2013;21(9):2011–8.
6. Miller MD, Kew ME, Quinn CA. Anterior cruciate ligament revision reconstruction. J Am Acad Orthop Surg. 2021;29:723–31.
7. Mitchell JJ, Chahla J, Dean CS, Cinque M, Matheny LM, LaPrade RF. Outcomes after 1-stage versus 2-stage revision anterior cruciate ligament reconstruction. Am J Sports Med. 2017;45:1790–8.
8. Cristiani R, Forssblad M, Edman G, Eriksson K, Stålman A. Age, time from injury to surgery and quadriceps strength affect the risk of revision surgery after primary ACL reconstruction. Knee Surg Sports Traumatol Arthrosc. 2021;29:4154–62.
9. Wright RW, Gill CS, Chen L, et al. Outcome of revision anterior cruciate ligament reconstruction: a systematic review. J Bone Joint Surg Am. 2012;94(6):531–6.
10. Mitchell JJ, Chahla J, Dean CS, Cinque M, Matheny LM, LaPrade RF. Outcomes after 1-stage versus 2-stage revision anterior cruciate ligament reconstruction. Am J Sports Med. 2017;45(8):1790–8.
11. Śmigielski R, Zdanowicz U, Drwięga M, Ciszek B, Williams A. The anatomy of the anterior cruciate ligament and its relevance to the technique of reconstruction. Bone Joint J. 2016;98-B(8):1020–6.
12. Werner BC, Gilmore CJ, Hamann JC, et al. Revision anterior cruciate ligament reconstruction: results of a single-stage approach using allograft dowel bone

grafting for femoral defects. J Am Acad Orthop Surg. 2016;24(8):581–7.
13. Shelbourne KD, Benner RW, Jones JA, Gray T. Posterior tibial slope in patients undergoing anterior cruciate ligament reconstruction with patellar tendon autograft: response. Am J Sports Med. 2021;49(10):NP53. https://doi.org/10.1177/03635465211025265.
14. Salmon LJ, Heath E, Akrawi H, Roe JP, Linklater J, Pinczewski LA. 20-year outcomes of anterior cruciate ligament reconstruction with hamstring tendon autograft: the catastrophic effect of age and posterior tibial slope. Am J Sports Med. 2018;46(3):531–43.
15. D'Ambrosi R, Meena A, Raj A, Ursino N, Formica M, Herbort M, Fink C. Multiple revision anterior cruciate ligament reconstruction: not the best but still good. Knee Surg Sports Traumatol Arthrosc. 2023;31(2):559–71.

Rehabilitation After ACL Reconstruction

8

Abstract

This review traces the evolution of anterior cruciate ligament (ACL) rehabilitation, highlighting its historical progression and modern practices. It covers the shift from standardized protocols to personalized approaches, emphasizing accelerated recovery and patient-specific modalities.

Key aspects such as prehabilitation's role in surgery preparation and a comparative study affirming its benefits are highlighted. Post-surgery, detailed insights into range of motion (ROM) exercises, bracing, cautious weight-bearing, and targeted strengthening exercises are provided, balancing early mobilization with potential risks.

The text emphasizes proprioception, neuromuscular control, and the integration of kinetic chain exercises in rehabilitation. It outlines a structured, staged rehabilitation protocol and delineates criteria for safe return to sports activities, emphasizing multifaceted assessments.

This concise review offers a comprehensive understanding of ACL rehabilitation's evolution, providing insights into historical foundations, contemporary practices, and evidence-based methodologies crucial for optimal recovery.

Keywords

Rehabilitation evolution • Prehabilitation • ROM exercise • Brace • Weight-bearing strategies • Strengthening exercises • Proprioception and neuromuscular control • Kinetic chain exercises • Staged rehabilitation protocol • Return to sports criteria

8.1 Introduction

Rehabilitation after anterior cruciate ligament reconstruction is becoming increasingly important. ACL rehabilitation protocols vary greatly, with little consensus among practitioners. Nonetheless, there has been agreement over the last decade to shift from conservative, standardized length protocols to more accelerated, individualized protocols that vary in length and modalities based on patient-specific findings and preferences.

8.2 A Brief History of ACL Rehabilitation

The rehabilitation of ACL reconstruction surgery has undergone significant developments over the past several decades. The earliest forms of reha-

Y. B. Jung et al., *Treatment of the Cruciate Ligaments Injuries*,
https://doi.org/10.1007/978-981-95-9039-1_8

bilitation focused primarily on immobilization of the knee joint and limited activity to promote healing. However, as the understanding of ACL injuries and surgical techniques improved, so too did rehabilitation strategies.

In the 1970s, early mobilization techniques were introduced, which emphasized the importance of early movement to prevent stiffness and promote circulation in the knee joint. By the 1980s, rehabilitation protocols began to incorporate exercises aimed at restoring strength and stability to the knee joint, such as quadriceps and hamstring strengthening exercises.

In the 1990s, a more structured approach to ACL rehabilitation was developed, which included specific phases of recovery and defined goals for each phase. This approach emphasized the importance of a comprehensive rehabilitation program that included a range of motion exercises, strength training, and functional activities, such as jumping and landing exercises.

Advancements in technology have also played a significant role in the evolution of ACL rehabilitation. In the 2000s, the use of motion analysis systems and force plates became more common in rehabilitation programs, allowing healthcare providers to better assess patient progress and tailor their rehabilitation programs to their individual needs.

In recent years, ACL rehabilitation has continued to evolve, with a greater emphasis on individualized treatment plans, more aggressive rehabilitation protocols, and the use of new technologies, such as virtual reality and wearable sensors.

8.3 Prehabilitation

Prehabilitation is an essential step before undergoing anterior cruciate ligament (ACL) reconstruction surgery. It refers to a series of exercises and activities that aim to improve the strength, flexibility, and stability of the knee joint before the operation. Prehabilitation is beneficial for several reasons. First, it can help reduce the swelling and pain in the knee, which can improve the range of motion and facilitate the recovery process. Second, prehabilitation can help improve the patient's overall fitness and strength, which can enhance their ability to cope with the postoperative rehabilitation process. Third, prehabilitation can help identify and address any underlying imbalances or weaknesses in the knee or surrounding muscles, which can help prevent future injuries.

The prehabilitation process typically involves a combination of exercises and activities that are designed to target specific muscle groups and improve joint mobility. These may include exercises such as squats, lunges, leg presses, and hamstring curls, as well as balance and stability exercises. Additionally, prehabilitation may also include activities, such as cycling, swimming, or other low-impact exercises, to improve cardiovascular fitness and overall endurance. The goal of prehabilitation is to prepare the knee joint and surrounding muscles for the stress of surgery, as well as to improve overall physical fitness, which can help facilitate a faster and more successful recovery. By participating in prehabilitation before ACL reconstruction surgery, patients can increase their chances of a successful outcome and reduce the risk of future knee injuries.

Mathew et al. reported a comparative effectiveness study. This study compared the functional outcomes and return-to-sport rates 2 years after ACL reconstruction in a cohort that underwent preoperative rehabilitation with a nonexperimental cohort. The preoperative rehabilitation included progressive strengthening and neuromuscular training. The study found that the cohort treated with additional preoperative rehabilitation had significantly better functional outcomes and a higher percentage of patients returning to preinjury sports compared to the nonexperimental cohort. The results suggest that preoperative rehabilitation should be considered as an addition to the standard of care to maximize functional outcomes after ACL reconstruction.

Rehabilitation after anterior cruciate ligament (ACL) reconstruction surgery is a critical component of the recovery process. The aim of rehabilitation is to restore full function and range of motion (ROM) to the knee joint while also strengthening the surrounding muscles and preventing reinjury. This chapter will discuss the key elements of ACL rehabilitation, including ROM exercises, bracing, weight-bearing, strengthening exercises, functional exercises, and return to sports.

8.4 Range of Motion (ROM) Exercises

ROM exercises are an essential component of ACL rehabilitation, and they typically begin within the first few days after surgery. The purpose of ROM exercises is to help restore full movement to the knee joint and prevent the formation of scar tissue. ROM exercises involve gently flexing and extending the knee joint, as well as rotating the foot to help improve mobility. ROM exercises are typically performed using a passive or active-assisted range of motion technique. In passive ROM, the patient relaxes their muscles, and the healthcare provider moves the joint through its full range of motion (Fig. 8.1). In active-assisted ROM, the patient uses their muscles to move the joint with assistance from their healthcare provider or by themselves (Fig. 8.2).

The timing of ROM exercises will depend on the patient's specific condition and the surgeon's recommendation. In general, ROM exercises typically begin within the first few days after surgery. The benefits of early ROM exercises include improved joint mobility, reduced swelling, and prevention of the formation of scar tissue. Early ROM exercises may also reduce the risk of developing knee stiffness and improve the patient's overall recovery outcomes.

However, early ROM exercise can also cause pain, swelling, or other complications if performed too aggressively or without proper guidance from a healthcare provider. Patients may also be at risk of reinjury if they push themselves too hard during early rehabilitation.

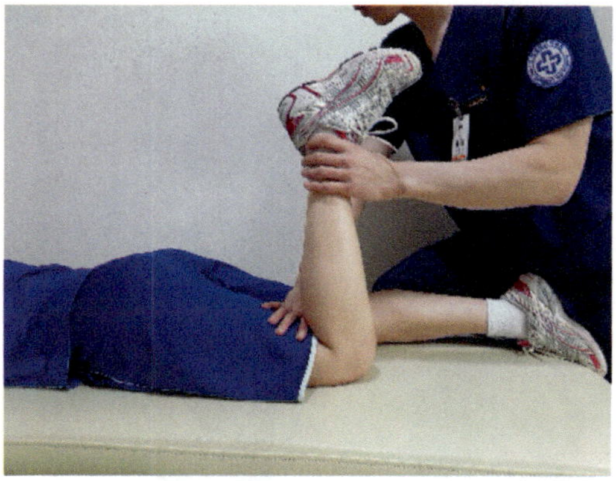

Fig. 8.1 Passive ROM exercise

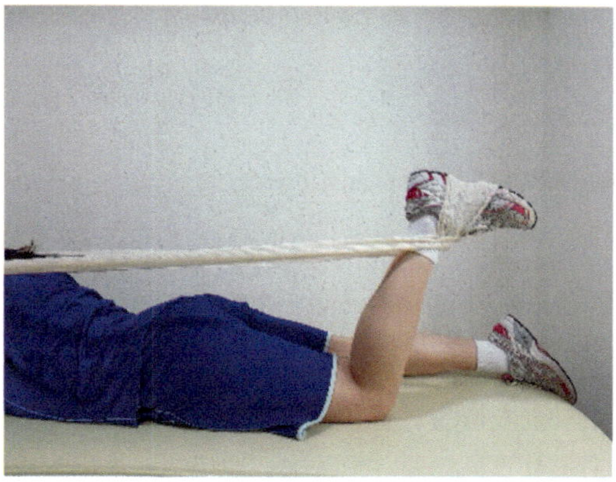

Fig. 8.2 Active-assisted ROM exercise

8.5 Bracing

Following ACL reconstruction surgery, patients may be prescribed a brace to help stabilize the knee joint and prevent reinjury. The type of brace prescribed will depend on the specific needs of the patient, but most braces are designed to limit motion in the knee joint and provide support during weight-bearing activities. Bracing is typically used in the early stages of rehabilitation but may be discontinued as the patient progresses (Fig. 8.3).

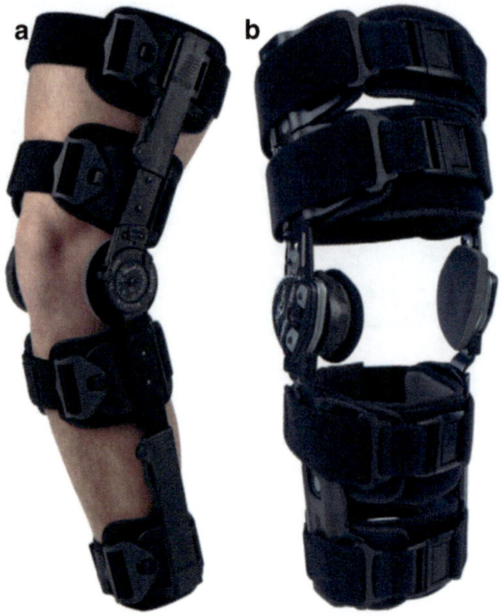

Fig. 8.3 ACL rehabilitation braces

Bracing is a commonly used tool in ACL rehabilitation to provide support and stability to the knee joint following surgery. The use of a brace can help patients improve their knee function, prevent reinjury, and facilitate the healing process. Bracing can be prescribed by a healthcare provider, and patients are usually advised to wear the brace during specific activities or for a specific duration.

One of the primary benefits of bracing is its ability to provide support to the knee joint, which can help patients feel more confident during activities such as walking, standing, and weight-bearing exercises. Bracing can also help to reduce the risk of reinjury to the knee joint by limiting the range of motion and providing additional stability during physical activities. Additionally, bracing can help to reduce swelling and inflammation in the knee joint, which can speed up the healing process.

Bracing can provide several benefits in ACL rehabilitation, such as supporting the knee joint, improving knee stability, reducing the risk of reinjury, and facilitating the healing process. Bracing can also provide a sense of security to patients, allowing them to participate in physical activities with more confidence. Furthermore, some patients may find bracing to be comfortable and easy to wear, making it a convenient and effective tool in their rehabilitation program.

Despite the benefits of bracing, there are also some potential drawbacks to consider. One of the main concerns with bracing is that it can limit the patient's range of motion, which can affect their ability to perform certain exercises or activities. Bracing can also be uncomfortable and may cause skin irritation or chafing. Additionally, some patients may feel self-conscious or uncomfortable wearing a brace, which can affect their overall confidence and willingness to participate in rehabilitation activities.

8.6 Weight-Bearing

Partial weight-bearing can be performed immediately after surgery. The timing and degree of weight-bearing will depend on the surgical condition of the articular cartilage or meniscus. Weight-bearing facilitates isometric activity to the muscles, decreases effusion and peripatellar fibrosis, and helps maintain subchondral bone strength.

In the absence of comorbid injuries or concomitant surgery, early postoperative weight-bearing is recommended, and full weight-bearing is allowed for 1–2 weeks. In a randomized trial comparing immediate versus delayed weight-bearing for 2 weeks, Tyler and coworkers found a decreased incidence of anterior knee pain in the weight-bearing group. This was thought to be secondary to earlier recruitment of the vastus medialis obliquus in the weight-bearing group.

Figure 8.4 shows how much shear force is generated in the anterior cruciate ligament depending on the angle of knee flexion and trunk flexion. From 0 to 60° of flexion, there is almost no shear force, regardless of the degree of trunk flexion. At flexion angles between 60 and 90°, the shear force increases rapidly, so attention should be paid to the instructions to avoid exercising at these angles in the early postoperative period.

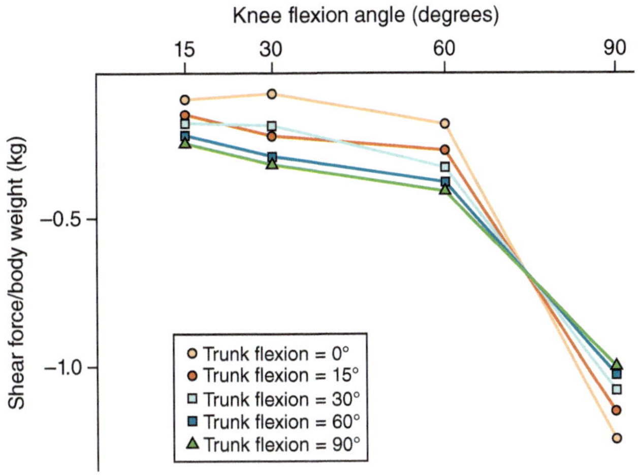

Fig. 8.4 FIG 10–4 Shear force (kilograms) per body weight (kilograms) while standing on both legs at various flexion angles of the knee and the trunk. (From Ohkoshi et al. [9])

8.7 Strengthening Exercises

Strengthening exercises play a crucial role in the rehabilitation process, and two common types of exercises used are closed kinetic chain (CKC) and open kinetic chain (OKC) exercises. CKC exercises involve the foot or hand being in contact with a stable surface, such as when performing squats or lunges. These exercises are advantageous as they mimic functional movements and engage multiple muscle groups simultaneously, promoting overall lower limb strength and stability. CKC exercises also help in improving proprioception and joint position sense, which are essential for returning to activities that require balance and coordination. On the other hand, OKC exercises involve moving a specific joint without the foot or hand being fixed, such as leg extensions or hamstring curls. OKC exercises allow isolated strengthening of specific muscles, enabling targeted muscle activation and rehabilitation of muscle imbalances. A well-rounded rehabilitation program after ACL reconstruction often incorporates a combination of CKC and OKC exercises to address both functional movement patterns and muscle-specific strength deficits, promoting a comprehensive recovery and reducing the risk of future injuries (Fig. 8.5).

The process of ACL graft maturation and healing is assumed to be influenced by strains and forces applied to the lower limb during weight-bearing and exercises. Based on the results of several studies, the following exercises are associated with low strain on the ACL: (1) isometric contractions of the hamstring muscles; (2) cocontractions of the quadriceps and hamstrings at 30, 60, and 90° of knee flexion; (3) isometric quadriceps contractions at 60 and 90° of knee flexion; and (4) passive flexion and extension of the knee. The activities that produced the highest ACL strain included (1) isometric quadriceps contractions at 15° of knee flexion with 30 N-m of extension torque, (2) squatting without and with resistance, and (3) active flexion and extension of the knee with a 45-N weight boot.

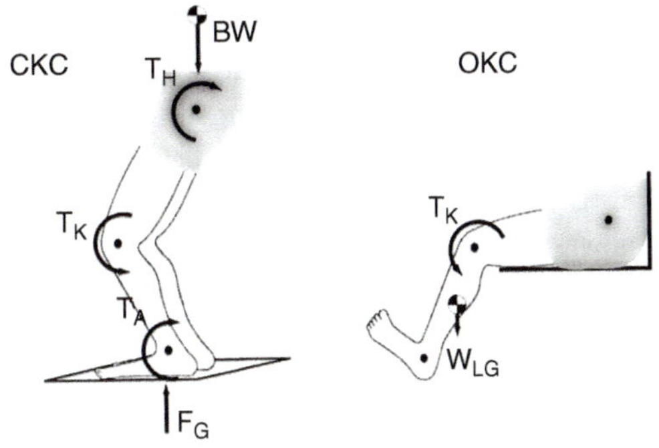

Fig. 8.5 The critical difference between CKC and OKC exercise. For OKC exercises, the resistive load (W_{LG})is applied to the tibia and transmitted to the knee (T_K). For CKC exercises, the ground reaction force(F_G) is transmitted to all joints of the leg (T_A, T_K, and T_H)

Given the above, it is important to be careful not to overstrain the graft in the early stages of rehabilitation. Excessive loading of the graft in the early stages of rehabilitation can have a negative impact on graft healing, but controlled loading is thought to help the graft incorporate. Although a general consensus exists that some strain is necessary to promote the process of ligamentization, questions remain regarding the amount of load that is safe and the amount that may produce graft elongation.

8.8 Proprioception and Neuromuscular Control

Regaining normal muscle function after ACL reconstruction is one of the most important factors in the process of returning to exercise and returning to daily activities. Proprioception is a key component of muscle performance and is known to be compromised when an ACL injury occurs. Several studies have shown that a decline in proprioception is observed 1–2 years after ACL reconstruction.

Dynamic postural control is another key component of proprioception, which is also known to be impaired with ACL injury. Restoration of proprioception and dynamic postural control is an important part of ACL reconstruction rehabilitation.

Exercises to improve proprioception and postural stability include joint repositioning, weight shifting, cup and cone walking, mini-squat, single-leg stance, and lateral and/or diagnostic lunge drills. It is important to provide instruction on how to perform these exercises with proper form and movement. Further ACL reinjury can be prevented by training the lower extremities to avoid pronation or supination, keeping the knees in flexion, avoiding hip adduction or internal rotation, maintaining overall balance, and minimizing ground reaction forces upon landing.

8.9 Rehabilitation Protocols

Table 8.1 shows rehabilitation protocols, which are organized into staged periods after surgery and describe the elements of rehabilitation needed at each stage [1–11].

Table 8.1 Rehabilitation protocols for primary anterior cruciate ligament reconstruction surgery

Phase	Goal

Prehabilitation	Pain control, decreased swelling
	ROM: 0–120
	Full WB
	Strengthening: Q muscle activation
	    CKC: single-leg-based exercise
	    OKC: Q set, SLR, leg extension, core, and hip
	Goal: normal walking, stationary bicycle

Phase I
(0–2 weeks)
	Pain control, decreased swelling
	ROM: 0–90, patella mobilization
	Tolerable WB (stand with double leg)
	Strengthening: Q muscle activation/low-load isometric
	    CKC: double-leg-based exercises (limited until 60)
	    OKC: Q set, SLR, core, and hip
	Goal: leg raise with full knee extension, stand

(continued)

Table 8.1 (continued)

Phase	Goal
Phase II (3–6 weeks)	Pain control, decreased swelling ROM: 0–130, patella mobilization Full WB, normal walking, stand with single leg Strengthening: endurance and strength—low to moderate load CKC: double-leg-based exercises (limited until 60), single-leg press (static-triphasic, 12–20 RM—50%BM, limited until 60), core, and hip OKC: Q set, SLR, leg curl (resisted by gravity) Proprioceptive function: single-leg standing (stable- unstable surface), movement retraining—double-leg-based exercise (symmetricity, joint coordination) Goal: normal walking, stationary bicycle, focus on the recovery of sagittal movement
Phase III	None or mild pain during daily living ROM: full Strengthening: hypertrophy and strength—low to moderate intensity, moderate volume CKC: single-leg-based exercises (limited by pain), single-limb leg press (8 ~ 12RM, 80%BM), hip bridge OKC: leg extension machine (limited until 60°), leg curl (machine, no pain, static-concentric contraction) Proprioception: single-leg stance (blind) on unstable surface, perturbation training (double leg), movement retraining—single-leg-based exercise (whole body control, especially lumbo-pelvic-hip control) Goal: stair climbing, coronal movement
Phase IV (10–12 weeks)	Pain and swelling control (pre-, during, post-exercise) Strengthening: hypertrophy and strength (knee extension strength to within 30% of contralateral limb)—low and moderate intensity, moderate to high volume CKC: single-limb leg press(8 ~ 12RM, 100%BM) OKC: leg extension machine(limited until 40°), leg curl (no pain, static and concentric contraction) Proprioception: perturbation training (single leg), maintaining bilateral lower extremity stability on unstable ground, responding to visual stimuli (visual-hand), retraining landing movements, and adapting to speed (whole body control, especially lumbo-pelvic-hip control) Goal: land on both feet, run in place, and start counter-rotating exercises
Phase V (13–18 weeks)	Pain and swelling control (pre, during, post exercise) Maximal strength(knee extension strength to within 20% of contralateral limb, symmetrical flexion)—moderate to heavy load, moderate volume CKC: 5 ~ 10RM, deadlift (low to moderate intensity), hip thrust OKC: leg extension machine (full), leg curl(no pain, eccentric) Proprioceptive functions: recovery of the explosive neuromuscular performance, retraining of sports-type movement skills, maintaining stability with a single lower limb on unstable ground, responding to visual stimuli (visual hand), and performing movements triggered by visual stimuli (visual foot) Goal Basic step: running, side step, cross over, sprint Jump—landing on bilateral limb, plyometric exercise on bilateral limb Counter-rotating movement, multidirectional movement Chronic training load increases
Phase VI	Pain and swelling control (pre, during, post-exercise) Strength—explosive neuromuscular performance—high intensity, low volume CKC: 3 ~ 8RM, high-speed power training, Nordic hamstring curl OKC: 3 ~ 8RM, leg extension leg Proprioceptive functions: recovery of maximal speed. Increased complexity during sports-type intense training (double task, planned-unplanned, fast reaction time) Goal Single-leg jump landing—acceleration, deceleration Single-leg plyometric—multidirectional running (planned, 45 cut, Figure 8, circle, 90 cut and turn) Sports-specific drill (unplanned, response, contact and indirect contact) 90% of the chronic training load of team training

8.10 Return to Sports

The ultimate goal of ACL rehabilitation is to return the patient to their preinjury level of activity. Before returning to sports, patients will typically undergo a series of tests and evaluations to ensure that their knee is fully healed and strong enough to handle the demands of their chosen sport. Patients may also work with a physical therapist or rehabilitation specialist to develop a customized training program that helps them safely return to their sport.

Return to sports (RTS) is based on a combination of subjective and objective measures, including the following. Some of the most commonly used criteria are as follows.

1. Knee examination
   - No effusion
     Full ROM
   - Lachman test, pivot shift test: Gr 0–I
2. Knee instability (KT-2000, stress X-ray)
   - Less than 3 mm from the contralateral side
3. Muscle strength test
   - Isokinetic test 60, 180: deficit within 10% compared to the contralateral side.
   - If there is no isokinetic test equipment, measure 1RM using bench press or leg press, etc.
4. Single-leg hop test
   - Less than 15% difference compared to the opposite side
5. Various functional tests
   - Shuttle run, carioca test, co-contraction test
   - Multiple hop test
6. Patient-reported outcomes
   - IKDC, Lysholm score
   - ACL RSI score

References

1. D'Amore T, Rao S, Corvi J, Jack RA 2nd, Tjoumakaris FP, Ciccotti MG, Freedman KB. The utility of continuous passive motion after anterior cruciate ligament reconstruction: a systematic review of comparative studies. Orthop J Sports Med. 2021;9(6):23259671211013841.
2. Failla MJ, Logerstedt DS, Grindem H, Axe MJ, Risberg MA, Engebretsen L, Huston LJ, Spindler KP, Snyder-Mackler L. Does extended preoperative rehabilitation influence outcomes 2 years after ACL reconstruction? A comparative effectiveness study between the MOON and Delaware-Oslo ACL cohorts. Am J Sports Med. 2016;44(10):2608–14.
3. Ghaderi M, Letafatkar A, Thomas AC, Keyhani S. Effects of a neuromuscular training program using external focus attention cues in male athletes with anterior cruciate ligament reconstruction: a randomized clinical trial. BMC Sports Sci Med Rehabil. 2021;13(1):49.
4. Hourston GJ, Kankam HK, McDonnell SM. A systematic review of anterior cruciate ligament primary repair rehabilitation. J Clin Orthop Trauma. 2022;25:101774.
5. Kruse LM, Gray B, Wright RW. Rehabilitation after anterior cruciate ligament reconstruction: a systematic review. J Bone Joint Surg Am. 2012;94(19):1737–48.
6. Lowe WR, Warth RJ, Davis EP, Bailey L. Functional bracing after anterior cruciate ligament reconstruction: a systematic review. J Am Acad Orthop Surg. 2017;25(3):239–49.
7. Mikkelsen C, Werner S, Eriksson E. Closed kinetic chain alone compared to combined open and closed kinetic chain exercises for quadriceps strengthening after anterior cruciate ligament reconstruction with respect to return to sports: a prospective matched follow-up study. Knee Surg Sports Traumatol Arthrosc. 2000;8(6):337–42.
8. Nagai T, Schilaty ND, Laskowski ER, Hewett TE. Hop tests can result in higher limb symmetry index values than isokinetic strength and leg press tests in patients following ACL reconstruction. Knee Surg Sports Traumatol Arthrosc. 2020;28(3):816–22.
9. Ohkoshi Y, Yasuda K, Kaneda K, Wada T, Yamanaka M. Biomechanical analysis of rehabilitation in the standing position. Am J Sports Med. 1991;19(6):605–11.
10. Ross MD, Denegar CR, Winzenried JA. Implementation of open and closed kinetic chain quadriceps strengthening exercises after anterior cruciate ligament reconstruction. J Strength Cond Res. 2001;15(4):466–73.
11. Yabroudi MA, Irrgang JJ. Rehabilitation and return to play after anatomic anterior cruciate ligament reconstruction. Clin Sports Med. 2013;32(1):165–75.

Part III

Posterior Cruciate Ligament (PCL)

Conservative Treatment of the Posterior Cruciate Ligament (PCL) Rupture

9

Abstract

Posterior cruciate ligament (PCL) rupture has naturally healing potential, in 72–86% of the ruptured PCL looks good continuity by MRI studies after 6 months. In our clinical experience, in the case of chronic posterior cruciate ligament injury, it is very rare that there is no continuity of the injured PCL, and almost 95% or more of them have good continuity in elongated posterior cruciate ligament. It is thought that a ruptured isolated PCL naturally heals over time, due to the fact that PCL is well-covered by synovial tissue and its blood supply is better than ACL's. The isolate PCL rupture is considered to be within 5–6%. In the PCL partially ruptured case, less than 1.5 ~ 2.0° clinically, we can treat it with immobilization, such as a long leg cast or cylinder cast in full extension of the knee for 6 weeks, and then, for 6 more weeks, take a PCL brace . The ruptured PCL will be healed and reduce posterior instability and improve stability by active conservative treatment (cast immobilization) and taking PCL brace, which prevents posterior sagging pad with a spring (Fig. 9.3). The active conservative treatment is done in an isolated PCL ruptured case, which is grade 2 posterior instability; it improves somewhat posterior instability, but in most cases, some instability remains, so surgical treatment can yield better results for young and active patients. Therefore, we recommend active conservative treatment for the isolated PCL injury of grade 1–1.5, which means an incomplete PCL injury, less than grade 2. The active conservative treatment, such as cylinder cast or long leg cast immobilization of the PCL injury, is a good indication, one of the treatment method, especially when the growth plate open in young children with an acute PCL injury.

Keywords

Isolate PCL rupture • Active conservative treatment

9.1 Principles of Conservative Treatment of Posterior Cruciate Ligament

The posterior cruciate ligament is anatomically composed of the anterolateral bundle (ALB), the posteromedial bundle (PMB), and the meniscofemoral ligaments, or Wrisberg's ligament. Posterior cruciate ligament (PCL) rupture has natural healing potential; in 72–85% of the ruptured PCL, continuity looks good by MRI studies after 6 months, and animal experiments (rabbits) show that PCL, artificially cut off 12 weeks after, is well connected at the cut surface of the PCL fibers (Fig. 9.1). In our clinical experience, in the

Y. B. Jung et al., *Treatment of the Cruciate Ligaments Injuries*,
https://doi.org/10.1007/978-981-95-9039-1_9

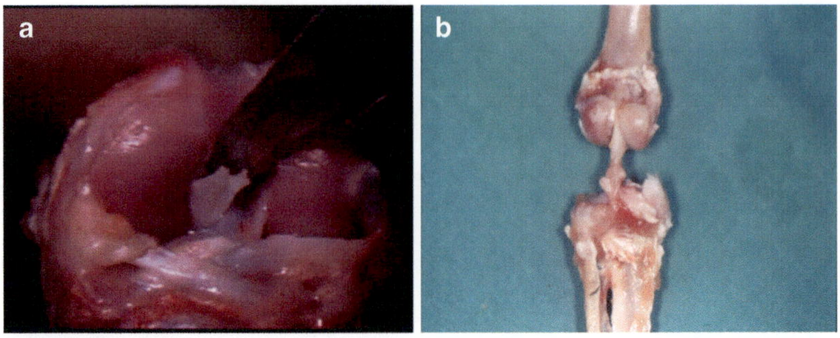

Fig. 9.1 (**a**, **b**) Animal experiments (rabbit) show that the PCL, artificially cut off after 12 weeks, is well connected at the cut surface of the PCL fibers

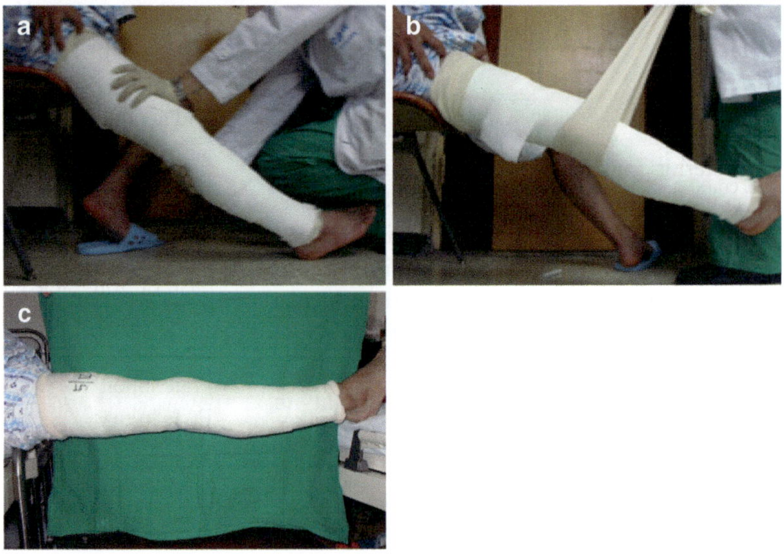

Fig. 9.2 (**a**) Applied a cast at reduced posterior sagging tibial plateau with manual for a while, presetting the cast in full extension of the knee as normal tibiofemoral stepping. (**b**, **c**) Cylindrical cast immobilization in full extension of the knee reduces posterior sagging of the tibial plateau

case of chronic posterior cruciate ligament injury, it is very rare that there is no continuity of the injured PCL, and almost 95% or more of them had good continuity in the stretched posterior cruciate ligament. However, MRI studies show that 70–86% of ruptured PCLs have good continuity, but the results can only be considered different, depending on when the scan is performed after the PCL injury. It is thought that isolated PCL ruptures heal naturally over time because the PCL is well covered by synovial tissue and has a better blood supply than the ACL. The isolated PCL rupture is considered to be within 5–6% to 10%. In the PCL partially ruptured case, less than 1.5–2° clinically, we can treat with immobilization such as a long leg cast or cylinder cast in full extension of the knee for 6 weeks (Fig. 9.2) and then for 6 more weeks, take a PCL brace (Fig. 9.3). The aim of active conservative treatment is to heal the PCL tear and reduce posterior instability and improve stability and function. In most cases, if the patient's knee moves inside the cylindrical cast immobilization (as swelling goes out after injury), then changing the cylindrical cast immobilization to full extension of the knee will be required once a week initially. Of course, we need to do muscle-strengthening exercises from the start of treatment. However, in our clinical experience, even if active conservative treatment is done in the case of isolated complete PCL rupture, which is grade 2 posterior instability, it improves the posterior instability somewhat, but in most cases, some instability remains, so surgical treatment may give better results in young and active patients. Therefore, we recommend active conservative treatment for the isolated PCL injury grade 1–1.5, which means incomplete PCL injury, less than grade 2 (Figs. 9.4, 9.5, and 9.6). The active conservative treatment, such as cylinder cast or long leg cast

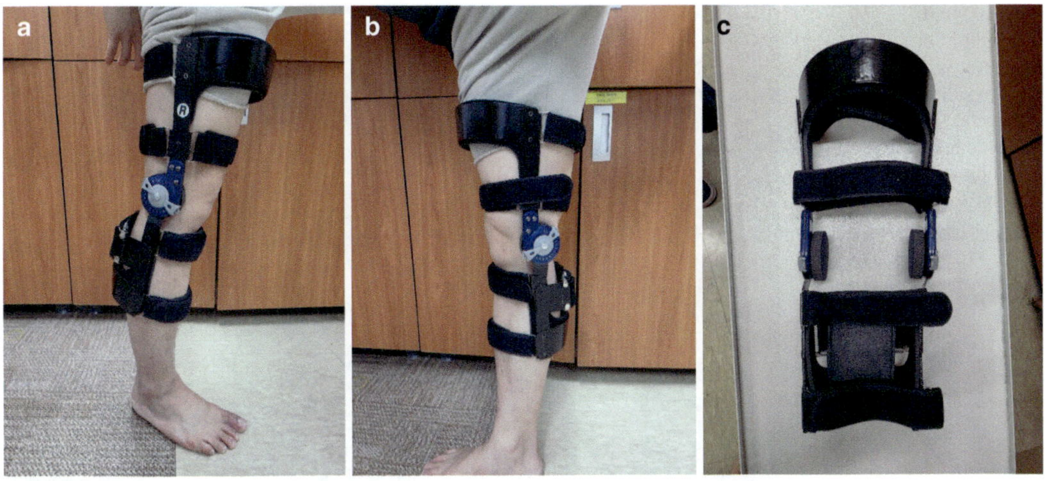

Fig. 9.3 (**a**, **b**) PCL brace with tibial support and a spring to prevent posterior sagging is used. Using this support, the PCL could be protected. (**c**) PCL brace with spring and pad to prevent posterior sagging of the proximal tibia

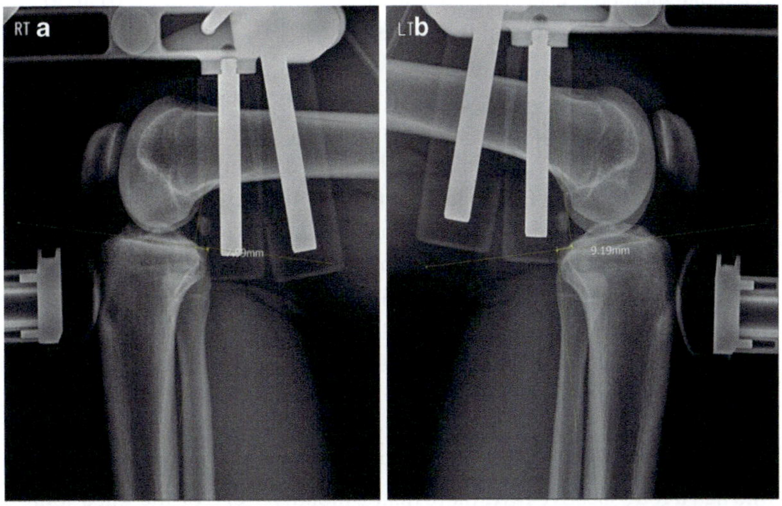

Fig. 9.4 (**a**, **b**) 1.5 mm side-to-side difference was checked compared to the unaffected side in the push stress test view

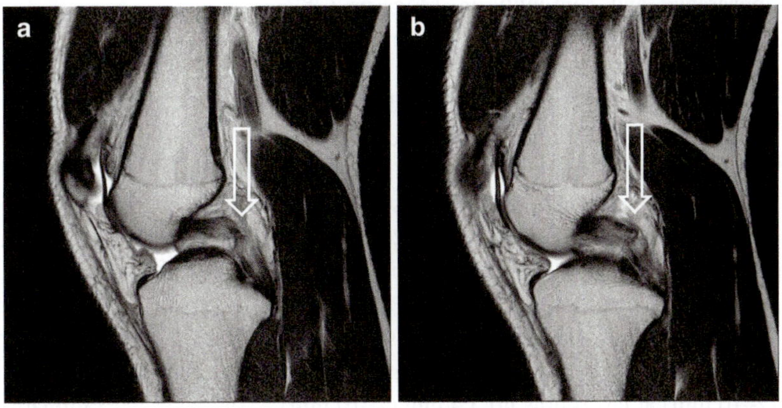

Fig. 9.5 (**a**, **b**) PCL rupture can be seen on MRI

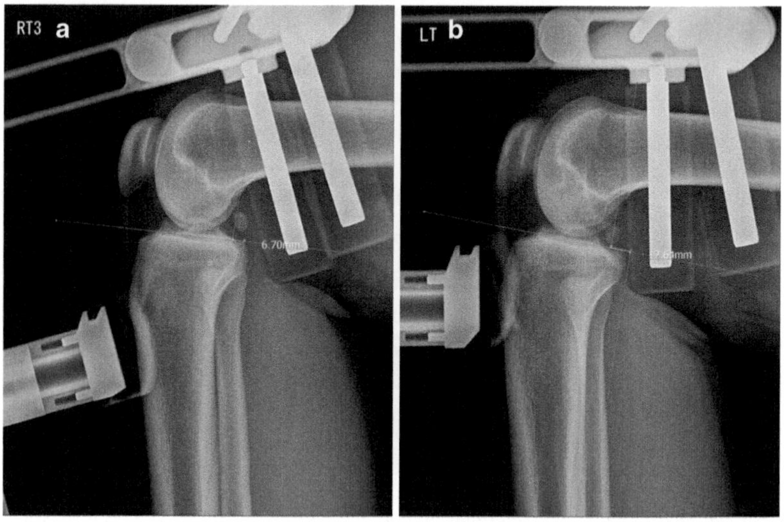

Fig. 9.6 (a, b) 3 months after conservative treatment. Side-to-side difference was increased up to 6 mm compared to the previous stress test imaging

immobilization, is a good indication, one of the treatment methods, especially when the growth plate is open, in young children's cases. In the MRI study of PCL injury, according to Shelbourne's report, PCL healed with continuity in all the low- and medium-grade injuries.

Nineteen (19) of 22 patients had high-grade injuries; four of them (22) healed with normal contour, and 15 of them had continuous healing with altered morphology. Three of them (high-grade injury patients, 22) did not regain continuity. They did a follow-up MRI study for a mean of 3.2 years; most nonoperatively treated PCL injuries, even in association with other knee ligament injuries, can heal with continuity. We performed MRI analysis in 46 cases of PCL injury who had a retrospective MRI more than 2 months after injury. Among them, almost normal PCL appearance and continuity in 13 cases (28%, Fig. 9.1), PCL healed with continuity but is deformed in 20 cases (44%, Fig. 9.2), discontinuity of PCL without bridging fibers and fluid or fat between two ends of torn PCL in 13 cases (28%, Fig. 9.3). In our experiences, we did active PCL conservative treatment in 15 patients with acute isolated PCL injuries, for 5 years (2001–2006). Mean follow-up was 23.8 months (range 12–56), 12 male, 3 female, mean age was 28.2 years. Using Telos stress device, push stress view, side to side differences, at pre-treatment 7.36 mm (2–10 mm) at last follow up 5.4 mm (1–10 mm), KT 1000 arthrometer (by maximum manual test) 3.6 mm (1–6) at 30* flexion and 3.5 mm (1–6) at 70* flexion of the patient's knee. Three patients underwent PCL reconstruction (as a tension and augmentation of the anterolateral bundle). At the last follow-up, the OAK (orthopedic knee working group) objective score was 85.6 (74–98), the IKDC (International Knee Documentation Committee) score at the last follow-up was A in 1 case, B in 7, C in 6, and D in 1. As another conservative treatment, rehabilitation treatment is attempted when you need to return as an athlete as soon as possible through muscle-strengthening exercises and rehabilitation treatment from the beginning. In this case, the aim is not to improve stability but to achieve a rapid functional recovery of the knee joint by strengthening the thigh muscles.

9.2 Cases of PCL Conservative Treatments

Case 1: PCL Rupture Conservative Treatment

A 15-year-old male patient with no history of knee problems presented to the outpatient clinic complaining of pain in his left knee. The pain started 1 week ago after slipping down while playing soccer. Posterior drawer test was positive on physical examination.

A long leg cast was applied for conservative treatment.

KT-2000 arthrometer maximum manual test (MMT); 10 mm right, 13 mm left were checked.

Case 2: PCL Rupture Conservative Treatment Failure, Which Led to PCL Reconstruction

A 20-year-old male patient with no history of knee problems presented to the outpatient clinic complaining of pain in his right knee. He got injured during skiing. Posterior drawer test was grade 1 ~ 1.5 and varus stress test was positive on physical examination (Fig. 9.7).

The MRI was taken on the date of trauma. PCL injury at the medial femoral condyle was observed. The posterior instability was mild, and no other instability was observed, so we decided to undergo conservative treatment(long leg cast applied).

After 2 months of cast, he converted to a PCL brace, showing good recovery. However, after 1 year, he presented again due to his recurrent right knee pain after slip down 3 days ago (Figs. 9.8, 9.9, and 9.10).

Therefore, we performed PCL reconstruction and MCL repair.

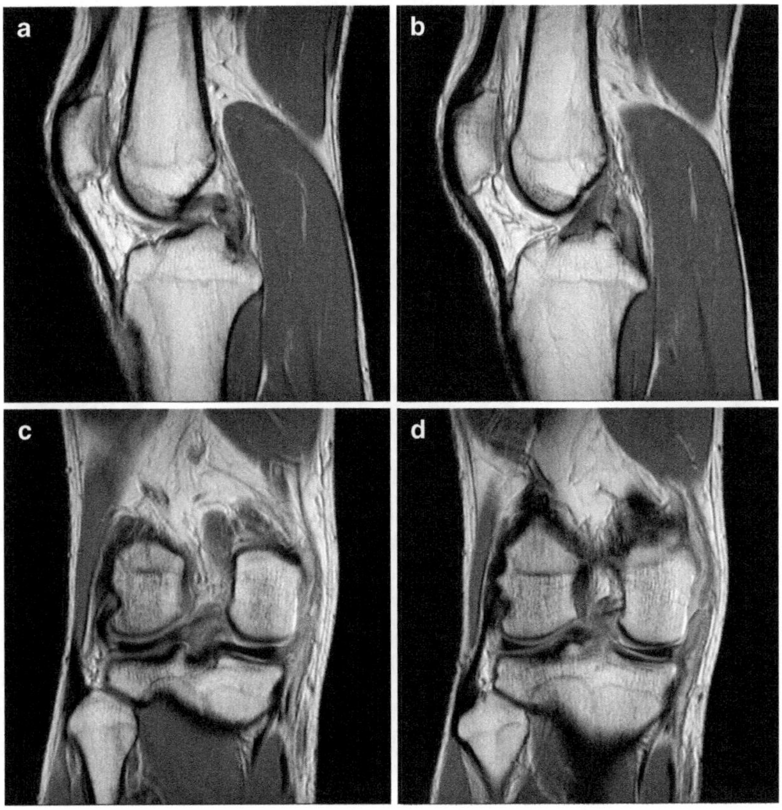

Fig. 9.7 (**a**, **b**) PCL rupture was shown on the MRI sagittal view. The continuity of PCL was good but the signal increased. (C,D) PCL ruptured at the femoral attachment site, with increased signal in the coronal view

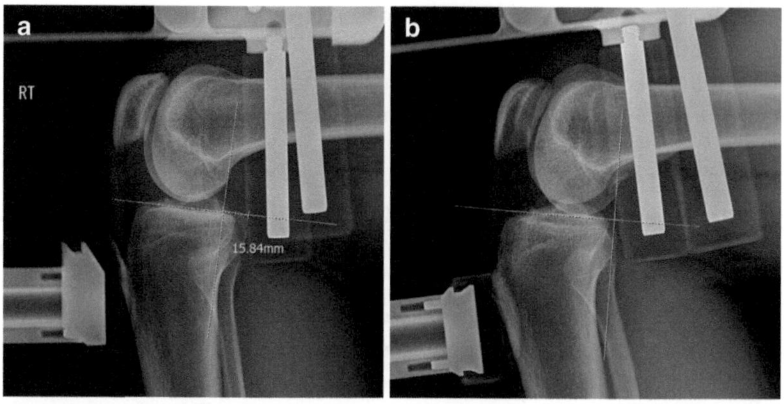

Fig. 9.8 (**a**, **b**) 15 mm side-to-side difference was checked compared to the unaffected side in the push stress test image

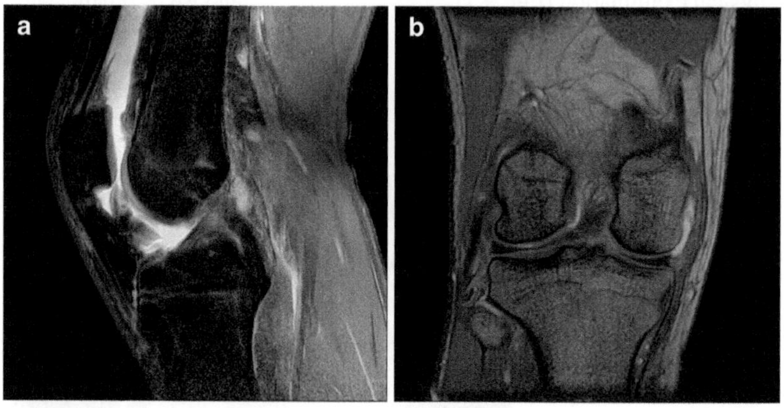

Fig. 9.9 (**a**, **b**) PCL and MCL ruptures were observed on MRI image

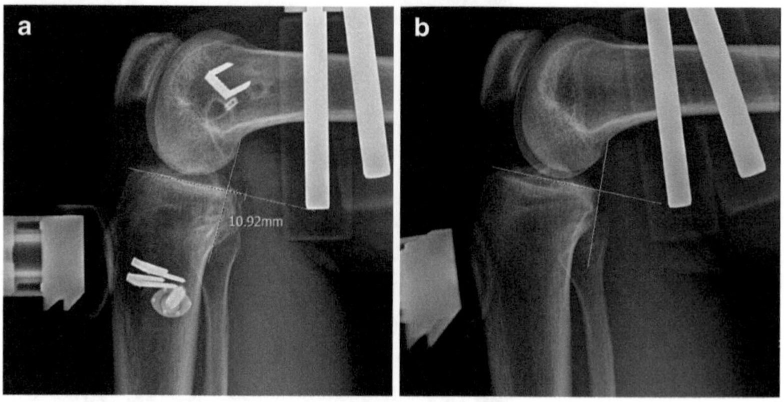

Fig. 9.10 (**a**, **b**) After 1 year 6 months post-operatively, a push stress view was taken showing a reduction of posterior instability. There was stepping anterior tibiofemoral condyle

Further Reading

1. Boynton MD, Tietjens BR. Long-term follow up of the untreated isolated posterior cruciate ligament-deficient knee. Am J Sports Med. 1996;24:306–10.
2. Cross MJ, Powell JF. Long-term follow up of posterior cruciate ligament rupture: a study of 116 cases. Am J Sports Med. 1984;12:292–7.
3. Fowler PJ, Messieh SS. Isolated posterior cruciate ligament injuries in athletes. Am J Sports Med. 1987;15:553–7.
4. Indelicato PA. Non-operative treatment of complete tears of the medial collateral ligament of the knee. J Bone Joint Surg Am. 1983;65:323–9.
5. Jung YB, Tae SK, Lee YS, Jung HJ, Nam CH, Park SJ. Active non-operative treatment of acute isolated posterior cruciate ligament injury with cylinder

cast immobilization. Knee Surg Sports Traumatol Arthrosc. 2008;16(8):729–33.
6. Jung YB, Jung HJ, Tae SK, Lee YS, Lee KH. Reconstruction of the posterior cruciate ligament with a mid-third patellar tendon graft with use of a modified tibial inlay method. J Bone Joint Surg Am. 2005;87(Suppl1):247–63.
7. Jung YB, Kwon YS, Jin WJ, Kim TH, Lee TJ. Healing potential of transected posterior cruciate ligament of the rabbit. J Korean Knee Soc. 2002;14:90–101.
8. Jung YB, Lee EW, Koo BH. Reliability of the manual maximal displacement test and quadriceps active test with KT-1000 Arthrometer in the assessment of posterior instability of the knee. J Korean Knee Soc. 1998;10:56–9.
9. Jung YB, Tae SK, Yang DL, Han JN, Song IS, Kang IK. Magnetic resonance imaging on posterior cruciate ligament injury – can the PCL heal? J Korean Knee Soc. 2000;12:172–8.
10. Keller PM, Shelbourne KD, McCarroll JR, Rettig AC. Nonoperatively treated isolated posterior cruciate ligament injuries. Am J Sports Med. 1993;21:132–6.
11. Muller W, Biedert R, Hefti F, Jacob RP, Munzinger U, Staubli HU. OAK knee evaluation. A new way to assess knee ligament injuries. Clin Orthop. 1998;232:37–50.
12. Shelbourne KD, Davis TJ, Patel DV. The natural history of acute, isolated, nonoperatively treated posterior cruciate ligament injuries. A prospective study. Am J Sports Med. 1999;27:276–83.
13. Shelbourne KD, Jennings RW, Vahey TN. Magnetic resonance imaging of posterior cruciate ligament injuries: assessment of healing. Am J Knee Surg. 1999;12:209–13.
14. Tewes DP, Fritts HM, Fields RD, Quick DC, Buss DD. Chronically injured posterior cruciate ligament: magnetic resonance imaging. Clin Orthop. 1997;335:224–23221.
15. Torg JS, Barton TM, Pavlov H, Stine R. Natural history of the posterior cruciate ligament-deficient knee. Clin Orthop. 1989;246:208–16.

Posterior Cruciate Ligament Reconstruction

10

Abstract

To achieve successful PCL reconstruction, we should know the correct surgical technique, especially the femoral tunnel position, and also as much as possible to preserve the remnant of the PCL. The tunnel position on the femoral side is more important than on the tibial side. The guide pin is inserted through the small-diameter hole 5–6 mm proximal to the edge of the articular cartilage of the medial femoral condyle. To obtain the longer tunnel length, use an oval or rounded rectangular shape dilator to better cover the anatomical PCL femoral and tibial attachment site. Preserve PCL remnant as much as possible, as this will work as a soft bumper cushion effect, and also, remnant lax PCL will shrink and heal with a new reconstructed graft. The edge of the tunnel opening should be chamfered with a rasp to reduce the killer turn effect of both tunnels. The tibial tunnel was created using a modified transseptal portal—the posteromedial portal was created using a standard arthroscopic technique. A Wissinger rod was inserted through the posteromedial portal to the posterolateral side of the knee, along just posterior to the PCL fiber to avoid neurovascular damage. (Using a modified transseptal technique). Using the PCL tibial angle guide (55–60° to make the tibial tunnel as oblique as possible, just distal to the center of the PCL tibial attachment fiber), insert through the anteromedial portal to the posterior compartment. Reaming with a 5 mm cannulated reamer along the guide pin and then using a rounded rectangular dilator 12 × 4mm, 13 × 5mm, 13 × 6mm, 14 × mm, depending on graft size, gradually increase. A wire loop and a No. 5 Ethibond suture loop were passed through the lower AMP to the femoral tunnel and tibial tunnel separately for passing the graft at each end. The graft was fixed after cyclic loading with an adjustable loop cortical suspension device (Tight Rope RT, Arthrex or Ultra-Button Inc., USA) and two transverse cross pins (Rigid Fix, DePuy Synthes Mitek Sports Medicine, USA) on the femoral side and a biodegradable interference screw as an IntraFix technique with an additional post-tie screw on the tibial side. I would like to do a backup fixation of the femur and the tibia on both sides. The surgeon should carefully evaluate and treat the combined injury, especially the posterolateral rotatory instability (PLRI) and also the posteromedial instability.

Quadriceps strengthening is important, starting preoperatively. Postoperative rehabilitation should be more gradual to achieve further knee flexion. The patient should be made aware of the importance of rehabilitation (gradual, gentle, passive flexion of the knee)

Supplementary Information The online version contains supplementary material available at https://doi.org/10.1007/978-981-95-9039-1_10.

Y. B. Jung et al., *Treatment of the Cruciate Ligaments Injuries*,
https://doi.org/10.1007/978-981-95-9039-1_10

and the importance of exercises to strengthen the quadriceps muscle. Active flexion of the knee should be performed at least 3–4 months after surgery, and flexion should be performed carefully so that the proximal part of the tibia does not have a posterior sagging force.

Keywords

PCL reconstruction · PLRI · slowly rehabilitation

10.1 The Principle of Operative Treatment for PCL Injury

Posterior cruciate ligament (PCL) rupture has natural healing potential. 72–85% of ruptured PCLs show good continuity on MRI at 6 months, and animal studies (rabbits) show that PCLs artificially cut 12 weeks later are well connected at the cut surface of the PCL fibers. Prior to 1995, attempts at isometric PCL reconstruction often resulted in postoperative posterior laxity.

Burn W.C. et al. reported that posterior laxity could be reduced if the femoral tunnel were placed distal to the isometric point. Subsequently, distal femoral tunnel placement has been a factor in the improvement of treatment outcomes.

Isolated posterior cruciate ligament (PCL) tears are relatively rare but are more common in multi-ligament knee injuries. Historically, isolated PCL injuries have been treated conservatively with good short to medium-term functional outcomes. However, a high incidence of articular cartilage degeneration, particularly in the medial and patellofemoral compartments, has been reported in chronic high-grade PCL-deficient knees. The most common causes of PCL reconstruction failure are neglected PLRI, followed by inappropriate femoral tunnel position, suboptimal physical therapy, or lower extremity malalignment. The generally accepted surgical technique for treating PCL tears is to drill the femoral tunnel for single-bundle reconstruction of the anterolateral (AL) bundle of the PCL. However, the femoral footprint of the PCL is relatively large, and the surgeon has considerable flexibility in choosing the location of the femoral tunnel to cover as much of the footprint as possible. The PCL has two functional bundles, the anterolateral (AL) and posteromedial (PM) bundles. These have co-dominant rather than reciprocal functions during knee movement. When performing a single-bundle PCL reconstruction, it would be important to cover the PCL footprint as much as possible in order to reproduce the normal kinematics of the knee.

There are many controversial issues regarding PCL reconstruction, i.e., transtibial tunnel, modified tibial inlay technique, single or double bundle reconstruction, and depending on PCL fiber remnant status and timing of surgery. Experimentally, biomechanical studies have reported that stretching or thinning of the reconstructed PCL is better using the tibial inlay technique compared to the transtibial tunnel technique. In our clinical experience, the timing of the PCL injury and the status of the remaining PCL have led to different treatment approaches. In acute or subacute injury (up to 3–6 months after injury), we try to preserve the PCL remnant and perform anterolateral bundle reconstruction as an augmentation; the damaged posterior cruciate ligament can heal with the graft. In the chronic stage, the PCL remnant looks good on the MRI film, tensioning the PCL remnant with augmentation of the ALB of the PCL reconstruction using the modified inlay technique. However, whether acute or chronic, if the remaining PCL was tiny and very weak or absent, especially if the torn PCL is not connected and has melted away on MRI images, double-bundle reconstruction will be better. If the use of a large, rounded rectangular or oval-shaped dilator will cover more of the normal PCL footprint, as is possible with the use of a larger graft, we could perform single-bundle reconstruction with a rounded rectangular or oval-shaped dilator instead of the double-bundle technique. Although double bundle reconstruction has been reported to have better results than single bundle reconstruction in biomechanical experiments (Race et al.), in clinical practice, there are not enough cases reported, and there are also no clinical differences between the two groups. The area of the femoral footprint of the PCL is three times larger than the cross-sectional area of the PCL mid-substance, and the size and shape of the PCL footprint have been reported as a "broad half-moon" with a curved distal edge adjacent to the articular cartilage.

Moreover, the area of tibial footprint of PCL was known as larger than that of femoral footprint, there might be advantages in using rounded rectangular dilator for the femoral and tibial tunnel establishment to cover the PCL footprint efficiently (more anatomically) with the larger covered cross-sectional area than using the conventional round reamer, if the long axis of rectangular dilator and PCL aligned parallel. In recent clinical results, the rate of excellent results, as grade A in IKDC objective scores in the rounded, rectangular dilator, 48.2% (13 out of 27 cases), was found to be higher than that of the conventional rounded reamer and dilator (32.4%,35 out of 108 cases). In addition, combined injuries to the posterolateral structures should be taken into consideration. Posterolateral rotatory instability (PLRI) can be observed in more than 12.5% of the ACL injuries and in 65–83% of the PCL injuries in our series. Considering that concomitant PLRI is an important determinant of ACL and PCL reconstruction, PLRI should be assessed prior to cruciate ligament reconstruction. Neglecting PLRI, cruciate ligament reconstruction will fail. In cases where PLRI is combined with a PCL injury, reduction of the knee to the normal position should be performed prior to assessment because PLRI may not be easier to detect at the posterior sagging position of the proximal tibia (Video 10.1). It is considered that the treatment for external rotational instability should also be treated differently depending on the acute, chronic, and degree of instability. In my opinion, pullout suture was effective when the ligament attachment area, bony avulsion situation. But for the substance or difficult evaluation of the torn sites, even for acute complex ligament injury, reconstruction will be better than repair. Anatomical reconstruction, as fibular head tunnel and tibial tunnel, was more complex technique, so anatomical reconstruction will be needed in severe injury such as grade 3 PLRI (by grade C, Fanelly et al.) otherwise grade 2 PLRI cases, through fibular head tunnel to the femoral lateral epicondyle area, such as PLCS sling through fibular head tunnel, obliquely was easier to do and good enough. The PLC injuries were classified according to varus and rotatory instability as assessed using the varus stress, dial, and posterolateral drawer tests. The classification of the PLC injuries and posterolateral rotatory instability (PLRI) was as follows: grade 1, increased external rotation by 5° to 10° as compared with the contralateral side, without any varus instability; grade 2, increased external rotation by ≥10° with posterolateral subluxation of the tibial plateau combined with grade 0 to 2 varus instability; and grade 3, increased external rotation by ≥10° without a firm end point, combined with grade 3 varus instability from lateral collateral ligament injury or over 20° external rotation.

10.2 Indication for PCL Reconstruction

*Posterior instability is more than grade II. Posterior drawer test, grade II, as no anteromedial step of the medial tibial plateau and femoral condyle at 90° knee flexion.

*Even with an isolated PCL injury grade II, a young active patient (If the surgeon has good experience with PCL reconstruction, PCL reconstruction will have better results than conservative treatment, even for an isolated PCL injury.).

*PCL injury with combined ligament injury, lateral collateral ligament, PLRI, MCL, and posteromedial instability.

10.3 Surgical Technique of Transtibial PCL Reconstruction

The PCL reconstruction was performed using the ipsilateral autogenous hamstring tendon with or without a tibialis allograft if the diameter of the autograft was<8–9 mm. The tip of the femoral guide pin was placed at 5–6 mm from the articular margin, near the midportion of the PCL anatomy of the femoral origin site, 10′30– 11 o'clock position, right knee (Fig. 10.1).

At first, a guide pin is inserted 5–6 mm from the medial femoral articular margin. A femoral tunnel was created using the inside-out technique with a 4.5 mm reamer, then 12 × 4 mm, 13 × 5 mm,13 × 6 mm, 14 × 7 mm rectangular dilator, depending on graft diameter. Usually we'd like more than 13 × 5 mm − 13 × 6 mm (same as 9–10 mm round tunnel) or a larger size. The skin incision was made at medial or just lateral to the patellar tendon lower side just above meniscus upper margin (to avoid medial femoral condyle fracture.), the femoral guide pin was inserted through small diameter guide pin such as a Rigid fix guide pin hole 4 mm diameter, 5–6 mm proximal to the margin of the articular cartilage of the medial femoral condyle. Preserve the PCL remnant as much as possible, which will work like a soft bumper cushion effect (Fig. 10.2).

The edge of the tunnel orifice should be chamfered with a rasp to reduce the killer turn effect of both tunnels. The tibial tunnel was made using a modified transseptal portal—the posteromedial portal was made using the usual arthroscopic technique. Through the anterolateral portal, the arthroscopic sheath and trocar were inserted into the posterior medial compartment to see the arthroscopically posteromedial wall. An 18-G needle was inserted through a posteromedial skin incision into the posterior compartment of the medial side capsule. A Wissinger rod was inserted through the posteromedial portal to the posterolateral side of the knee (skin incision was made at the protruding site), along just posterior to the PCL fiber to avoid neurovascular damage. (Using modified transseptal technique Video 10.2) The arthroscopic sheath is inserted over the Wissinger rod from the posterolateral side to the posteromedial compartment. Under arthroscopic viewing control, a power shaver or a vapor (electric cautery instrument) is inserted through the posteromedial portal and resection of the soft tissue just over the PCL insert area to identify the PCL tibial attached fiber and the inferior posterior capsule. During the tibial tunneling procedure, a Wissinger rod was inserted to protect neurovascular structures. Then, the PCL tibial guide was inserted from the anterior compartment through the anteromedial portal over the posterior horn of the medial meniscus to the PCL tibial insertion area. (tibial angle guide 55–60° to make the tibial tunnel as oblique as possible). Reaming with a 5 mm cannulated reamer along the guide pin and then using a rounded rectangular dilator 12 × 4 mm, 13 × 5 mm, 13× 6 mm, 14 × 7 mm, depending on the graft size (Fig. 10.3).

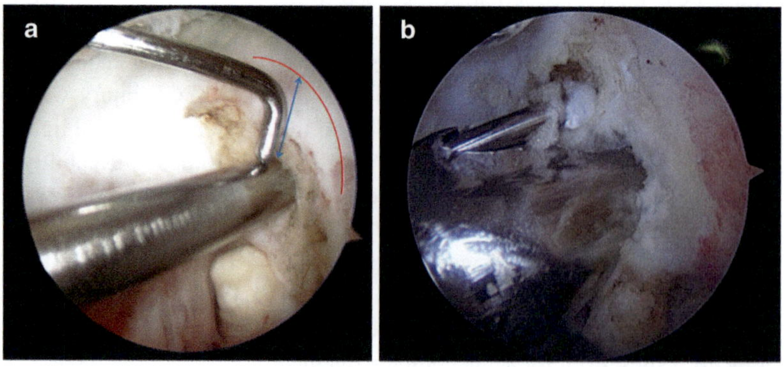

Fig. 10.1 (**a**) Femoral tunnel was established by a guide pin insert, (**b**) oval dilator

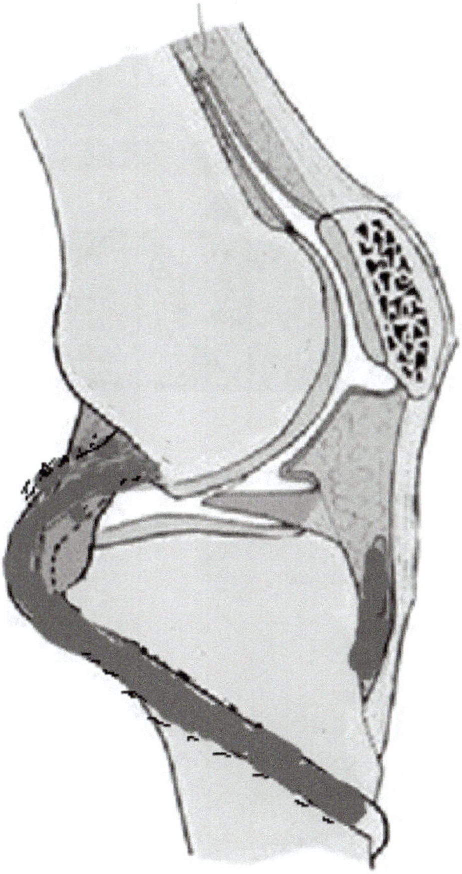

Fig. 10.2 PCL tibial tunnel was made just distal to the center of the PCL tibial attachment fiber. PCL remnant fiber works as a bumper cushion effect for the graft

The direction of the long axis of the rectangular dilator was slightly oblique to match the anatomy of the PCL tibial footprint. A no.5 Ethibond suture loop was passed from the lower accessory AMP to the femoral tunnel, and a wire loop was inserted from the anterior medial side of the tibial tunnel to the posterior PCL tibial angle guide hole (PCL tibial angle guide, Arthrex Co., USA). The wire loop was pulled out of the AMP with the tibial angle guide or with a curved pituitary rongeur and then separately to pass each end of the graft. The graft was pulled from the lower AMP to the femoral tunnel first, then the wire loop with the distal part of the graft was passed to the tibial tunnel.

The graft was fixed after cyclic loading with an adjustable loop cortical suspension device (TightRope RT, Arthrex or Ultra-Button Inc., USA) and Rigid Fix (DePuy Synthes Mitek Sports Medicine, USA) cross pin on the femoral side and a biodegradable interference screw (IntraFix technique, Depuy Co.) with an additional post-tie screw on the tibial side. A long leg splint was applied postoperatively with full extension of the knee position (Figs. 10.4 and 10.5).

PS: We can do the outside-in technique to make the femoral tunnel or the inside-out technique, the surgeon's choice.

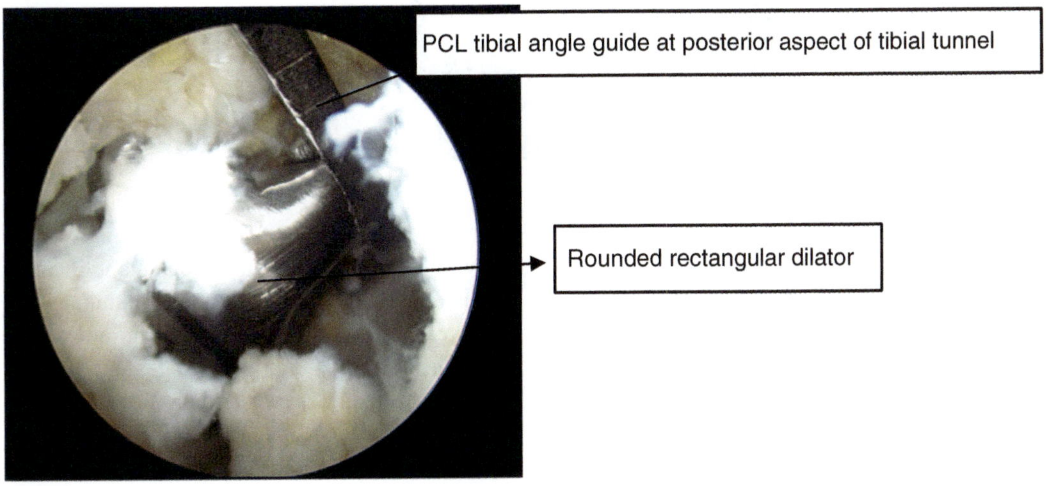

Fig. 10.3 Posterior of the tibial tunnel. Tibial tunnel was established by an oval or rectangular dilator

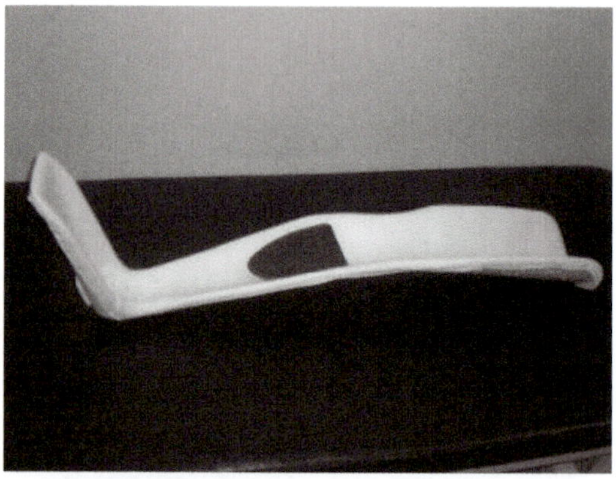

Fig. 10.4 A long leg splint with a tibial support in full extension prevents posterior sagging and is used for 2 weeks postoperatively

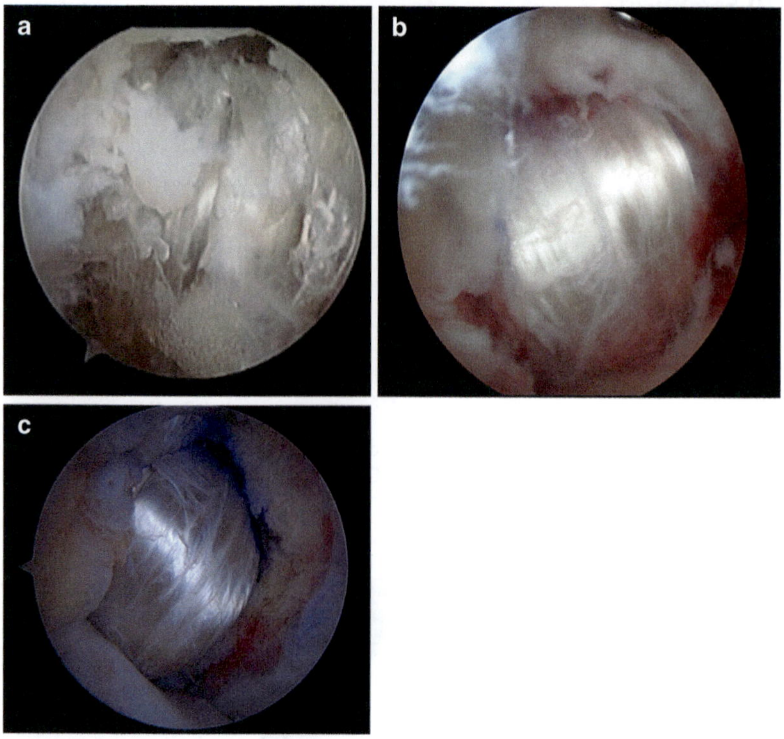

Fig. 10.5 (**a**) Round tunnel using round reamer and round dilator, there was a larger gap between the femoral tunnel edge and graft, however. (**b**) Rectangular tunnel with a rounded rectangular dilator, there was less gap between the femoral tunnel margin and graft. (**c**) Arthroscopic picture, using an oval-shaped dilator, there is less gap between the articular margin and the graft

10.4 Surgical Technique of Modified Tibial In-Lay PCL Reconstruction (Video 10.3)

When we do the modified in-lay technique:

1. PCL revision, especially the tibial tunnel, was widened and overlapped a new tunnel; a bone graft will be needed, and a two-stage situation will be needed. We can do one-stage revision using the modified tibial inlay technique.
2. In chronic case, the PCL remnant looks good in the MRI image. In order to get better stability, we'd like to do tensioning of the PCL remnant at the tibial attachment site detached with a bone block and tensioning and augmentation. In our clinical experience, if the PCL remnant fiber looks normal in MRI, which

was usually 6–9 months post-trauma or more, just tensioning the PCL tibial bone block detached, and fixation was good enough; however, it was a very rare case. Usually, we can do tensioning and augmentation with autologous hamstring tendon or allograft.

3. In chronic case, posterior sagging grade 3 and not reduced as normal position, even anterior drawer forces applied to the posterior of the proximal tibia, due to posterior capsule contracture, some release of the posterior capsule will be needed.

10.5 Surgical Technique of Tensioning the Remnant PCL and Reconstruction of the AL Bundle

The patient is placed in the supine position and general or spinal anesthesia is induced. The end of the operating table is lowered so that the patient's knee can be flexed to 90°. The arthroscope is introduced through the anterolateral portal and the intra-articular structures are examined. Meniscus surgery is performed when needed. The authors harvest the hamstring tendon from the affected side or the contralateral side, and the 4 bundles of hamstring tendon are prepared for reconstruction of the AL bundle of the PCL. Without removing the remnant PCL, using anteromedial portal, the tip of the guide hole is placed 5- to 6-mm proximal to the margin of the articular cartilage of the medial femoral condyle at approximately the 12:30 o'clock to 1 o'clock position on the right knee and at the 11 to 11:30 o'clock position on the left (Fig. 10.1). The distal femoral cortex medially is exposed through a 3- to 5-cm long skin incision and the vastus medialis is elevated subperiosteally. After placing the guide pin, a tunnel is made through the medial femoral condyle using a cannulated drill. We begin to make a femoral tunnel with a 6-mm cannulated drill, then dilate the femoral tunnel manually in 0.5–1 mm increasements of dilator size (Linvatec, Largo, FL), to avoid damage to the remnant PCL, sequentially according to graft diameter, and then the tunnel edge is chamfered with rasps(recently we'd like to do rounded rectangular dilator or oval-shaped dilator, as same as transtibial tunnel technique, we can do inside-out technique usually). A 21-gauge wire loop is passed through the femoral tunnel, directed toward the medial side of the remnant PCL of the tibia, and later used to pass the graft from the PCL tibial insertion area into the femoral tunnel. For the posterior approach to the knee, the leg and foot are placed on a side table, and the hip is flexed about 80°, abducted, and externally rotated as much as possible. The knee is flexed 70° to 90° to provide easier access to the popliteal area. The operating table is tilted over 30° so that the operated knee is lower than the contralateral knee (Fig. 10.6).

A 5- to 8-cm long, gently curved longitudinal incision is made in the posteromedial aspect of the knee. The interval between the medial head of the gastrocnemius muscle and the semimembranosus tendon is identified and developed bluntly. The semimembranosus and semitendinosus tendons are retracted toward the medial side. The

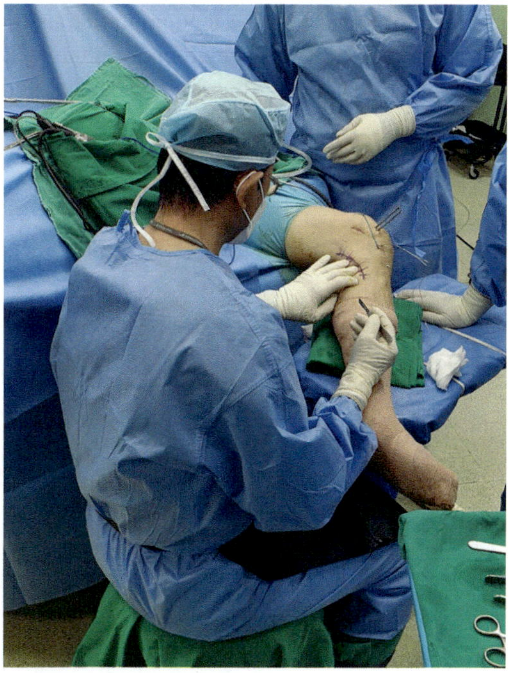

Fig. 10.6 The operating table is tilted as much as possible so that the posteromedial aspect of the knee can be approached (Video 10.3)

gastrocnemius muscle is retracted laterally, protecting the popliteal neurovascular structures. If the branches of the inferior medial geniculate artery and vein are encountered near the mid-posterior capsule, they are ligated securely. The popliteus muscle is detached subperiosteally from the posteromedial surface of the proximal tibia, and the posterior slope of the proximal tibia is palpated. The posterior knee capsule is incised adjacent to the medial femoral condyle, and the remnant PCL fibers are preserved. A tibial attachment of the PCL is demarcated as a 1.5 × 2-cm area using an osteotome, and a 7-mm thick bone block is detached from distal to the proximal area using a 1.2- to 1.5-cm wide curved osteotome (Fig. 10.7).

At the junction of bone and the remnant PCL bundle, a stitch of No. 5 nonabsorbable Ethibond suture (Ethicon, Somerville, NJ) is placed for easy distal traction of the remnant PCL. A bony trough is made at the medial side of the PCL tibial insertion just distal to the portion of bone block detached site, to which the detached bone block and graft are to be fixed with a cannulated screw and washer and additional fixation using a staple or post and tie. The tendon graft traction sutures are passed with a wire loop from the PCL tibial insertion area into the femoral tunnel, and the graft for augmentation (hamstring four bundles or allograft) is pulled up through the knee joint into the femoral tunnel. Then, the remnant PCL is tensioned by pulling the bone block distally. The knee joint is flexed 70–90° to check the step-off as an anatomic reduction between the anteromedial femoral condyle and the medial tibial plateau. The remnant PCL bone block is temporarily fixed on the hamstring graft using 1 or 2 K-wires, and a 5- or 6.5-mm cannulated screw with a spiked washer is used to secure fixation of the bone block to the tibia. During insertion of the cannulated screw, care is taken to avoid damage to the graft. When the fixation is not firm, additional fixation is accomplished with a staple (Fig. 10.8).

The operating table is changed back to the neutral position, and the range of motion of the knee joint is checked for full extension. The tibial fixation should be readjusted if the knee joint does not get full extension. After the tension and the accurate position of the graft are assessed arthroscopically, the graft is cyclically loaded in tension with 15–20 lbs. and is fixed with a biodegradable interference screw at the femoral tunnel with the knee joint in 70–90° of flexion and additionally fixed with a 10-mm staple or post-tie on the femoral side. Finally, the knee joint is assessed once more to check if full extension and flexion are possible without any resistance.

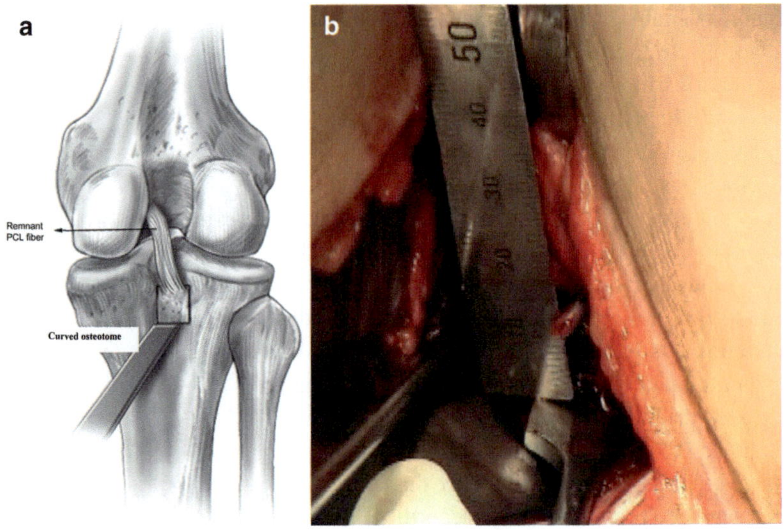

Fig. 10.7 (**a**, **b**) Detached PCL tibial insertion with bone block, usually 17 × 20 × 7 mm

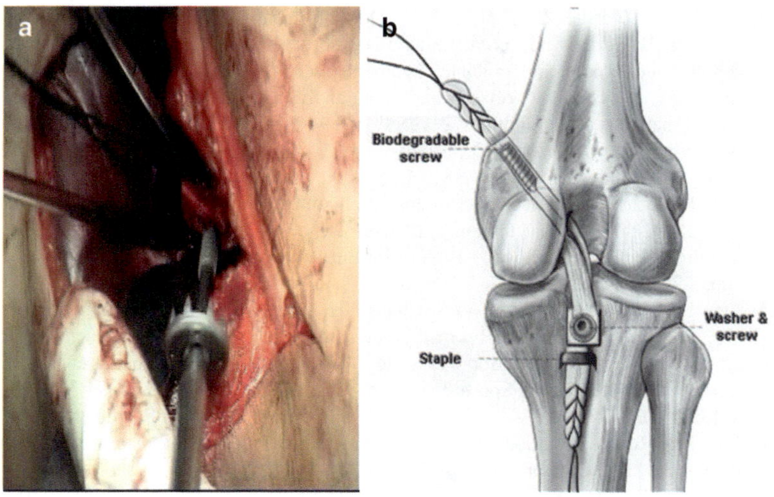

Fig. 10.8 (**a**) Screw and washer fixation of the tibial bone block and augmentation graft, (**b**) additional fixation with a staple

10.6 Rehabilitation After Surgery

For the first 2 or 3 weeks after surgery, a long leg splint is used to hold the knee in full extension. It has a posterior pad that prevents the tibia from sagging posteriorly (Fig. 10.9). Straight leg raising and quadriceps setting exercises are begun the day after the surgery, and the patient is allowed partial or non-weight-bearing using crutches. Starting on the third postoperative day, the splint is removed once or twice a day, and the patient is encouraged to perform a passive range of motion at 30–90° of flexion; he or she uses both hands to support the proximal part of the tibia or performs these exercises in the prone position to prevent tibial sagging by a physiotherapist. The range of flexion is allowed to 90° by the fourth to sixth postoperative week and to 120–130-° by 12 postoperative weeks. Full weight-bearing is begun by the sixth week. At 3–6 weeks after the surgery, a PCL brace with a tibial supporter is applied. Three to six months postoperatively, a progressive program of running is initiated if the knee is asymptomatic with this activity. By 8–10 months, sports activities such as soccer can be resumed if rehabilitation has progressed satisfactorily and quadriceps muscle power or thigh circumferences are nearly the same on both sides as nearly normal.

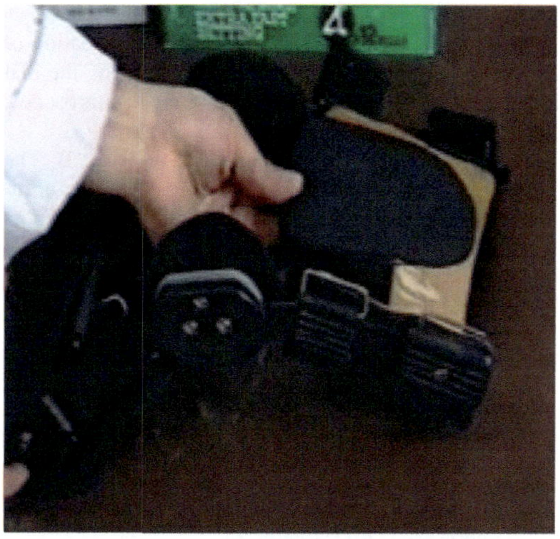

Fig. 10.9 PCL brace with tibial supporter and spring to prevent posterior sagging and is used for 6–8 weeks postoperatively

Further Reading

1. Ahn JH, Yang HS, Jeong WK, Koh KH. Arthroscopic transtibial posterior cruciate ligament reconstruction with preservation of posterior cruciate ligament fibers: clinical results of minimum 2-year follow-up. Am J Sports Med. 2006;34:194–204.
2. Apsingi S, Bull AM, Deehan DJ, Amis AA. Review: femoral tunnel placement for PCL reconstruction in relation to the PCL fiber bundle attachments. Knee Surg Sports Traumatol Arthrosc. 2009;17:652–9.

3. Chahla J, Moatshe G, Cinque ME, Dornan GJ, Mitchell JJ, Ridley TJ, et al. Single-bundle and double-bundle posterior cruciate ligament reconstructions: a systematic review and meta-analysis of 441 patients at a minimum 2 years' follow-up. Arthroscopy. 2017;33:2066–80.
4. Jung YB, Jung HJ, Tae SK, Lee YS, Lee KH. Reconstruction of the posterior cruciate ligament with a mid-third patellar tendon graft with use of a modified tibial inlay method. J Bone Joint Surg Am. 2005;87(suppl 1):247–63.
5. Jung HJ, Kim JH, Lee HJ, Koo S, Chang SH, Jung YB, et al. The isometry of two different paths for remnant-preserving posterior cruciate ligament reconstruction. Knee Surg Sports Traumatol Arthrosc. 2013;21:1029–35.
6. Jung YB. Recent evolution of cruciate ligament surgery of the knee. Clin Orthop Surg. 2012;4:103–6.
7. Jung YB, Jung HJ, Song KS, Kim JY, Lee HJ, Lee JS. Remnant posterior cruciate ligament-augmenting stent procedure for injuries in the acute or subacute stage. Arthroscopy. 2010;26:223–9.
8. Jung YB, Lee YS, Jung HJ, Nam CH. Evaluation of posterolateral rotatory knee instability using the dial test according to tibial positioning. Arthroscopy. 2009;25:257–61.
9. Jung YB, Nam CH, Jung HJ, Lee YS, Ko YB. The influence of tibial positioning on the diagnostic accuracy of combined posterior cruciate ligament and posterolateral rotatory instability of the knee. Clin Orthop Surg. 2009;1:68–73.
10. Kernkamp WA, Jens AJT, Varady NH, van Arkel ERA, Nelissen R, Asnis PD, et al. Anatomic is better than isometric posterior cruciate ligament tunnel placement based upon in vivo simulation. Knee Surg Sports Traumatol Arthrosc. 2019;27:2440–9.
11. Kim YM, Lee CA, Matava MJ. Clinical results of arthroscopic single-bundle transtibial posterior cruciate ligament reconstruction: a systematic review. Am J Sports Med. 2011;39:425–34.
12. Lee KH, Jung YB, Jung HJ, Jang EC, Song KS, Kim JY, et al. Combined posterolateral corner reconstruction with remnant tensioning and augmentation in chronic posterior cruciate ligament injuries: minimum 2-year follow-up. Arthroscopy. 2011;27:507–15.
13. Lee SH, Jung YB, Lee HJ, Jung HJ, Kim SH. Remnant preservation is helpful to obtain good clinical results in posterior cruciate ligament reconstruction: comparison of clinical results of three techniques. Clin Orthop Surg. 2013;5:278–86.
14. Markolf KL, Feeley BT, Jackson SR, McAllister DR. Where should the femoral tunnel of a posterior cruciate ligament reconstruction be placed to best restore anteroposterior laxity and ligament forces? Am J Sports Med. 2006;34:604–11.
15. Nakase J, Toratani T, Kosaka M, Ohashi Y, Numata H, Oshima T, et al. Technique of anatomical single bundle ACL reconstruction with rounded rectangle femoral dilator. Knee. 2016;23:91–6.
16. Narvy SJ, Pearl M, Vrla M, Yi A, Hatch GF 3rd. Anatomy of the femoral footprint of the posterior cruciate ligament: a systematic review. Arthroscopy. 2015;31:345–54.
17. Petrillo S, Volpi P, Papalia R, Mafulli N, Denaro V. Management of combined injuries of the posterior cruciate ligament and posterolateral corner of the knee: a systematic review. Br Med Bull. 2017;123:47–57.
18. Schlumberger M, Schuster P, Eichinger M, Mayer P, Mayr R, Immendörfer M, et al. Posterior cruciate ligament lesions are mainly present as combined lesions even in sports injuries. Knee Surg Sports Traumatol Arthrosc. 2020;28:2091–8.
19. Mcallister DR, Markolf KL, Oakes DA, Young CR, Mcwilliams J. A biomechanical comparison of tibial inlay and tibial tunnel posterior cruciate ligament reconstruction techniques. Am J Sports Med. 2002;30(3):312–7.
20. Jung YB, et al. Biomechanical effect of cyclic loading on the reconstructed posterior cruciate ligament - comparison between inlay and transtibial technique. J Korean Orthop. 2002;37(4):19.
21. Jung YB, et al. Tensioning of remnant posterior cruciate ligament and reconstruction of anterolateral bundle in chronic posterior cruciate ligament injury. Arthroscopy. 2006;22(3):329–38.
22. Burns WC, et al. The effect of femoral tunnel position and graft tensioning technique on posterior laxity of the posterior cruciate ligament-reconstructed knee. Am J Sports Med. 1995;23(4):424–30.
23. Seong Hwan Kim, Woo Sung Kim, Boo Seop Kim,·Hyun Soo Ok,· Jong Heon Kim Jeuk Lee, Young Bok Jung . Clinical outcomes of rectangular tunnel technique in posterior cruciate ligament reconstruction were comparable to the results of conventional round tunnel technique. Knee Surg Sports Traumatol Arthrosc 2021 29(11):3724–3734.
24. Fink C, Farinelli L, Abermann E, Meena A, Smigielski R, Herbort M. Posterior cruciate ligament reconstruction using flat soft-tissue grafts. Arthrosc Tech. 2023;12(2):e261–71.
25. Kato T, Śmigielski R, Ge Y, Zdanowicz U, Ciszek B, Ochi M. Posterior cruciate ligament is twisted and flat structure: new prospective on anatomical morphology. Knee Surg Sports Traumatol Arthrosc. 2018;26(1):31–9.

Management of the PLC Injury 11

Abstract

Posterolateral complex injury (PLC): The incidence of the PLC was reported to be 5.8–16% among knee ligament injuries.

According to Delee et al. and Laprade et al., the isolated PLC injury was about 1.6–2.1% of the knee ligament injuries. Most of the PLC injuries are associated with cruciate ligament injuries, especially combined PCL, 80–83% more. To avoid neglect of the PLC injury, the physician should have a high suspicion and routinely physically examine the PLRI and take history carefully. PLRI is identified as posterolateral subluxation and external rotation of the lateral tibial plateau in relation to the lateral femoral condyle as a consequence of injury to structures of the PLC of the knee. It is easy to miss PLRI and also the difficulty of relying on physical examination for the diagnosis of PLRI; no objective quantitative test exists for assessing increased external rotation. This makes an accurate diagnosis of PLRI difficult. The physician should check the reduced position of the medial tibial plateau to the femoral condyle as normal and then check PLRI or not; otherwise, it easily leads to misdiagnosis, especially in PCL with PLRI combined cases. The most common cause of the failure of the cruciate ligament reconstruction, especially PCL reconstruction, is neglected PLRI.

Most of the PLC injuries are associated with cruciate ligament injuries; 43–80% (Hughston 1976), 59% (Baker 1983), 65% (DeLee 1983), and 80% (Hughston and Jacobson 1985). To avoid neglect of the PLC injury, the physician should have a high suspicion and routinely perform a physical examination of PLRI and take history carefully. Take a history about varus and hyperextension injury, tenderness, and ecchymosis around the knee, and also check gait, especially for varus thrust gait or not. In a cadaver study, sectioning the PLC increased in situ force in the PCL 2–6 times, and the PCL with PLC cut resulted in 21 * external rotation and 14* varus rotational instability increase, but in isolated PCL loss, there is a small amount of the rotatory or varus and valgus laxity.

PLRI is identified as posterolateral subluxation and external rotation of the lateral tibial plateau in relation to the lateral femoral condyle as a consequence of injury to structures of the PLC of the knee. It is easy to miss PLRI and also the difficulty of relying on physical examination for the diagnosis of PLRI, and no objective quantitative test exists for assessing increased external rotation. This makes accurate diagnosis of PLRI difficult. As is known, a positive dial test may result from either pos-

Supplementary Information The online version contains supplementary material available at https://doi.org/10.1007/978-981-95-9039-1_11.

Y. B. Jung et al., *Treatment of the Cruciate Ligaments Injuries*,
https://doi.org/10.1007/978-981-95-9039-1_11

terolateral or medial knee injuries, and the results of rotatory instability tests should be carefully interpreted.

Keywords

Posterolateral corner injury · PLRI · Combined injury

11.1 The Principle of Treatment for PLRI

Posterolateral corner (PLC) injuries are usually combined with cruciate ligament injuries. These types of injury were frequently overlooked in the past but are now widely acknowledged as a major factor contributing to poor results in the overall treatment process, particularly if there is a concomitant cruciate ligament injury. Several physical examinations, radiographic, and magnetic resonance imaging (MRI) tests have been developed to assess injuries to the posterolateral structures. Physical examinations include the 30° of flexion external rotation-dial test, reverse pivot shift test, external rotation recurvatum test, posterolateral drawer test, and adduction stress test. However, each test has its limitations in diagnosing PLC injuries. The physical examinations are inevitably vulnerable to subjective judgments, and the reverse pivot shift test has a false positive rate of 35%. With posterior cruciate ligament (PCL) stress radiographs (Figs. 11.7, 11.11, 11.12, 11.13, 11.16, 11.17, 11.21, 11.22a, b) more than 12 mm of side-to-side difference with respect to posterior tibial translation has been suggested to indicate a combined PCL-PLC injury until proven otherwise (Figs. 11.7, 11.8, 11.13, and 11.14). We can see PCL-PLRI even if there is less than 12 mm of side-to-side difference in posterior tibial translation (Figs. 11.17, 11.18, and 11.19). MRI with the coronal oblique view has been shown to have an accurate diagnostic rate and, particularly in the case of an acute injury, is highly reliable (Fig. 11.9a–d). A problem with MRI, however, is that it has low reliability in chronic injury cases.

The dial test is commonly used to evaluate the PCL-PLC injury with settings of 30° and 90° of knee flexion. The medial border of the foot is used as the reference measurement. Therefore, it is important to note that this measurement only correlates indirectly with the tibial rotation at the knee. Increased external rotation at 30°, but not 90°, indicates an isolated injury to posterolateral structures, whereas increased external rotation at both angles suggests injury to both posterolateral structures and the PCL. If external rotation of the injured tibia exceeds 10° in a side-to-side comparison with the uninjured tibia, posterolateral corner injury is suggested. The dial test is easy to perform and has been found to provide a good assessment of the amount of posterolateral knee injury. Moreover, although it has been shown to reliably assess PLC injuries in the laboratory, the dial test is difficult to accurately apply in a clinical situation. There is also some controversy as to whether the dial test should be performed with the patient in the supine position or in the prone position. Especially in the supine position dial test, we should do it at the normal position of the tibiofemoral joint, which means the anterior force is applied, such as reduced as the normal position (medial tibiofemoral stepping (about 10 mm at 90° flexion of the knee) of the tibia in PCL-combined injured cases.

We classified PLC injuries according to varus and rotatory instability, as assessed by the varus stress, dial, and posterolateral external rotation tests.

For varus instability, the difference in the lateral joint space distance and the presence or absence of a firm end point were assessed and classified as follows: grade I, when the difference was less than 5 mm; grade II, 5 to 10 mm with a firm end point; and grade III, more than 10 mm without a firm end point. To assess the degree of rotatory instability, we conducted the posterolateral external rotation test at 30° and 90° of knee flexion as follows: the TFA and PTA were measured with a goniometer after applying an external rotation stress to the tibia at both 30° and 90° of knee flexion in two different positions (reduced and posterior subluxed).

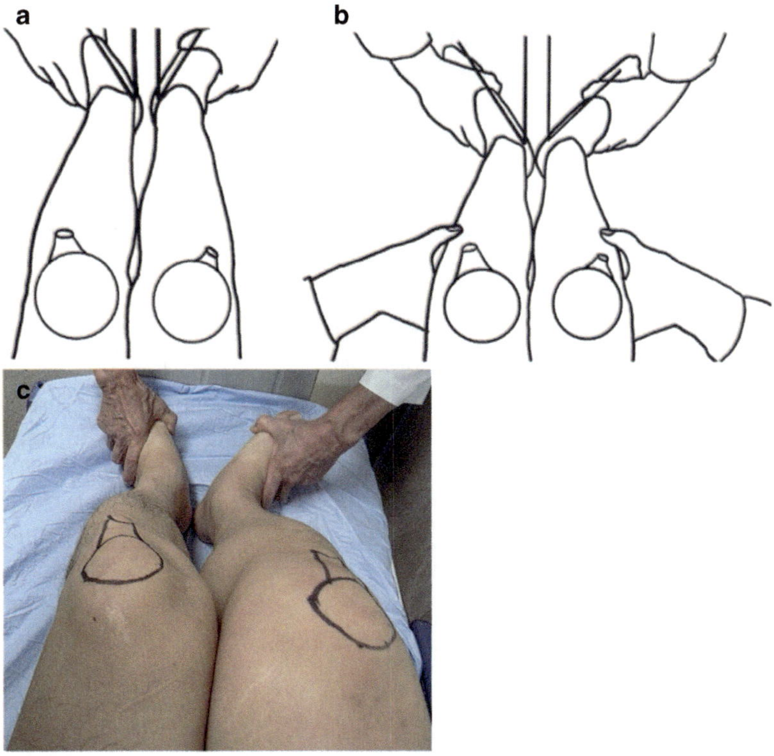

Fig. 11.1 The thigh-foot and patella-tubercle angles were measured with external rotation stress applied to the tibia at both 30° and 90° of knee flexion. Before the torque was applied, a neutral force (**a**) and an anterior force (**b**) were applied to the tibia. (**c**) Lt knee shows a positive dial test (PLRI)

The test was performed with the patient in the supine position, and the AP force was applied to the tibia (Fig. 11.1).

The degree of rotation was compared to that of the contralateral side, and the side-to-side difference was investigated. The classification of PLC injuries was as follows: grade I, increased external rotation of 5–10° compared with the contralateral side, without any varus instability; grade II, increased external rotation of more than 10°, or posterolateral subluxation of the tibial plateau combined with grade 0–2 varus instability; and grade III, increased external rotation of more than 10° without a firm end point, combined with grade III varus instability from lateral collateral ligament injury or increased external rotation of more than 20°.

In combined PCL-PLC injuries, we should first do the reduction of a posteriorly partially displaced knee to correctly check for the PLRI or not (Video 10.1). Strauss et al. (2007) reported that knees tested with the application of an anterior force showed a mean external rotation of 25.9°, which was significantly greater than that observed in the neutral position (mean, 21.4°) and with the application of a posterior force (mean, 18.7°). In our study series, the mean differences in TFA between the subluxed and reduced positions at 30° and 90° of knee flexion were 5.9° and 6.2°, respectively.

The addition of the anterior force to the dial test, which is the same as performing the test in the prone position, reduces the posterior tibial subluxation often seen in the PCL-deficient knee.

We have done a dial test with a maximal manual torque and compared it to that of the contralateral side because only the relative difference is important.

In varus stress radiography, side-to-side differences are >2.7 mm in isolated fibula collateral ligament injury (FCL) and > 4.0 mm in FCL + PLC (LaPrade 2008) (Table 11.1).

The patient who has a tibial plateau posterior inclination of nearly zero degree, PCL with PLRI injury has occurred; the patient has genu recurvatum with varus thrust gait. In this case, we should first medial anterior open wedge osteotomy was done to correct posterior inclination of the tibial plateau. Then, PCL reconstruction should be done or not. Some of them only require medial open wedge osteotomy and correct gait and alignment; also, we don't need PCL reconstruction (Genu recurvatum case, Video 11.1).

Table 11.1 The classification of PLRI was shown (Fanelli, Oper Tech Sport Med, 1999)

Classification	Injury description	Damaged structures
PLRI-A	Increased tibial external rotation only (>10′)	PFL, popliteus tendon only
PLRI-B	Increased tibial external rotation and mild varus laxity (~5 mm increased lateral joint line opening)	PFL, popliteus tendon, attenuation of FCL
PLRI-C	Increased tibial external rotation and severe varus laxity(>10 mm increased lateral joint line opening)	PFL, popliteus tendon, FCL, lateral capsular avulsion, cruciate ligament disruption

11.2 Surgical Technique and Current Concept of Operative Treatment of PLC Injury

In an experimental study, PCL and PLC cut compared to PLCS through fibular head tunnel (modified Larson) vs. anatomical reconstruction (popliteal reconstruction with LCL, Laprade), there was no difference between the two groups (Apsingi et al., KSSTA, 2009). My clinical experiences in grade 2 PLRI, PLCS through fibular head tunnel (modified Larson technique), are enough to correct PLRI (Fig. 11.2). However, grade 3 PLRI, maybe we should do anatomical reconstruction (fibular head tunnel and popliteal tendon reconstruction). Sometimes, even additional reinforcement of the LCL will be needed (Fig. 11.6).

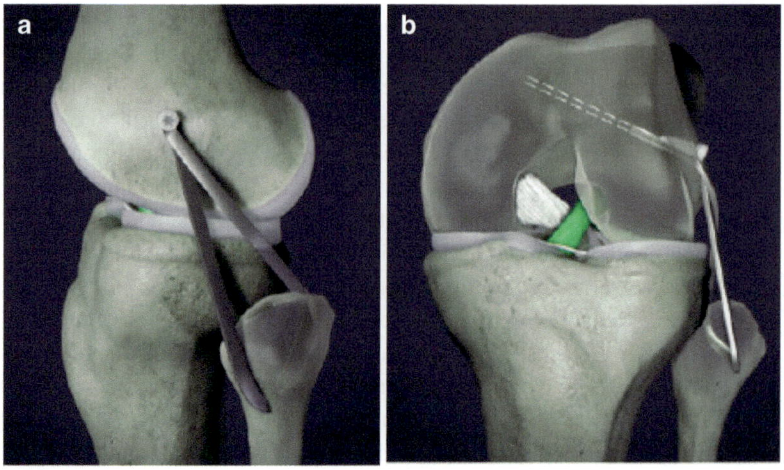

Fig. 11.2 (**a**, **b**) Schematic depictions of how the modified posterolateral corner sling is passed through the fibular head tunnel and the oblique tunnel configurations employed to reduce a killer turn effect. Both ends of the grafts were passed through the femoral tunnel in a figure-of-eight pattern

11.3 Anatomic Reconstruction of LCL/PLT/PFL ("Versailles Technique")

For the anatomical PLC reconstruction, the long lateral incision was applied, then the peroneal nerve exploration was performed (Fig. 11.3).

The apex of the fibula (anterior and posterior aspects) is released using a monopolar electrocautery to allow identification of the attachments of the PFL and LCL. A guide wire is then inserted in the distal-to-proximal and anterior-to-posterior direction into the head of the fibula. A guide wire is sequentially positioned along the directions of the anatomic attachments of the FPL and LCL. A tunnel is then drilled using a 6 to 7-mm bit. It may be positioned slightly more distally (in the wide part of the fibular head). An anteroposterior 7- to 8-mm tibial tunnel is then drilled for the popliteal tendon. The tunnel starts at Gerdy's tubercle and ends at the popliteal depression located about 1 cm below the lateral edge of the lateral tibial plateau. This depression can be readily identified by finger palpation. A ligamentoplasty aiming system can be used for this step. A guide wire is used to check proper tunnel position (with a retractor placed behind the tibial plateau to protect the soft tissues), and the cannulated drill bit is then introduced. A metal wire is finally used to retrieve the loop from the anterior orifice. The last tunnel is curved and connects the popliteus tendon attachment site anterior to the lateral femoral epicondyle to a hole created immediately behind the epicondyle (at the LCL attachment site). The tunnel is drilled using two 6-mm drill bits, one at each end, then completed using a curved rasp (Fig. 11.4a,b).

The spaces under the fascia lata and LCL are released using a Kelly forceps to facilitate the passage of the graft. The tendon graft should be prepared in a Y shape, with about 10-cm-long-whip-stitched common portion that divides into two strands. Reconstruction is achieved by introducing the two strands together into the tibial tunnel from anterior to posterior using wire graft passers. The two strands are retrieved and then passed through the femoral tunnel in the anterior-to-posterior direction. The femoral bony bridge is reinforced by a staple to limit the risk of collapse and secure the graft to the femur. The leg is then extended (in neutral rotation), and the common tibial strand, held taut by an aide, is fixed using an absorbable tibial interference screw to form the popliteal portion of the reconstruction. The LCL can then be reconstructed using the two strands exiting from the posterior part of the condylar tunnel. The thicker strand is introduced into

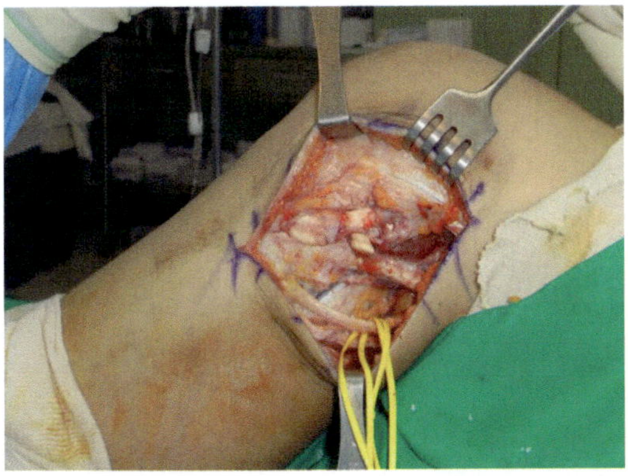

Fig. 11.3 Torn PLC ligaments and peroneal nerve exploration were shown

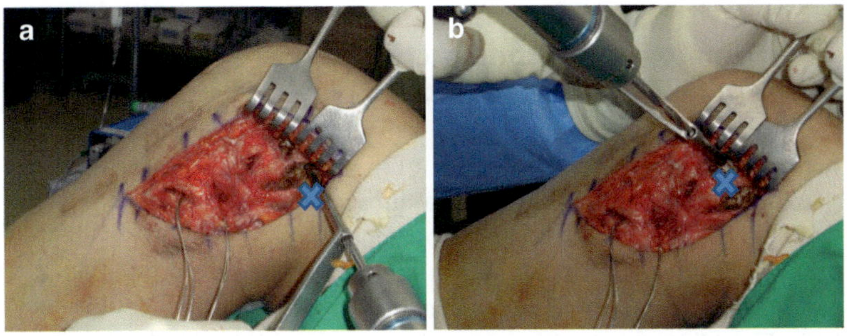

Fig. 11.4 (a, b) Femoral tunnel was made from posterior to anterior around the lateral epicondyle

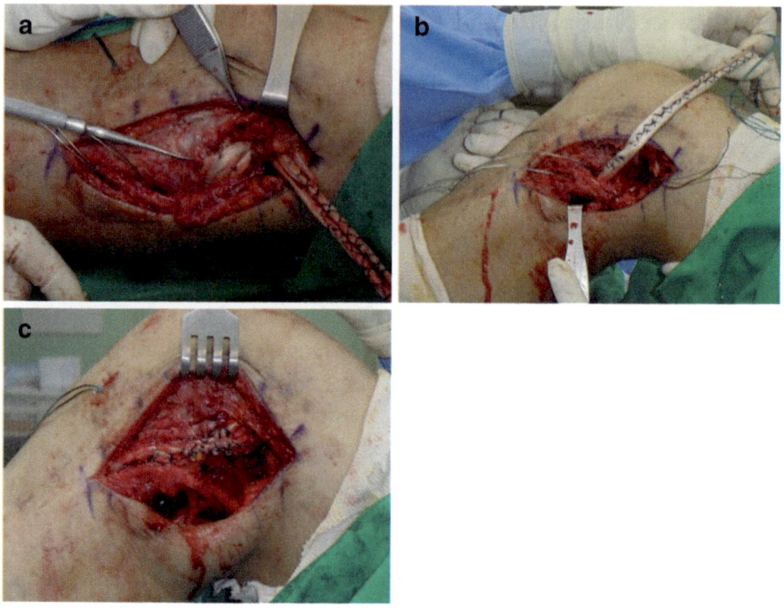

Fig. 11.5 The graft was passed from the femoral to the tibial side. (**a**) The graft was passed to the tibial side first, then passed through the femoral tunnel from posterior to anterior. This graft has the function of the popliteus and posterolateral complex. (**b**) Then, the passed graft could be turned down to the fibular head. The separated ends of the graft were passed anterior to posterior and posterior to anterior for each end. (**c**) Finally, a suture was done for the final passed graft. This graft has the function of the LCL

the fibular tunnel from anterior to posterior and the thinner strand from posterior to anterior. These strands are fixed into the fibular tunnel using an absorbable screw, with the knee flexed at 30° (neutral rotation), then stitched to each other. Tension must be sufficient but not excessive to avoid postoperative stiffness. The excess tendon threaded from posterior to anterior is stitched to the reconstruction. Reconstruction of the PFL is achieved using the excess tendon threaded from anterior to posterior, which is stitched to the middle third of the popliteal portion of the reconstruction (Fig. 11.5a–c).

11.4 Anatomical Reconstruction of LCL/PLT/PFL (Laprade RF)

LaPrade et al., AJSM (2004) (Fig. 11.6).

When the PCL is ruptured, three arthroscopic findings can be identified, which are pseudolaxity of the ACL (Figs. 11.10a and 11.15a) a widened gap between the medial femoral condyle and the PCL (Fig. 11.10b) and a drive-through sign.

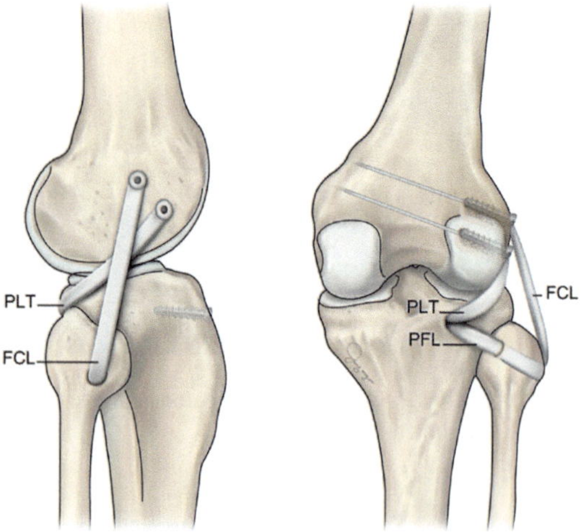

Fig. 11.6 Femoral tunnels (9 mm)
- Proximal 1/5 popliteus sulcus (PLT)
- Proximo-posterior to lateral epicondyle (LCL)
- 7 mm interference screws

In this patient, pseudolaxity of the ACL and a widened gap (black arrow) between the medial femoral condyle and the PCL were observed (Fig. 11.10a, b).

After PCL reconstruction, the pseudolaxity of the ACL was resolved (Fig. 11.10d).

In this patient, during femoral tunneling (using our first-generation rectangular dilator), the femoral condyle was fractured, so we performed two cannulated screw fixation (Fig. 11.11b, d, f).

11.5 Cases of PCL Reconstruction Combined with PLCS

Case 1: PCL Reconstruction Combined with PCLS

A 57-year-old female patient with no history of knee problems presented to the outpatient clinic complaining of pain in her left knee. The pain started 1 week ago after slipping on an icy road. Posterior drawer test (gr 3), PLRI (gr 2), and varus stress were positive on physical examination. KT-2000 arthrometer maximum manual test (MMT): 7 mm right and 13 mm left were checked (Figs. 11.7, 11.8, and 11.9).

Therefore, PLCS was performed along with A/S PCL reconstruction (Figs. 11.10, 11.11, and 11.12).

KT-2000 arthrometer maximum manual test (MMT); 7 mm right and 8 mm left were checked on physical examination.

Case 2: PCL Reconstruction Combined with PCLS

A 27-year-old male patient with a history of knee problems presented to the outpatient clinic complaining of right knee pain. He had an injury to his right knee 2 years ago during a soccer game. The pain was tolerable at first but became worse. He was a young man, with some discomfort when walking downhill and jumping. The posterior drawer test was positive, PLRI gr 2, varus stress test grade 0–1, and the dial test was positive on physical examination. KT-2000 arthrometer maximum manual test (MMT); 12 mm right and 7 mm left were checked (Figs. 11.13 and 11.14).

Therefore, PCL reconstruction with PLCS was done (Figs. 11.15 and 11.16).

KT-2000 arthrometer maximum manual test (MMT); 8 mm right and 7 mm left were checked on physical examination.

Case 3: PCL Rupture with PLRI

A 41-year-old female patient with right knee pain presented to the outpatient clinic with no history of knee problems. 1 month ago, she injured her left knee when she fell on it while walking. The pain was tolerable at first but became worse. Physical examination revealed a positive poste-

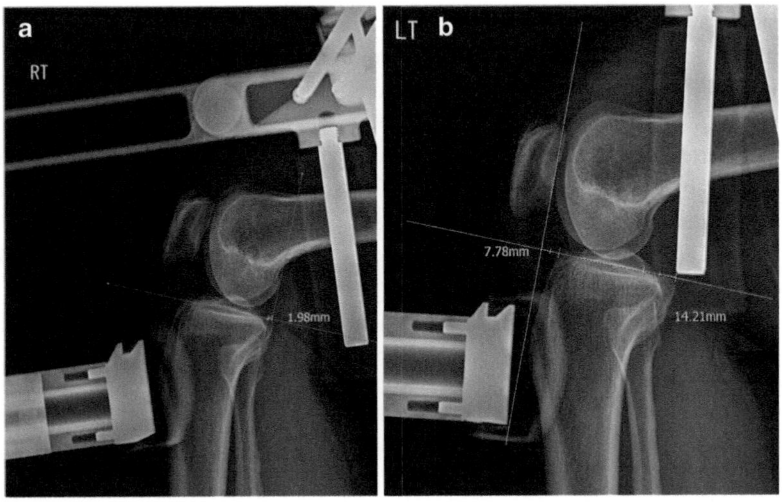

Fig. 11.7 (a, b) 10.6 mm side-to-side difference was checked compared to the unaffected side in the push stress test imaging

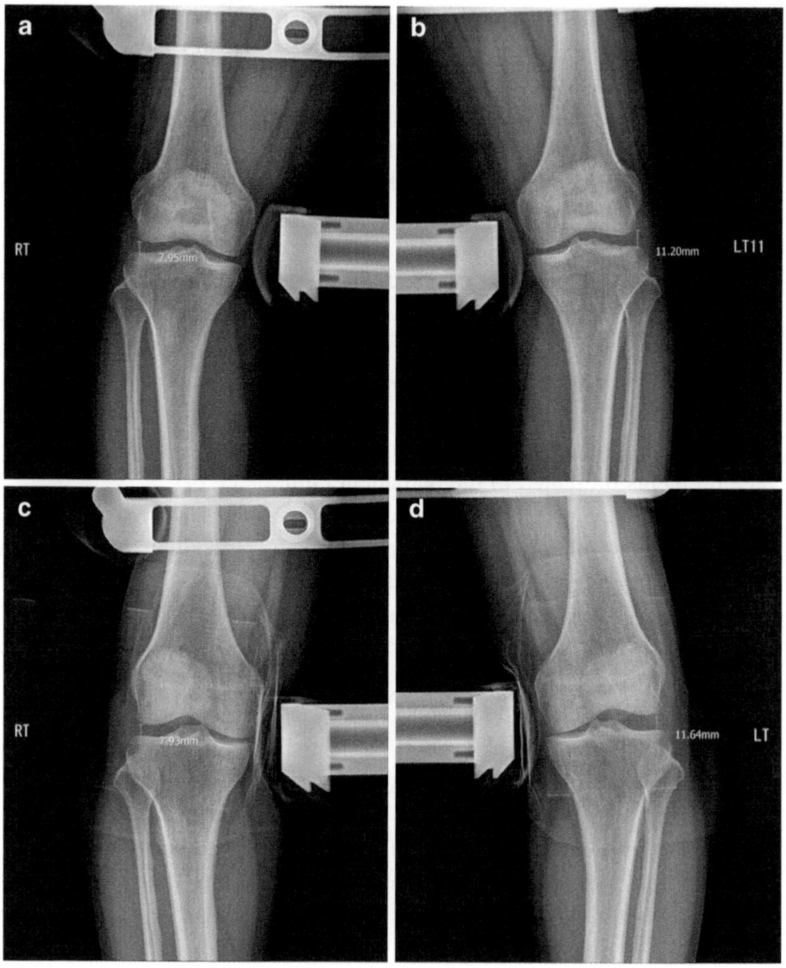

Fig. 11.8 (**a**, **b**) 0° varus stress view (**c**, **d**) 30° flexion varus stress view; left knee lateral joint space is wider than right knee

rior drawer test, PLRI grade 2, varus stress test grade 1–2. KT-2000 arthrometer maximum manual test (MMT); 10 mm right and 8 mm left were checked (Figs. 11.17, 11.18, and 11.19).

Therefore, PLCS was performed along with arthroscopic PCL reconstruction at 30° flexion, varus stress view of both knees. There is no laxity in the varus stress and push views (Figs. 11.20 and 11.21).

KT-2000 arthrometer maximum manual test (MMT); 9 mm right and 9 mm left were checked on physical examination (Fig. 11.22).

Case 4

A 52-year-old lady had fallen down in an accident about 3 years ago.

Preoperative stress film. PUSH VIEW; posterior sagging grade 3, varus stress test ++. Physical examination: posterior drawer test grade 2.5–3, varus stress test grade 2, and PLRI grade 2. I have done PCL reconstruction as a modified inlay technique with a bone block attached to the Achilles allograft. The femoral tunnel was made inside-out technique using a rounded rectangular dilator, PLCS as the fibular head tunnel to just anteroposterior to the lateral femoral epicondyle (modified Larson's PLCS). 21 months postoperative stress film and physical test; her knee was very stable; posterior drawer test, negative; varus stress test, negative; dial test, negative. KT-2000, maximum manual test; RT 9 mm and LT 9.5 mm thigh circumferences were nearly the same in

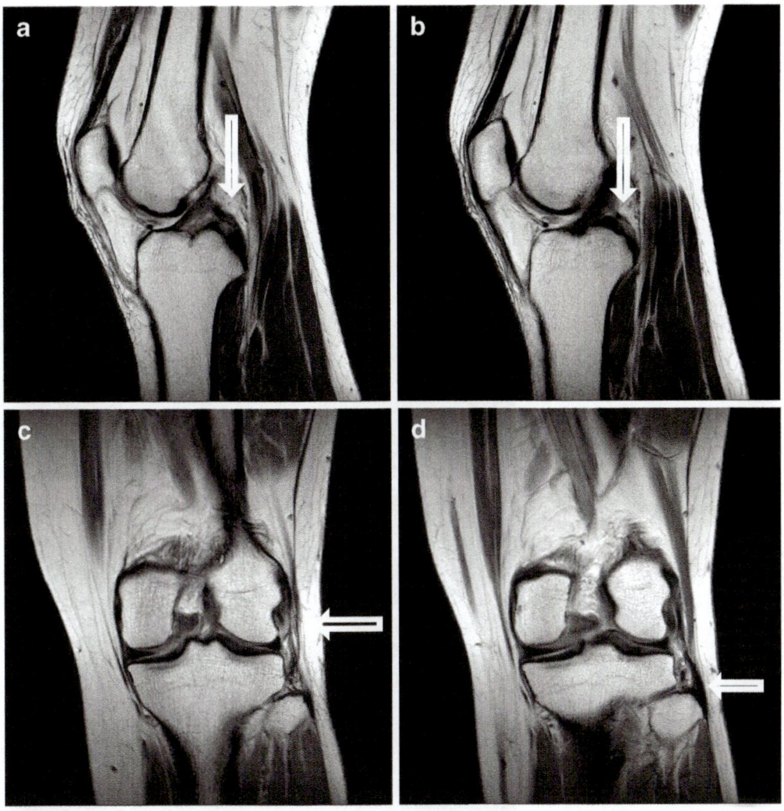

Fig. 11.9 (**a**, **b**) PCL rupture and lateral collateral ligament injury can be seen. (**c**, **d**) lateral collateral ligament and posterolateral complex injury

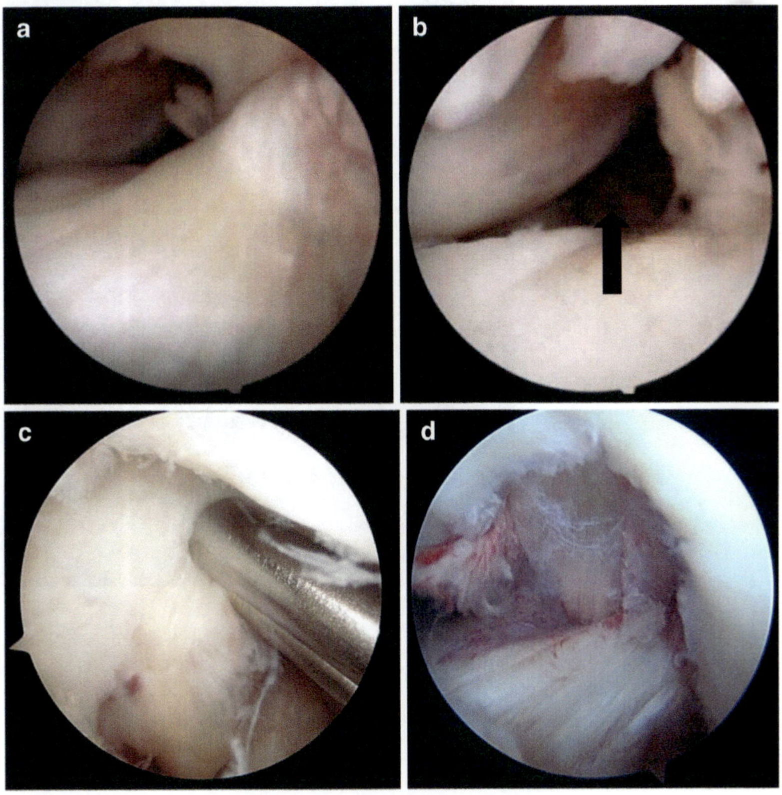

Fig. 11.10 (**a**) ACL pseudolaxity (**b**) wider gap between the PCL and medial femoral condyle inner wall (**c**) A guide pin insert to create a femoral tunnel (**d**) After PCL graft fixation with preserved remnant PCL. The ACL pseudolaxity was not seen

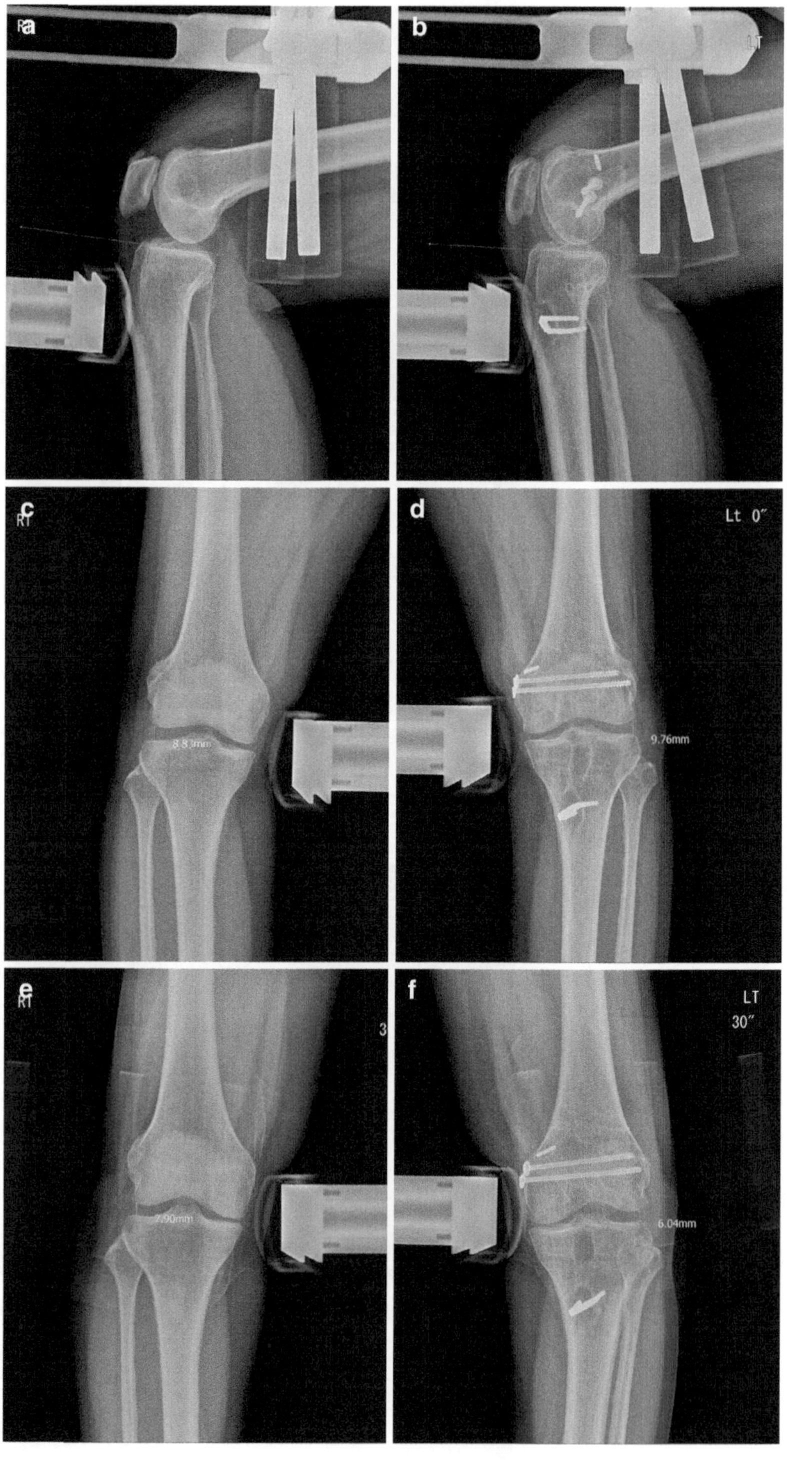

Fig. 11.11 12 months after PCL reconstruction and PLCS. (**a**, **b**) Push view. (**c**, **d**) 0° Varus stress view. (**e**, **f**) 30° flexion varus stress view of both knees. There is no instability in the varus stress and push views

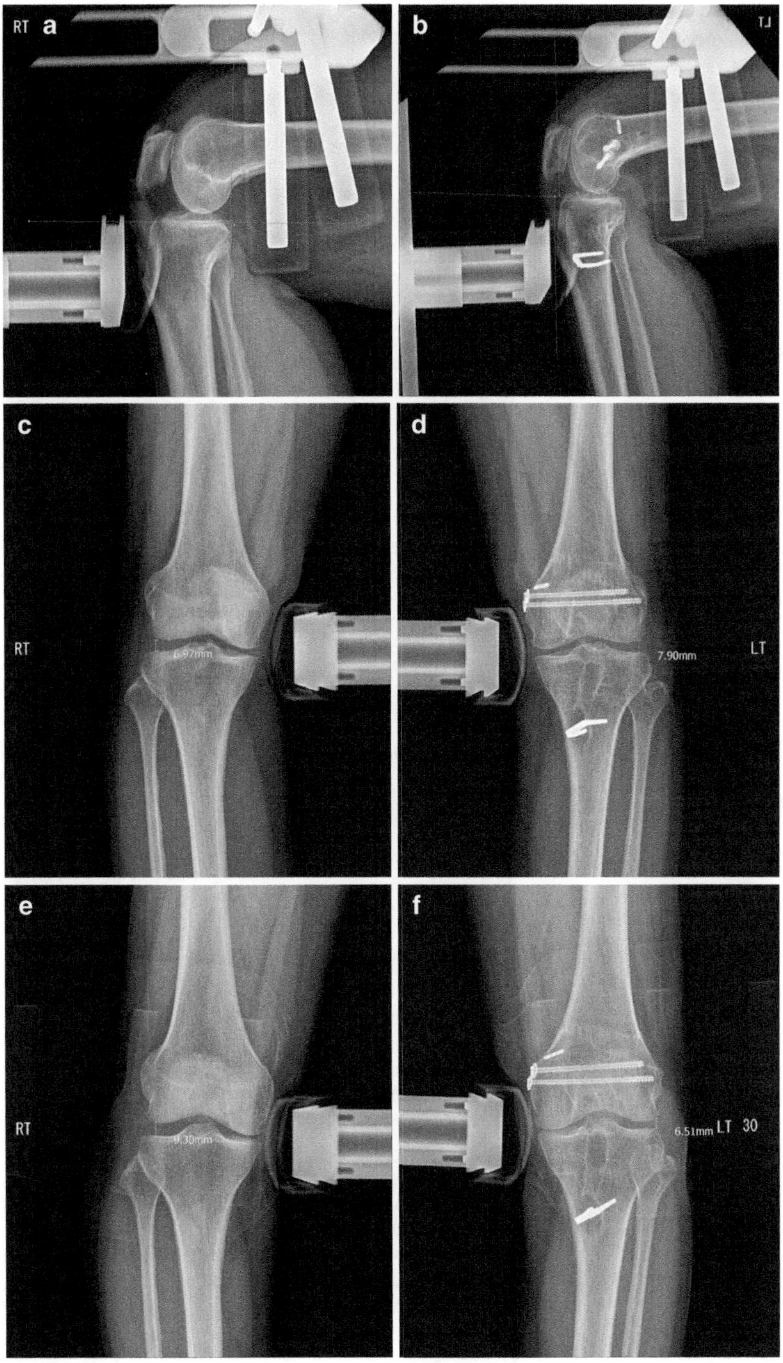

Fig. 11.12 (**a**, **b**) Push view, 24 months after PCL reconstruction and PLCS. (**c**, **d**) 0° varus stress view. (**e**, **f**) 30° flexion varus stress view of both knees. There is no instability in the varus stress and push views

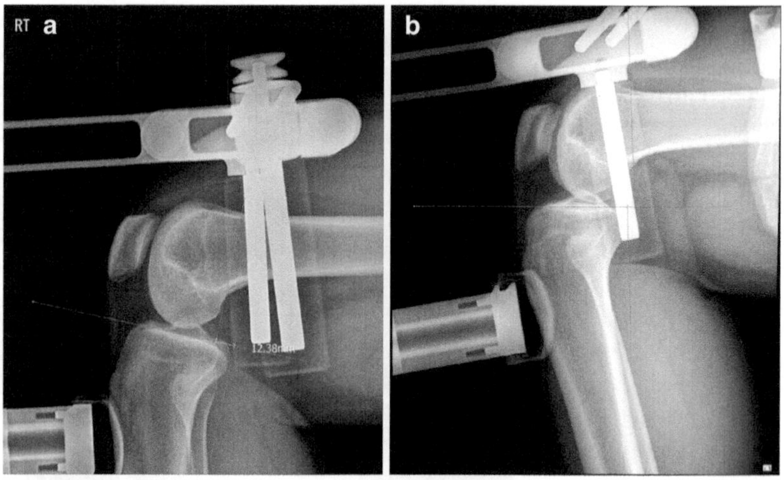

Fig. 11.13 (**a**, **b**) 12.4 mm side-to-side difference was checked compared to the unaffected side in the push stress test view. (**a**) There was no anterior stepping of the tibiofemoral condyle and posterior displacement of the tibia plateau

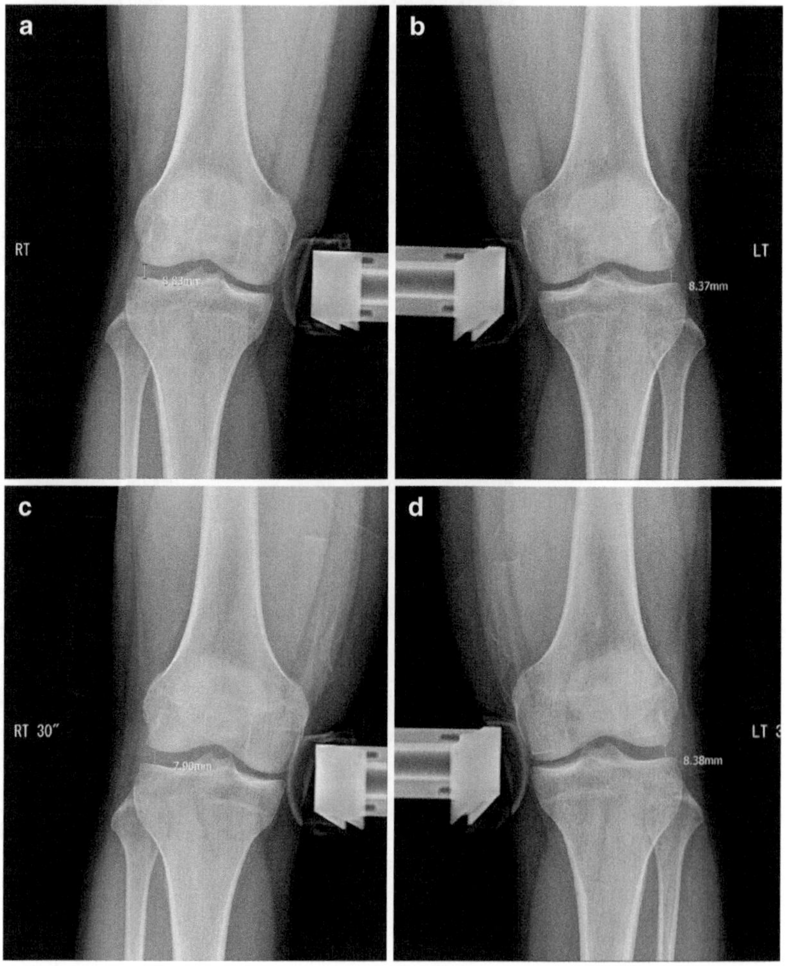

Fig. 11.14 (**a**, **b**) 0° and (**c**, **d**) 30° flexion varus stress view; no significant difference between both knees

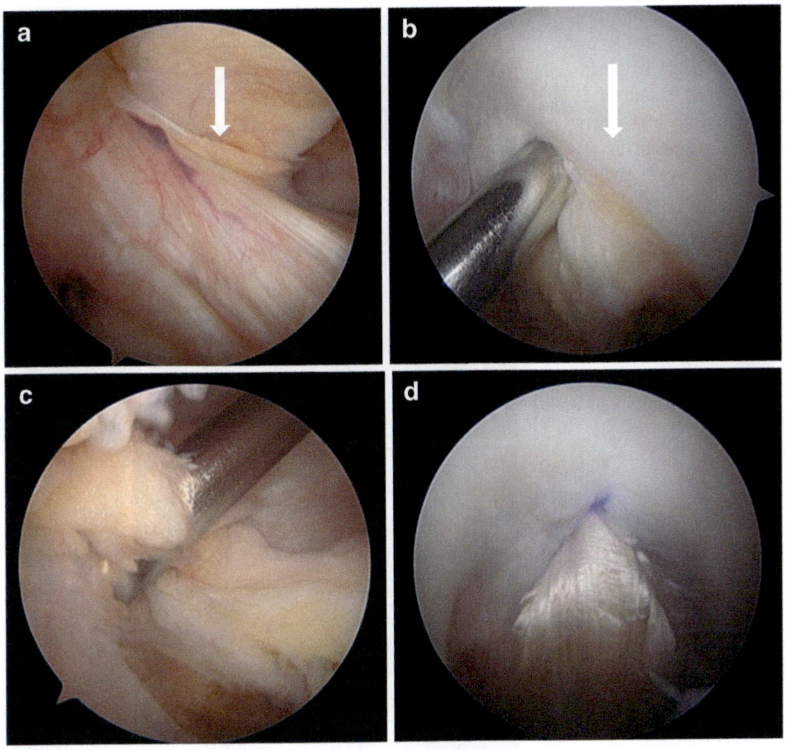

Fig. 11.15 (**a**) ACL pseudolaxity was mild, and PCL looks not bad in gross. (**b**, **c**) A guide pin was inserted anterior to the PCL remnant at the femoral attachment site to preserve the remnant PCL as much as possible. (**d**) The PCL graft over the remnant PCL after fixation of the graft. These are the intraoperative arthroscopic

both sides. RT 40 cm, LT 41 cm. The result was excellent. In the senior author's experience, like this patient with posterior sagging grade 2.5–3, doing the modified inlay technique will yield better results, especially since the PCL remnant looks good in the MRI film and the remnant PCL tensioning and augmentation will have better stability and easier neurovascular coverage of the graft (better synovialization) (Figs. 11.23, 11.24, and 11.25).

Fig. 11.16 12 months after PCL reconstruction and PLCS. (**a**, **b**) push view (**c**, **d**) 0° and (**e**, **f**) 30° flexion varus stress view; no significant difference between both knees. Varus stress and push view of both knees. There is no instability in the varus stress and push views

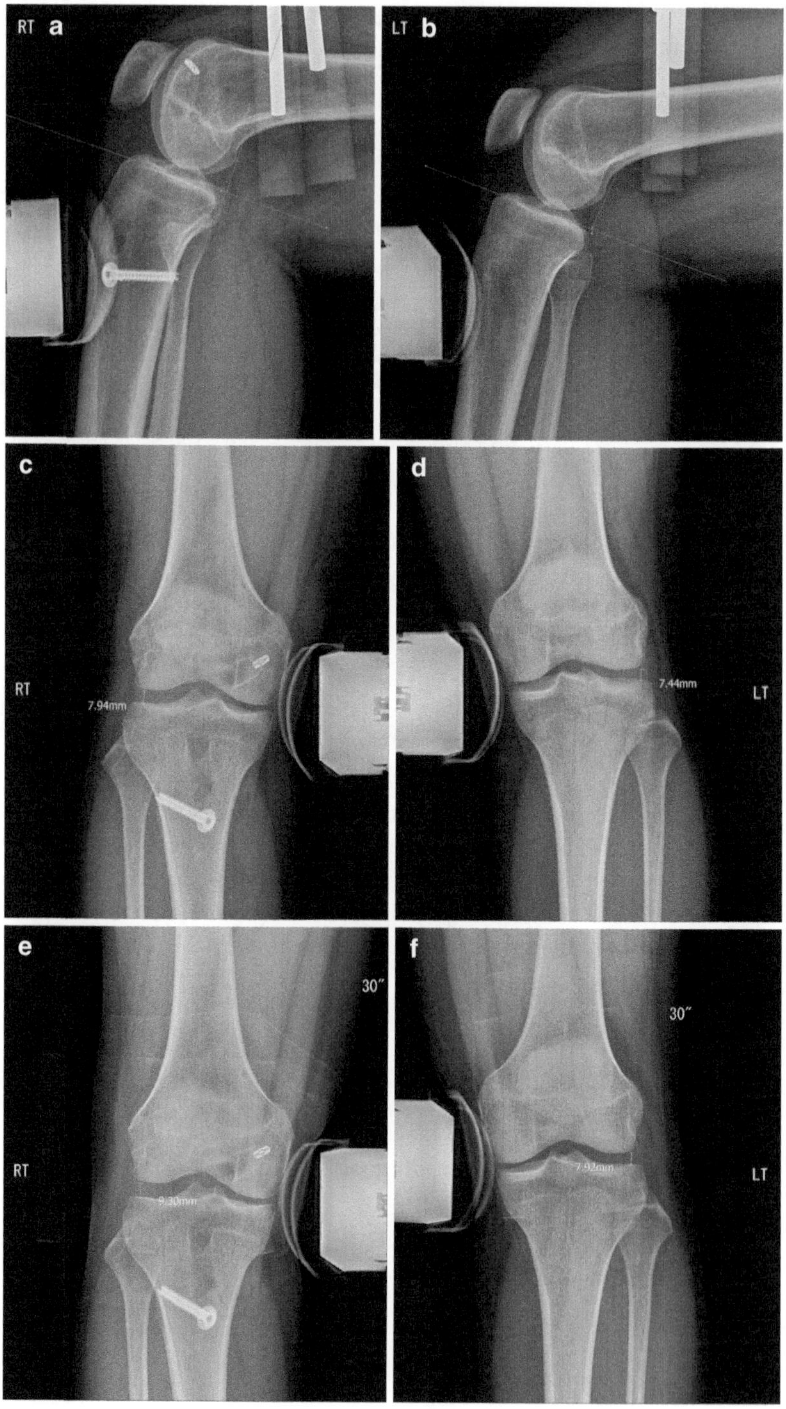

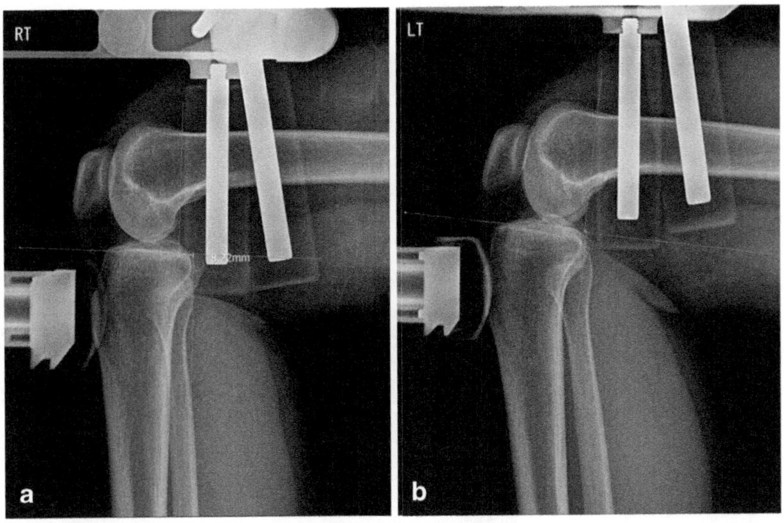

Fig. 11.17 (**a**, **b**) 8.2 mm side-to-side difference was checked compared to the unaffected side in the push stress test imaging

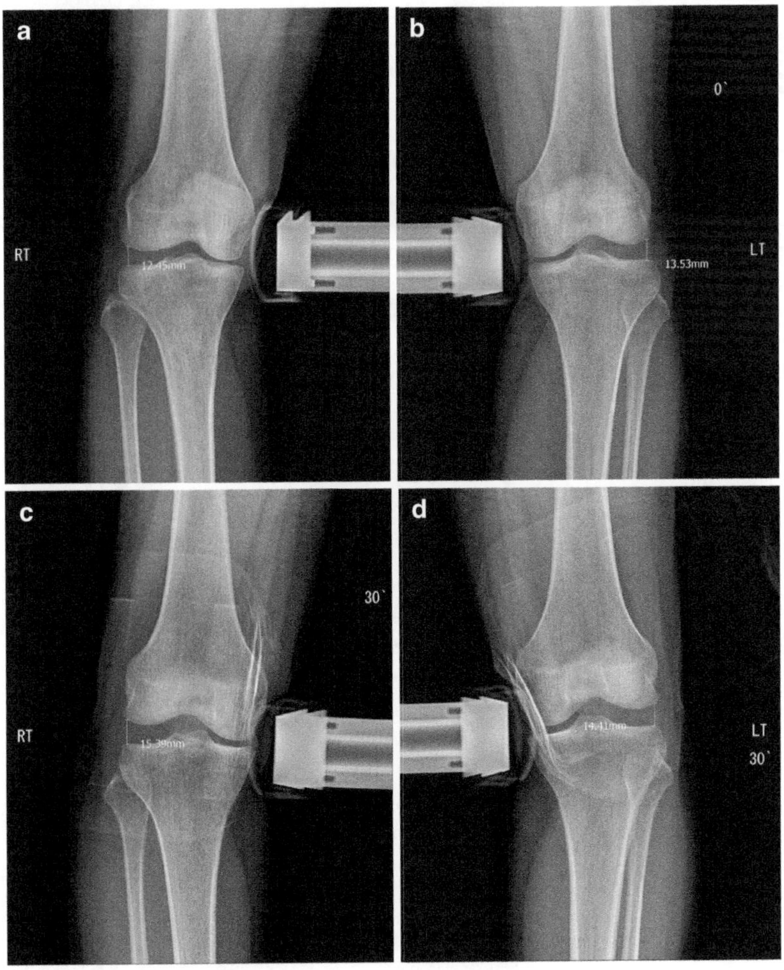

Fig. 11.18 (**a**, **b**) 0° varus stress view, (**c**, **d**) 30° flexion, varus stress view: there was no significant difference between both knees

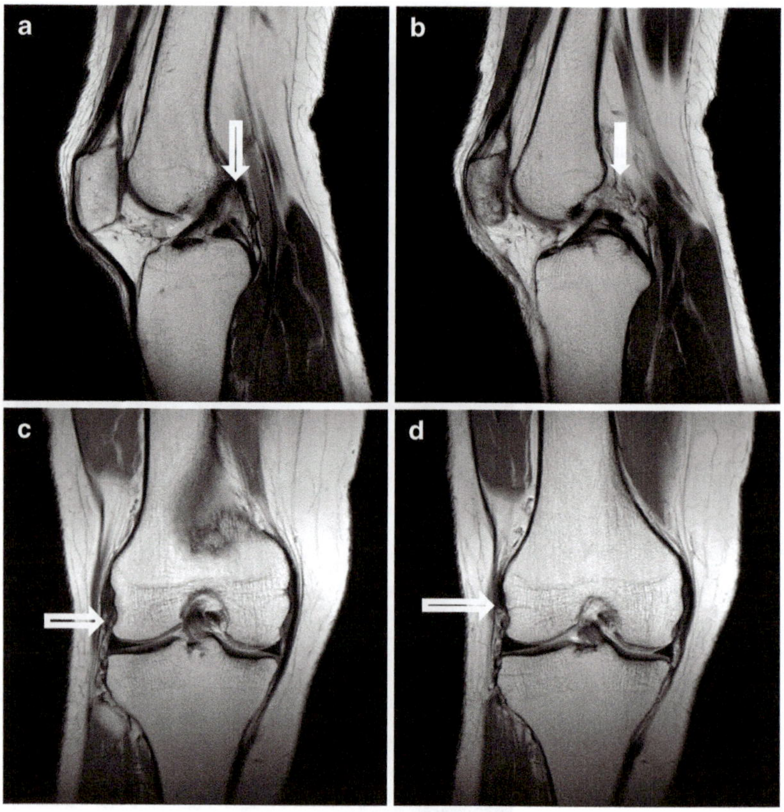

Fig. 11.19 (**a**, **b**) PCL rupture at the proximal substance, (**c**, **d**) lateral collateral ligament injury is seen

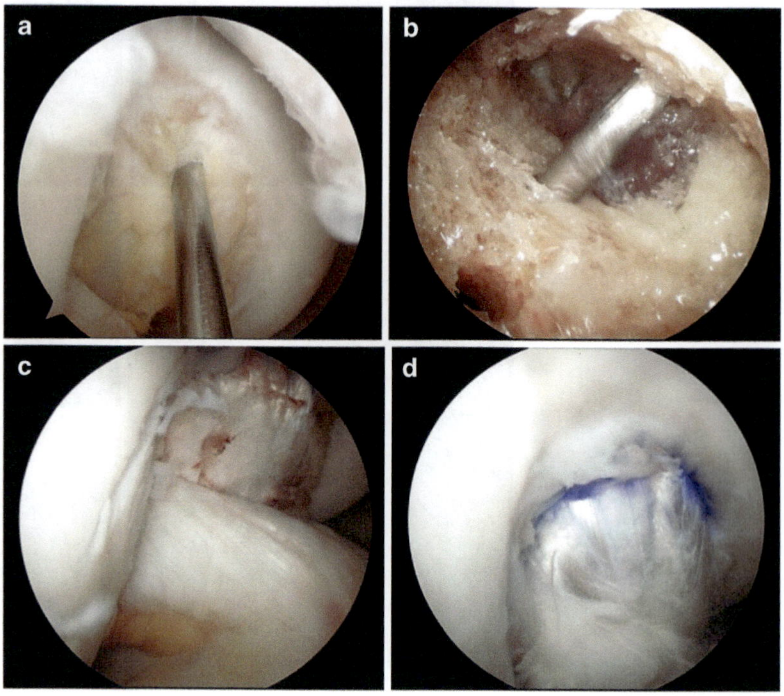

Fig. 11.20 These are the intraoperative arthroscopic findings: (**a**) guide pin from articular margin 5–6 mm 1 o'clock, (**b**) shows cross pin guide for double fixation, (**c**) there was no pseudolaxity of the ACL after PCL reconstruction, and (**d**) the PCL graft looks good in shape and wider cover of the normal PCL using a rounded rectangular dilator

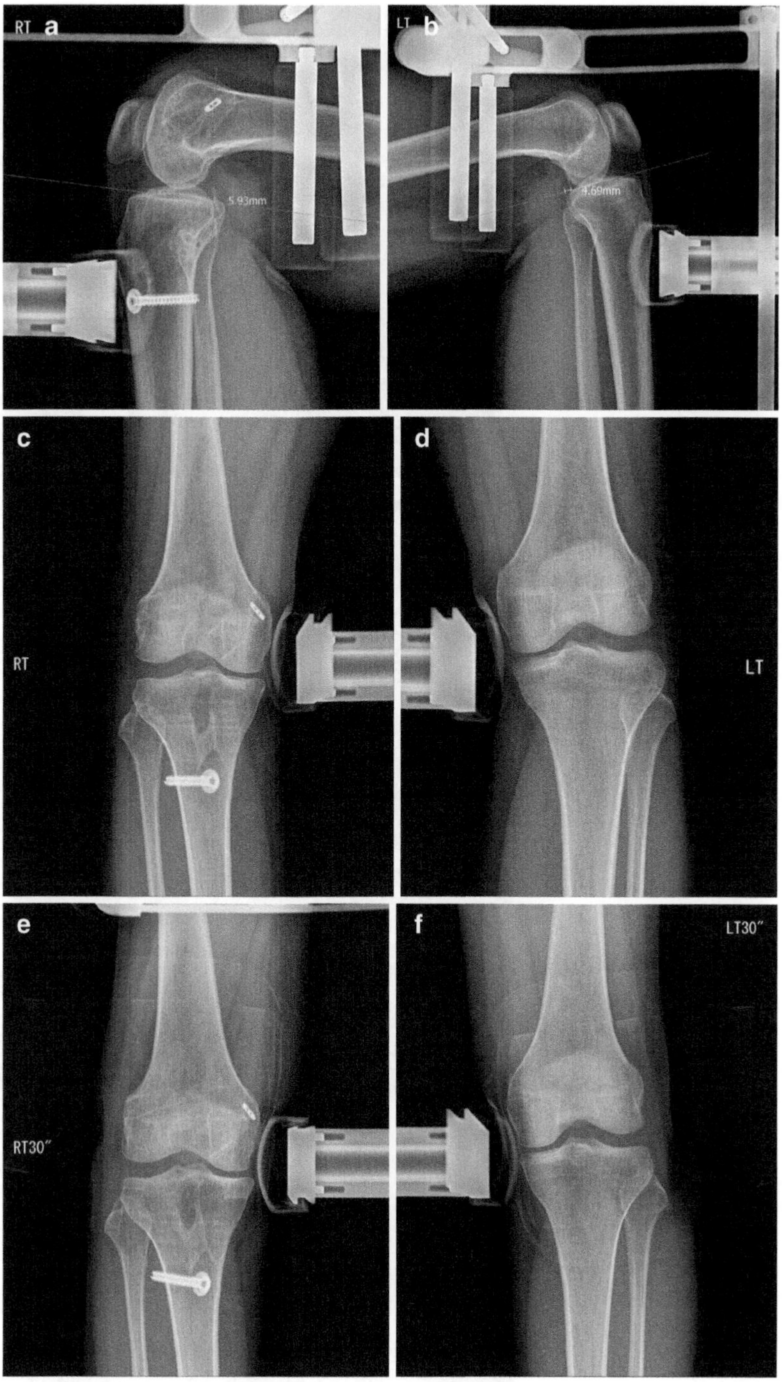

Fig. 11.21 21 months after PCL reconstruction and PLCS. (**a**, **b**) Push view (**c**, **d**) 0° varus stress view (**e**, **f**)

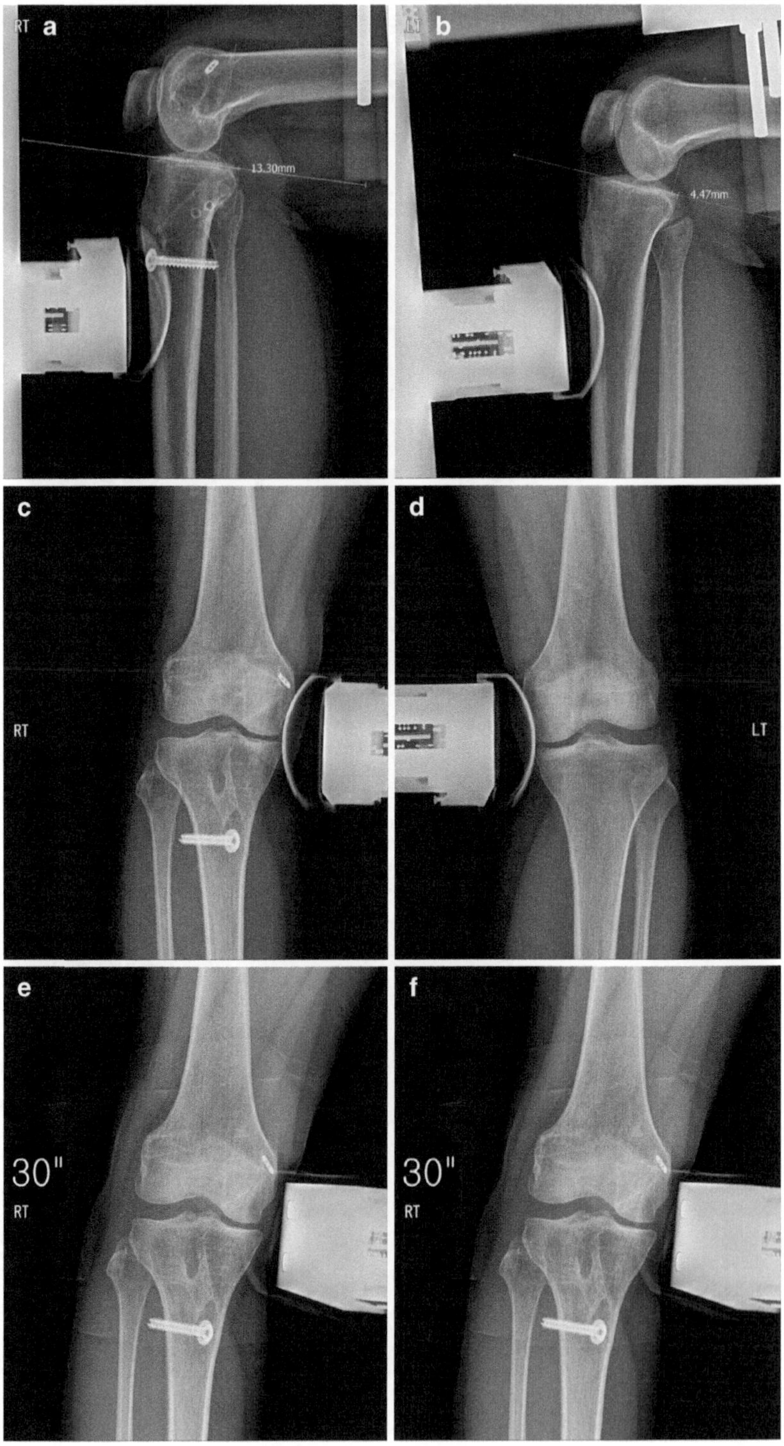

Fig. 11.22 35 months after PCL reconstruction and PLCS. (**a**, **b**) Push view: 8.9 mm posterior displacement difference compared to the unaffected side in the push stress image. (**c**, **d**) 0° varus stress view. (**e**, **f**) 30° flexion, varus stress view of both knees. There is no instability in the varus stress view

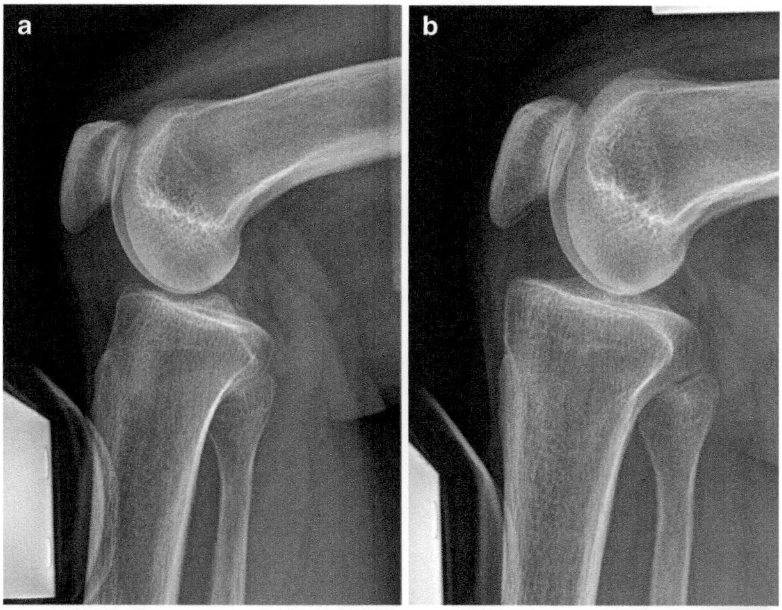

Fig. 11.23 Push stress view; grade 3 posterior sagging rt

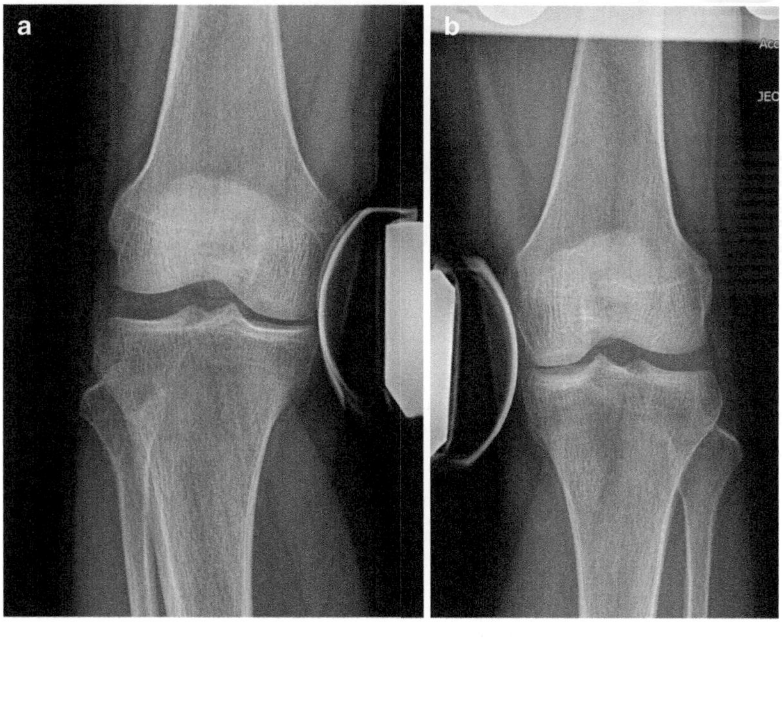

Fig. 11.24 (**a**, **b**) 0° varus stress view, (**c**, **d**) 30° flexion, varus stress view: there was no significant difference between both knees

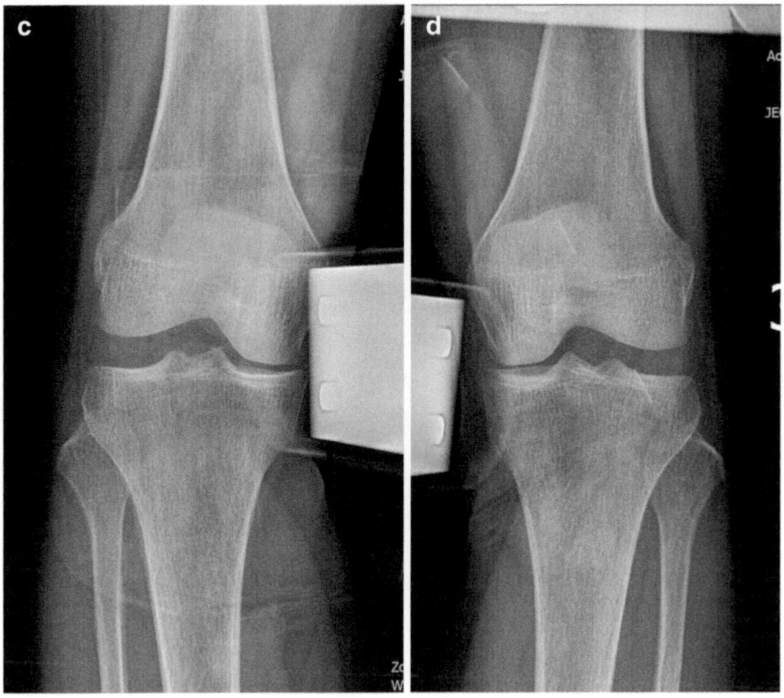

Fig. 11.24 (continued)

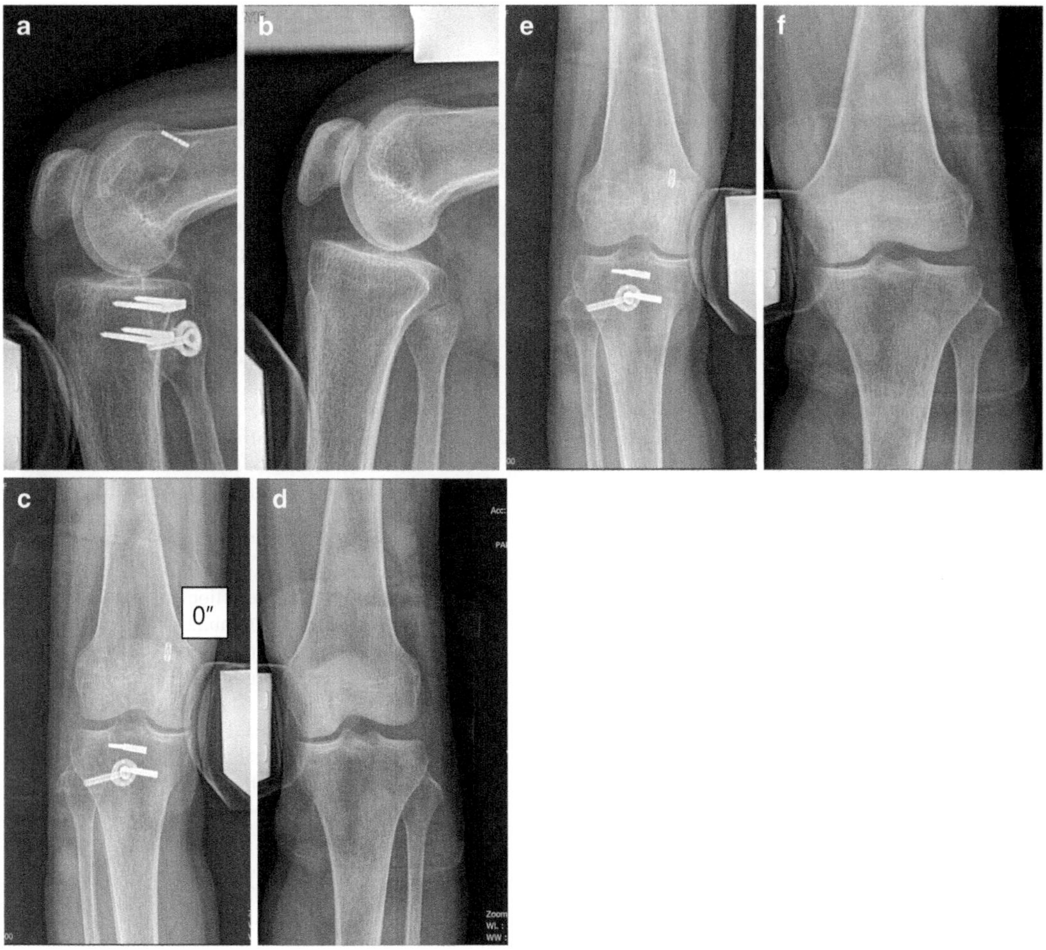

Fig. 11.25 21 months after PCL reconstruction and PLCS. (**a**, **b**) Push view: 8.9 mm posterior displacement difference compared to the unaffected side in the push stress image. (**c**, **d**) 0° varus stress view. (**e**, **f**) 30° flexion, varus stress view of both knees. There is no instability in the varus stress view

Further Reading

1. Veltri DM, Warren RF. Posterolateral instability of the knee. Instr Course Lect. 1995;44:441–53.
2. Veltri DM, Deng XH, Torzilli PA, Warren RF, Maynard MJ. The role of the cruciate and posterolateral ligaments in stability of the knee. A biomechanical study. Am J Sports Med. 1995;23:436–43.
3. Ross G, Chapman AW, Newberg AR, Scheller AD Jr. Magnetic resonance imaging for the evaluation of acute posterolateral complex injuries of the knee. Am J Sports Med. 1997;25:444–8.
4. Hughston JC, Andrews JR, Cross MJ, Moschi A. Classification of knee ligament instabilities. Part II. The lateral compartment. J Bone Joint Surg Am. 1976;58:173–9.
5. Cooper DE. Tests for posterolateral instability of the knee in normal subjects. Results of examination under anesthesia. J Bone Joint Surg Am. 1991;73:30–6.
6. Margheritini F, Mancini L, Mauro CS, Mariani PP. Stress radiography for quantifying posterior cruciate ligament deficiency. Arthroscopy. 2003;19:706–11.
7. Yu JS, Salonen DC, Hodler J, Haghighi P, Trudell D, Resnick D. Posterolateral aspect of the knee: Improved MR imaging with a coronal oblique technique. Radiology. 1996;198:199–204.
8. Hassine D, Rougereau G, Feron JM, et al. MR imaging of posteromedial and posterolateral stabilisers of

the knee: anatomic basis and patterns of lesions in knee injuries. Surg Radiol Anat. 1994;16:293–301.
9. Noyes FR, Stowers SF, Grood ES, Cummings J, VanGinkel LA. Posterior subluxations of the medial and lateral tibiofemoral compartments. An in vitro ligament sectioning study in cadaveric knees. Am J Sports Med. 1993;21:407–14.
10. Bae JH, Choi IC, Suh SW, et al. Evaluation of the reliability of the dial test for posterolateral rotatory instability: a cadaveric study using an isotonic rotation machine. Arthroscopy. 2008;24:593–8.
11. Loomer RL. A test for knee posterolateral rotatory instability. Clin Orthop Relat Res. 1991;264:235–8.
12. Bleday RM, Fanelli GC, Giannotti BF, Edson CJ, Barrett TA. Instrumented measurement of the posterolateral corner. Arthroscopy. 1998;14:489–94.
13. LaPrade RF, Wentorf F. Diagnosis and treatment of posterolateral knee injuries. Clin Orthop Relat Res. 2002;402:110–21.
14. Larsen MW, Toth A. Examination of posterolateral corner injuries. J Knee Surg. 2005;18:146–50.
15. Gollehon DL, Torzilli PA, Warren RF. The role of the posterolateral and cruciate ligaments in the stability of the human knee. A biomechanical study. J Bone Joint Surg Am. 1987;69:233–42.
16. Grood ES, Stowers SF, Noyes FR. Limits of movement in the human knee. Effect of sectioning the posterior cruciate ligament and posterolateral structures. J Bone Joint Surg Am. 1988;70:88–97.
17. Tibone JE, Antich TJ, Perry J, Moynes D. Functional analysis of untreated and reconstructed posterior cruciate ligament injuries. Am J Sports Med. 1988;16:217–23.
18. Jung YB, Jung HJ, Kim SJ, et al. Posterolateral corner reconstruction for posterolateral rotatory instability combined with posterior cruciate ligament injuries: Comparison between fibular tunnel and tibial tunnel techniques. Knee Surg Sports Traumatol Arthrosc. 2008;16:239–48.
19. Jung YB, Lee YS, Jung HJ, Young-Bok NCH, Jung YS, Lee H-JJ, Nam C-H. Evaluation of posterolateral rotatory knee instability using the dial test according to tibial positioning. J Arthrosc Relat Surg. 2009;25(3):57–261.
20. Strobel MJ, Schulz MS, Petersen WJ, Eichhorn HJ. Combined anterior cruciate ligament, posterior cruciate ligament, and posterolateral corner reconstruction with autogenous hamstring grafts in chronic instabilities. Arthroscopy. 2006;22:182–92.
21. LaPrade RF, Ly TV, Griffith C. The external rotation recurvatum test revisited: Reevaluation of the sagittal plane tibiofemoral relationship. Am J Sports Med. 2008;36:709–12.
22. Lee HJ, Park YB, Ko YB, Kim SH, Kwon HB, Yu DS, et al. The necessity of clinical application of tibial reduction for detection of underestimated posterolateral rotatory instability in combined posterior cruciate ligament and posterolateral corner deficient knee. Knee Surg Sports Traumatol Arthrosc. 2015;23:3062–9.
23. Moulton SG, Geeslin AG, LaPrade RF. A systematic review of the outcomes of posterolateral corner knee injuries, part 2: surgical treatment of chronic injuries. Am J Sports Med. 2016;44:1616–23.

12 Revision of the Posterior Cruciate Ligament Reconstruction

Abstract

The failure rate of posterior cruciate ligament reconstruction is reported to be 10–25%. The cause of PCL failure is reported as a single factor (44%) and multiple factors (56%) in our series. The most common cause of failure is failure to treat posterolateral rotational instability (PLRI) (40–67.6%) (cases 2 and 3); the next most common cause is tunnel misplacement (femoral and tibial tunnel) (case 3), more in femoral tunnel (31–44%), suboptimal rehabilitation, varus malalignment, primary repair, meniscal injury and cartilage lesion, etc. To achieve a successful PCL revision, the cause of the failure should first be carefully analyzed. If the location of the femoral-tibial tunnel is well analyzed and the placement of the tunnel is completely misplaced, a new tunnel can be created, but if the placement of the tunnel overlaps, the treatment method is more complicated. First, if the femoral tunnel is overlapping and widening, after 3–6 months of bone grafting (autogenous cortico-cancellous is better than allograft), the grafted bone is well incorporated, and the revision of PCL reconstruction is done. Second, with the use of a large enough bone block, an attached allograft could be used to cover the tunnel widening and overlap bone defect site in revision of PCL reconstruction with one stage. In addition, to get a successful revision of PCL reconstruction, we should not overlook associated ligament injury, such as posterolateral rotatory instability (PLRI) (case 2) and posteromedial instability (Case 2). Another thing was that if there was a previously grafted PCL or remnant PCL, it should be preserved as much as possible, as this is helpful to get stability, proprioception, blood supply to the new graft, etc. The alignment of the knee joint or lower extremity should also be carefully checked, and furthermore, if there is no posterior slope of the tibial plateau or reverse slope of the tibial plateau, the reconstructed PCL graft will be highly stressed (decreased posterior slope of the tibial plateau increases the loads on the reconstructed PCL graft) and may fail. In addition, if there was a PCL deficiency and PLRI in patients with a zero-degree posterior slope of the tibial plateau, genu recurvatum will occur, especially with a varus thrust gait when walking, so proximal tibial osteotomy should be performed first (case 4). If the tibial tunnel was good enough, it could be used to preserve the residual PCL graft. The recent use of rounded rectangular dilators or oval-shaped dilators is very helpful in preserving the graft or residual PCL as much as possible. Modified tibial inlay techniques are relatively easier to use in cases of poor tunnel

Supplementary Information The online version contains supplementary material available at https://doi.org/10.1007/978-981-95-9039-1_12.

Y. B. Jung et al., *Treatment of the Cruciate Ligaments Injuries*,
https://doi.org/10.1007/978-981-95-9039-1_12

position or malpositioning. If the location of the tunnel is not so good or malpositioned, it can be solved relatively easily with the modified tibial inlay technique, especially in tibial tunnel malposition. Combined injuries can be easily resolved by creating a posterolateral corner sling (PLCS) with a fibular head tunnel, especially if the grade of PLRI was 1–2°. However, for grade 3 PLRI, the stronger the ligament graft, the better, and a tibial tunnel will also be required, known as anatomic reconstruction. Sometimes, severe instability (grade 3 PLRI) of the lateral collateral ligament (LCL) with PLRI requires more reinforcement of the LCL, which will be better. When choosing a graft, a sufficiently strong ligament should be used whenever possible. In particular, the ALB reconstruction of the PCL uses the ligament diameter of at least 8–9 mm or larger and, at this time, a thickness of at least 8 mm, which is used by the tibialis allograft, Achilles allograft, or a mixture of allograft plus autogenous graft and PMB; another allograft should be used. The more the PCL bony insertion area is covered, the more we use a rounded rectangular dilator. Therefore, we can achieve good results even with a single-bundle PCL reconstruction. It is recommended to perform the interference screw fixation in the anatomically reduced anteromedial tibiofemoral condyle after 20–25 cycle loads with approximately 10–15 lbs. of tension. We can check the anteromedial step as on the normal side, usually 1 cm protrusion of the medial tibial condyle articular margin to the medial femoral condyle articular margin. In principle, the tibial side is also fixed with a post and tie after rigid fixation. It is recommended to use a double fixation (backup fixation) with a 5–6.5 mm screw and washer as the post and tie. For revision reconstruction of the posterior cruciate ligament, it is necessary to decide whether to use the tibial tunnel, i.e., the transtibial tunnel technique, or the modified tibial inlay technique. The transtibial tunnel technique can be used, but especially if the proximal tibia has a locally weakened bone or if there are too many tunnels, the modified tibial inlay technique is easier to perform. You should also consider when to perform a double-bundle reconstruction. If there is no remaining posterior cruciate ligament or graft and also if the patient's bone size is very large, a double-bundle reconstruction will give better results. In our experience, when a tunnel is created with a rounded rectangular dilator, much more bone can be preserved and the tunnel is not enlarged as much as in the case of a conventional round tunnel (round tunnel—tunnel enlargement is about 110%, but when a rounded rectangular dilator is used, a rectangular tunnel is created, about 73% tunnel enlargement is reported in the cadaver study).

Keywords

PCL revision · Posterolateral rotatory instability(PLRI)

12.1 The Principle of Treatment for PCL Revision

The use of the modified tibial inlay technique allows arthroscopic revision of the posterior cruciate ligament (PCL) without the need to change the patient's position from the supine to the prone position (Fig. 12.3).

There are many reported arthroscopic techniques for reconstructing the PCL. Most of them are modifications of a transtibial tunnel method through an anterior approach. However, the acute angular turn of the graft at the posterior opening of the tibial tunnel, which has been called the "killer turn," can lead to graft failure and stretching. Therefore, the tibial inlay technique was introduced for PCL reconstruction to avoid the problem of graft abrasion at the tunnel edge and to allow the graft to pass easily through the femoral tunnel. The advantages of the tibial inlay technique: Firstly, it is possible re-tensioning of the remnant fibers of the PCL (Figs. 10.7 and 10.8). The remnant PCL fibers are interposed between the tunnel edge bone and the graft, thus protecting the graft by cushioning it against abrasion on the posterior tibial edge of the tunnel entrance in transtibial tunnel technique (Fig. 10.2). The tibial inlay technique is preferentially indicated for surgical revision of primary failed PCL reconstruction (case 1.2.3. Figs. 12.8a,b. 12.11, 12.16, 12.17, 12.21, and 12.22a,b) and for the primary PCL augmentation and a good quality of the PCL remnant fibers with tensioning. In addition, this technique has been advocated for patients with chronic PCL rupture with scanty remnant fibers who need double-bundle PCL reconstruction. (If PCL remnant fibers are absent, we prefer to do double-bundle reconstruction (Fig. 12.2) rather than single-bundle reconstruction.) Modified the tibial inlay technique to eliminate the need to change the patient's position during surgery (Fig. 12.3).

12.2 Surgical Technique of Revision Posterior Cruciate Ligament Reconstruction with a Modified Tibial-Inlay Double-Bundle Technique

Graft Preparation

Prepare the Achilles tendon allograft as a tibial bone block with two femoral bundles (Fig. 12.1).

Transect the Achilles tendon allograft sagittally into two strands, and suture each strand to a diameter of 8–9 mm with a locking whipstitch using number-five nonabsorbable sutures. The strand consisting of the anterolateral bundle is usually prepared to a diameter of 8–9 mm, and the strand consisting of the posteromedial bundle is prepared to a diameter of 7–8 mm. The other method is a relatively large Achilles tendon PCL revision.

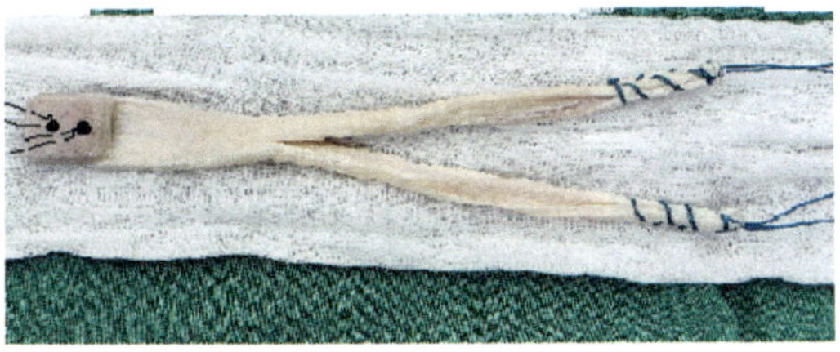

Fig. 12.1 The Achilles tendon allograft consists of a tibial bone block and two tendon tails secured with a locking whipstitch with a number 5 nonabsorbable suture

12.3 Patient Position

With the patient in the supine position, flexion, abduction, and external rotation of the hip and flexion of the knee 60–90° can provide easier access to the popliteal area.

For the modified tibial inlay technique, perform the arthroscopic operation with the patient in the supine position first. Then, tilt the operating table 30°, so that the operatively treated knee is lower than the contralateral knee, and place the lower limb on a side-table with the hip flexed, abducted, and externally rotated, and the knee flexed (Fig. 12.3).

12.4 Femoral Tunnel Preparation

Make anterolateral and posteromedial femoral tunnels in a shallow-shallow position using an outside-in or inside-out (depending upon the surgeon's choice)technique for the anterolateral bundle and the inside-out technique for the posteromedial bundle (Video 12.1).

Place the center of the anterolateral femoral tunnel 5–6 mm proximal to the margin of the articular cartilage of the femoral condyle at approximately the 1 to 1:30 o'clock position in a Right knee.

Place the center of the posteromedial femoral tunnel 8–9 mm proximal to the edge of the distal articular cartilage of the femoral condyle at the 3 o'clock position in a right knee (Fig. 12.2).

Make the femoral tunnel for the anterolateral bundle using the outside-in technique by inserting a guide pin through the medial-side incision under the vastus medialis, or the inside-out technique from the lower anterolateral or anteromedial portal just beside the patellar tendon, taking care to avoid damaging the anterior horn of the meniscus (surgeon's choice). Recently, I'd like to use a rounded rectangular dilator, in-out technique, starting point is just anterior-inferior medial side of the patellar tendon to make a lon-

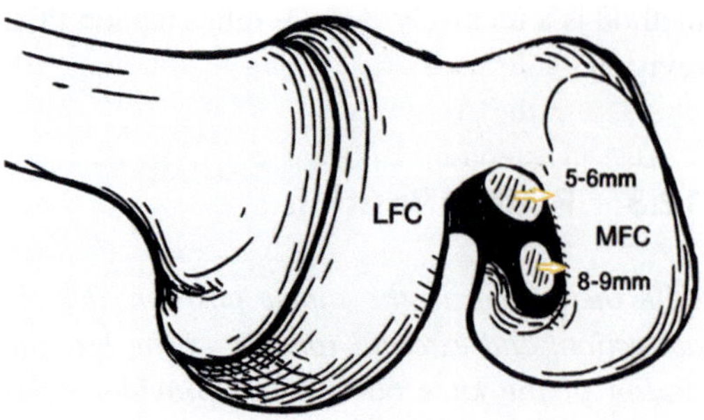

Fig. 12.2 The center of the anterolateral femoral tunnel is placed 5–6 mm proximal to the articular cartilage at the one o'clock position. The posteromedial tunnel is placed 8–9 mm proximal to the margin of the distal articular cartilage, at the 3 o'clock position in a right knee. *MFC* medial femoral condyle, and *LFC* lateral femoral condyle

ger tunnel and also if a femoral condyle fracture happens, the fracture fragment will be a larger size rather than smaller due to the fixation will be easier and strong enough. Create the femoral tunnel for the posteromedial bundle from an anterolateral accessory portal using an inside-out technique.

Remove the hardware, preserving the previous PCL graft or the original PCL remnant bundle if possible. Reuse the primary tunnel if the tunnel position for the anterolateral bundle is correct. If the tunnel position is completely incorrect, create a new tunnel in the correct position. The most difficult cases are those where the tunnel position is slightly, but not completely, incorrect. In these cases, a tunnel is first created with a dilator to avoid creating a large bone defect and to preserve the original graft. Occasionally, an autogenous cortico-cancellous bone graft will be impacted between the graft and the tunnel when the tunnel is widened. The other way is to use an impacted bone graft to widen the tunnel and then remake the tunnel with a rounded rectangular dilator, or to use a bone block attached allograft plus autogenous hamstring as a mixed graft.

If possible, use an autogenous quadriceps bone block or autogenous BPTB. The autogenous bone block attached graft to use was technically more demanding and take more loner operation time. Using a rounded rectangular dilator or oval shape dilator, it is easier to do because less bone is removed, just enlarge the tunnel with a dilator instead of reaming with a power reamer. And also the PCL graft is more well pitted at the tunnel than using a round reamer, because the tunnel shape and ligament's shape are rounded, rectangular, and a flat oval shape, not a round shape. Chamfer the inner opening of the femoral tunnel edge with rasps to prevent acute-angle impingement, which can lead to premature graft wear. Pass a 21-gauge wire loop through the femoral tunnel and direct it to the just medial side of the PCL remnant on the tibia. It will later be used to guide the graft from the tibial insertion of the PCL into the femoral tunnel (Video 12.3).

The femoral tunnel for the anterolateral bundle is prepared with an outside-in technique, and the femoral tunnel for the posteromedial bundle is made with an inside-out technique.

12.5 Tibial Side Preparation

Prepare the tibial tunnel with the patient supine, with the hip flexed, abducted, and externally rotated and the knee flexed 60° to 90° to provide easier access to the popliteal area.

After arthroscopic surgery on the anterior aspect of the knee, the operating table is tilted by 30° so that the operated knee is lower than the contralateral knee, and the lower limb is then placed on a side table with the hip flexed, abducted, and externally rotated and the knee flexed at 60–90° (Fig. 12.3).

Identify the interval between the medial head of the gastrocnemius muscle and the semimembranosus tendon and develop it bluntly. Retract the semimembranosus and semitendinosus tendons medially. Retract the gastrocnemius muscle laterally, protecting the popliteal neurovascular structures (Fig. 12.4).

If the branches of the inferior medial geniculate artery and vein are encountered near the mid -posterior portion of the capsule, ligate them securely. Detach the popliteus muscle subperiosteally from the posteromedial surface of the proximal part of the tibia, and palpate the PCL tibial attachment site. Move the previously inserted wire loop that you inserted to confirm the PCL insertion site. Then, incise the posterior

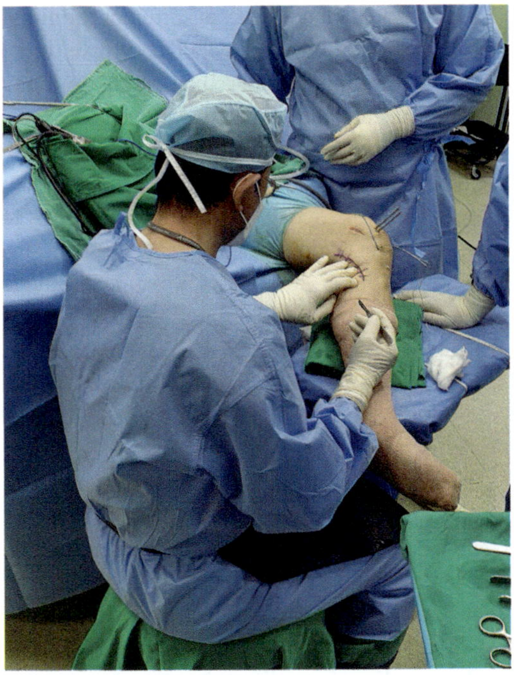

Fig. 12.3 The operating table is tilted down on the affected side for the posterior approach. Posteromedial approach between the gastrocnemius muscle and the posterior tibial plateau was performed (Video 12.2)

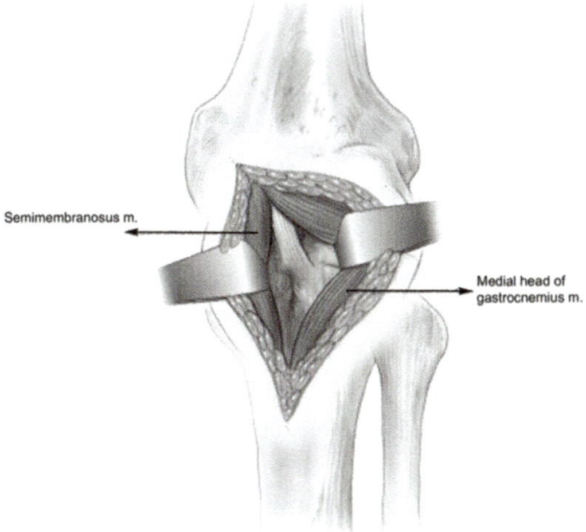

Fig. 12.4 The medial border of the medial head of the gastrocnemius muscle is identified, and the interval between it and the hamstring tendon with the semimembranosus tendon is developed, exposing the posterior aspect of the joint capsule

aspect of the knee capsule adjacent to the medial femoral condyle, and preserve the remnant PCL fibers with the graft.

Use an osteotome to delineate the tibial attachment of the PCL as a 1.5 × 2 cm area, and remove a 7 mm thick bone block from the distal to the proximal area using a 1.2–1.5 cm wide curved osteotome (Fig. 12.5).

At the junction of bone and the remnant PCL, place a number-5 non-absorbable Ethibond suture for easy distal traction of the remnant PCL.

The operating table is tilted 30–40° to access the popliteal area, PCL tibial insertion site (Video 12.2).

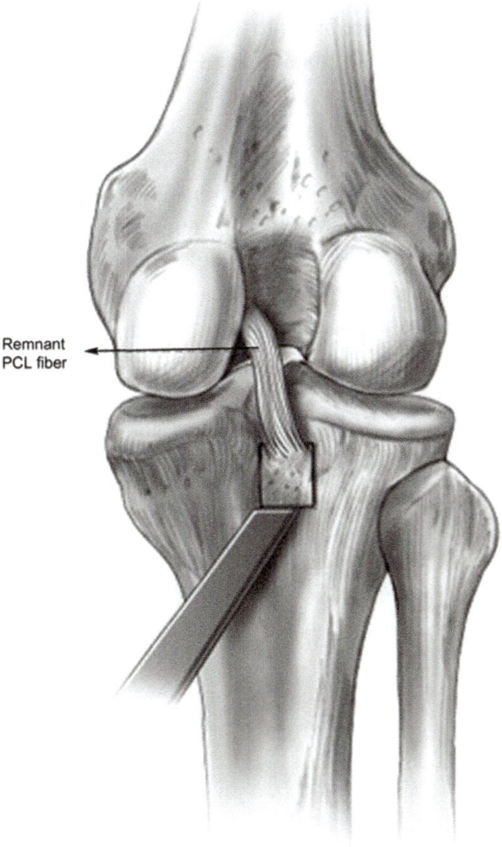

Fig. 12.5 The bone block of the tibial attachment site of the PCL is detached with the use of a curved osteotome, and a trough is created

12.6 Graft Passage

Pass the graft through the knee joint posterior to the intercondylar notch into the femoral tunnel using a wire loop.

Make a bony trough at the site of the bone block detachment (Fig. 10.7). Pass the tendon graft traction suture for the anterolateral bundle with a wire loop first, then pass the suture for the posteromedial bundle from the tibial PCL insertion site into the femoral tunnel. Pull the graft up through the knee joint into the femoral tunnel.

12.7 Graft Fixation

Use a cannulated screw with a pointed washer to secure the bone block to the tibia.

Usually, the tibial side of the bone block is fixed first.

Place the Achilles graft bone block in the bony trough and pull the detached native host tibial bone block with the remaining PCL fiber under tension over the Achilles graft bone block.

Use a 5 or 6.5 mm cannulated screw with a spiked washer to secure the bone block to the tibia (Figs. 12.6 and 10.8).

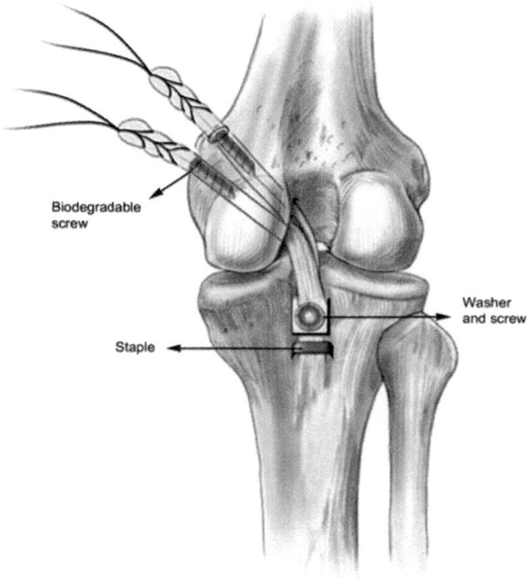

Fig. 12.6 6.5-mm cannulated screw and a spiked washer are used to fix the graft to the tibia

Care should be taken to ensure that the tibial side does not protrude beyond the screw tip. If the tibial side of the fixation of the bone block with washer and screw protrudes too much, this will result in compression of the neurovascular bundle.

Cyclically load the graft with 10–15LBS of tension by moving the knee through a passive range of motion 20 times. Fix biodegradable interference screws to the femoral tunnels with anteriorly directed force applied to the proximal part of the tibia and the knee joint flexed 70–90°. Additionally, backup fixation with a staple or post and tie. If you use the inside-out technique, nowadays we can use a Ultra-Button (Smith & Nephew Co.) with two cross pins (rigid fix, Depuy Co. Fig. 12.20b) or post and tie as backup fixation. Nowadays, I'd like a backup fixation of the tibia and femoral on both sides, especially in revision cases.

Apply a long leg splint to hold the knee in full extension (0°).

Look at the full video of the inlay technique (Video 12.3).

12.8 Postoperative Rehabilitation

Rehabilitation after PCL reconstruction is generally more conservative than after ACL reconstruction. For the first 2 weeks after surgery, a long leg splint or PCL brace with tibial support is used to keep the knee in 0° full extension to prevent posterior sagging of the graft. The patient is encouraged to gradually perform passive flexion exercises from the fourth or fifth postoperative day until the sixth postoperative week. The patient performs these exercises with both hands to support the proximal part of the tibia, or the exercises may be performed by another person with the patient in the prone position to prevent posterior translation of the tibia due to gravity. Soon after surgery, because of the agonistic function of the quadriceps on the PCL, straight leg raising and quadriceps strengthening exercises are started (routinely when we first meet the patient, outpatient clinic teaching quadriceps muscle strengthening exercise, half squat exercise). The patient remains partially weight-bearing with the use of crutches until the sixth postoperative week, and full weight-bearing is allowed with the limb in as extended a position as the pain permits (usually we start at 6–8 weeks post-op.). Jogging can be started at 6–9 months post-op if the knee is asymptomatic with this activity (thigh muscle power is similar in both sides, especially quadriceps muscle power, which will be judged by thigh circumference differences).

12.9 Results

In our study, 34 patients (20 males and four females; mean age 37.4 years) underwent revision PCL reconstruction using the described technique and were followed for a mean of 39.6 months (range, 24–72 months). Side-to-side differences on posterior stress radiographs improved from 9.9 ± 2.8 mm preoperatively to 2.8 ± 1.8 mm at the last follow-up ($p < 0.001$). The subjective and objective clinical scores at the latest follow-up evaluation were significantly better than the preoperative scores ($p < 0.001$). IKDC objective score at preoperative B 1, C 15, D 13. At follow-up, A 11, B 13, C 4, D 1. IKDC, subjective score preoperative 38.7, last follow-up 65.8. Fanelli et al. reported 75% of patients returned to preinjury activity, Tegner activity scale level of function. In addition, mean HSS and Lysholm scores were 81.5 and 87.3, respectively.

12.10 Surgical Indications

Recurrent pathological laxity (a side-to-side difference of >5 mm in posterior translation as demonstrated by posterior stress radiography with a TELOS stress device) that is painful during activities of daily living or athletic activities. There is no medial stepping, which means posterior sagging, or posterior drawer test grade II, above grade II or grade III, and neglected PLRI or other combined ligament injury.

Failure of conservative treatment consisting of physiotherapy and quadriceps-strengthening exercises for at least 2 months.

Persistent pain, functional disability, and instability prevent the patient from returning to activities such as sprinting and stair climbing.

Contraindications
Advanced osteoarthritis of the knee
Severe arthrofibrosis
Active infection
Severe malalignment of the affected limb

12.11 Pitfalls and Challenges

The most serious complication of the tibial inlay technique or transtibial tunnel technique is injury of the popliteal artery and vein during the operation. The surgeon needs to take a more cautious approach for posterior knee dissection, especially in the case of revision surgery, as postoperative scar formation and adhesion of the primary PCL reconstruction might have caused an anatomically abnormal position of the popliteal artery and vein. Posterior knee incision and dissection of deep layers can result in deep scar and adhesion formation and consequently delay the restoration of range of motion due to flexion contracture or limitation of flexion to 120°. However, this problem can usually be solved by constant passive range-of-motion exercise. Associated posterolateral rotatory instabilities should be surgically corrected during PCL reconstruction to prevent graft failure due to abnormal posterior subluxation of the lateral tibial plateau and lateral tibiofemoral joint opening.

12.12 Author's Comments

The most common cause of PCL reconstruction failure is neglected PLRI; the next common cause is tunnel misplacement, especially when the femoral tunnel is too proximal. The advantages of the modified tibial inlay technique: (1) There is no need for the patient's position change, just operating table tilting to approach the PCL tibial attachment area. (2) When there is tibial tunnel misplacement or a severe widening case, it is easier to do revision surgery using the modified tibial inlay technique.

PCL reconstruction or revision, postoperative slow recovery, ROM, and gentle passive flexion to prevent PCL graft stretching and posterior sagging forces due to leg gravity. Prevent active hamstring flexion for 3–4 months after PCL revision or reconstruction. The previous PCL graft or original PCL remnant bundle should be preserved as much as possible, as revision usually shows preserved contour and continuity of the PCL. A bifid Achilles tendon allograft is currently our first choice for PCL revision surgery. However, in some cases, the Achilles tendon is not thick enough, and in these cases, an additional mixed semitendinosus autograft is a good option for augmentation in revision PCL surgery. Recently, PCL reconstruction or revision surgery, using a rounded, rectangular, or oval-shaped dilator, more widely covered the PCL footprint and was more similar in shape to the normal PCL compared to the round tunnel.

12.13 Cases of PCL Reconstruction Revision

Case 1: PCL Revision and PLCS

A 32-year-old male patient with a history of PCL reconstruction of the left knee presented to the outpatient clinic complaining of persistent left knee discomfort postoperatively. Physical examination revealed posterior drawer test grade 2, varus stress test grade 2, and PLRI grade 2. KT-2000 arthrometer maximum manual test (MMT); 8 mm right, 13–14 mm left were checked (Figs. 12.7, 12.8, and 12.9).

KT-2000 arthrometer maximum manual test (MMT); 7 mm right, 9 mm left were checked.

Case 2: PCL Revision Combined with PLCS and MCL Reconstruction

A 31-year-old male patient with a history of PCL reconstruction presented to the outpatient clinic. He complained of instability of his right knee, especially during gait. Posterior drawer test, PLRI, varus and valgus stress were all positive on physical examination, and a varus thrust gait (Video 12.4) was observed on ambulation (Fig. 12.10).

Therefore, we performed a medial open wedge osteotomy with a plate. After medial open wedge osteotomy, varus thrust gait improved, but instability remained. After 1 year of open wedge osteotomy, we planned PCL revision and PLCS to overcome posterior/posterolateral instability (Figs. 12.11, 12.12, and 12.13).

Therefore, PCL revision with PLCS and MCL reconstruction was done (Figs. 12.14, 12.15, and 12.16).

KT-2000 arthrometer maximum manual test (MMT); 8 mm right and 5–6 mm left were checked.

Case 3: PCL Revision

A 29-year-old male patient presented to the outpatient clinic with a history of PCL reconstruction and PLCS. He complained of right knee pain. The pain started after hearing a cracking noise while lifting a heavy object. Posterior drawer test was positive while varus, valgus stress were negative on physical examination (Figs. 12.17, 12.18, 12.19, 12.20, and 12.21).

Case 4: Anterior Medial Open Wedge Tibial Osteotomy

A 60-year-old male patient with no history of knee surgery presented to the outpatient clinic complaining of right knee pain and gait disturbance. Pain started after a fall 2 years ago. Posterior drawer test was positive on physical examination with varus thrust gait (Video 12.5, Figs. 12.22 and 12.23).

This case requires an anteromedial open wedge osteotomy or postero close wedge out osteotomy with tibial tubercle osteotomy to correct the posterior tibial slope.

Intraoperative physical examination revealed posterior sagging, genu recurvatum, and posterolateral rotatory instability.

This patient initially underwent a posterior close wedge out osteotomy with tibial tubercle osteotomy (Figs. 12.24, 12.25, and 12.26).

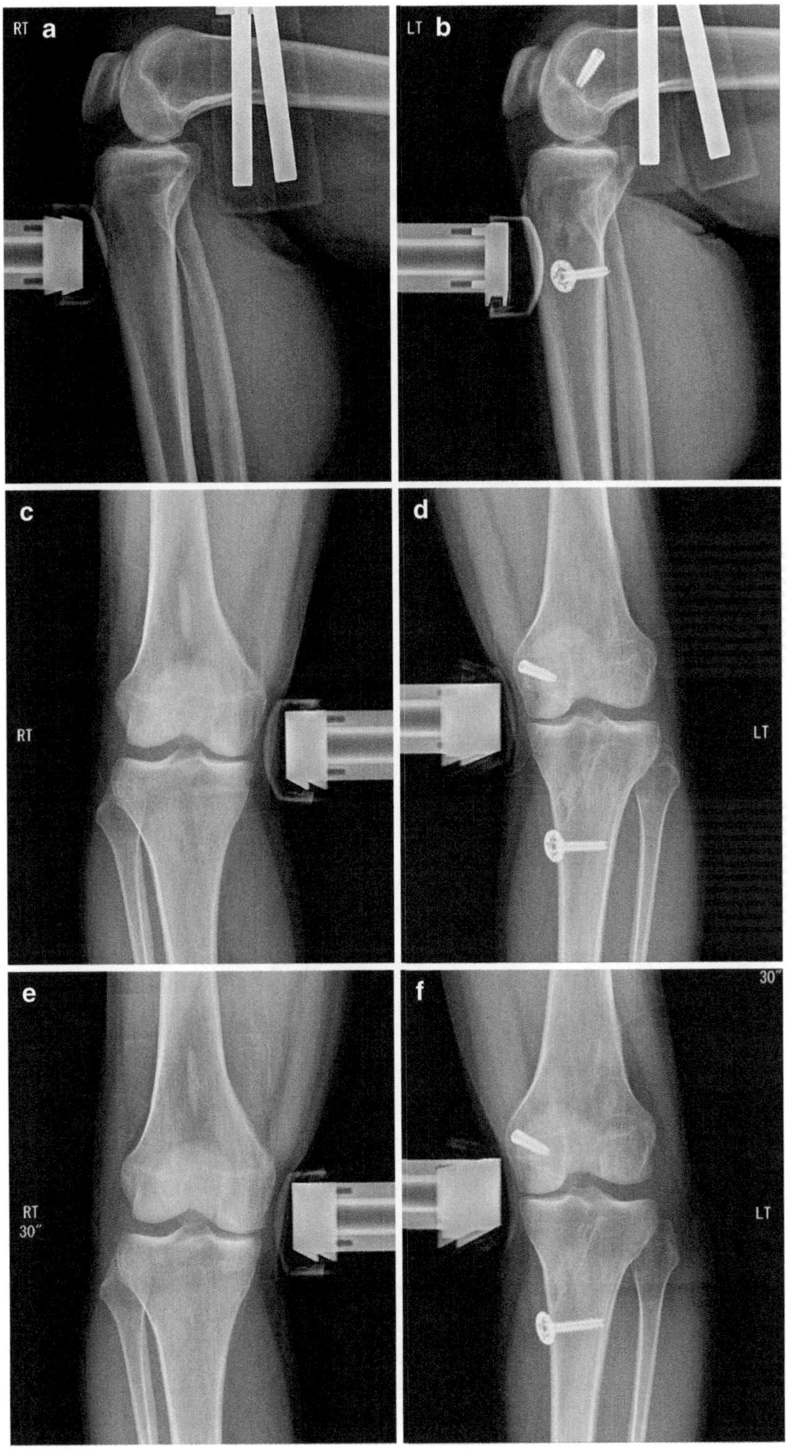

Fig. 12.7 (**a**, **b**) On push stress, the significant posterior translation, grade 2 posterior sagging was checked compared to the unaffected side. (**c**, **d**) 0° varus stress view. (**e**, **f**) 30° flexion view; there is grade 1.5- 2 lateral laxity in the varus stress views

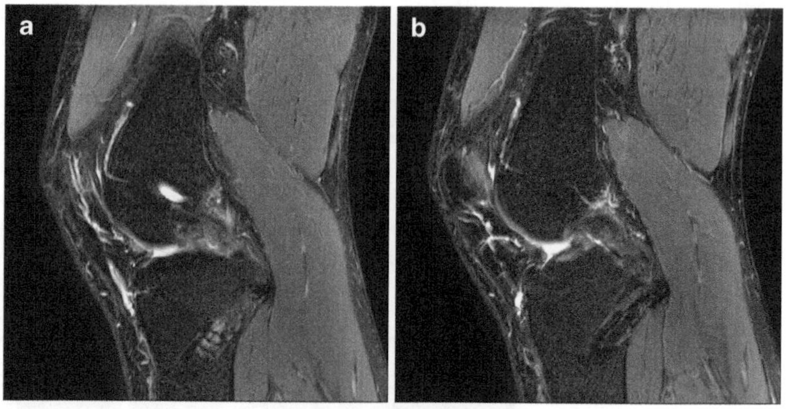

Fig. 12.8 (**a**, **b**) On MRI, the PCL graft quality was not so good and laxed

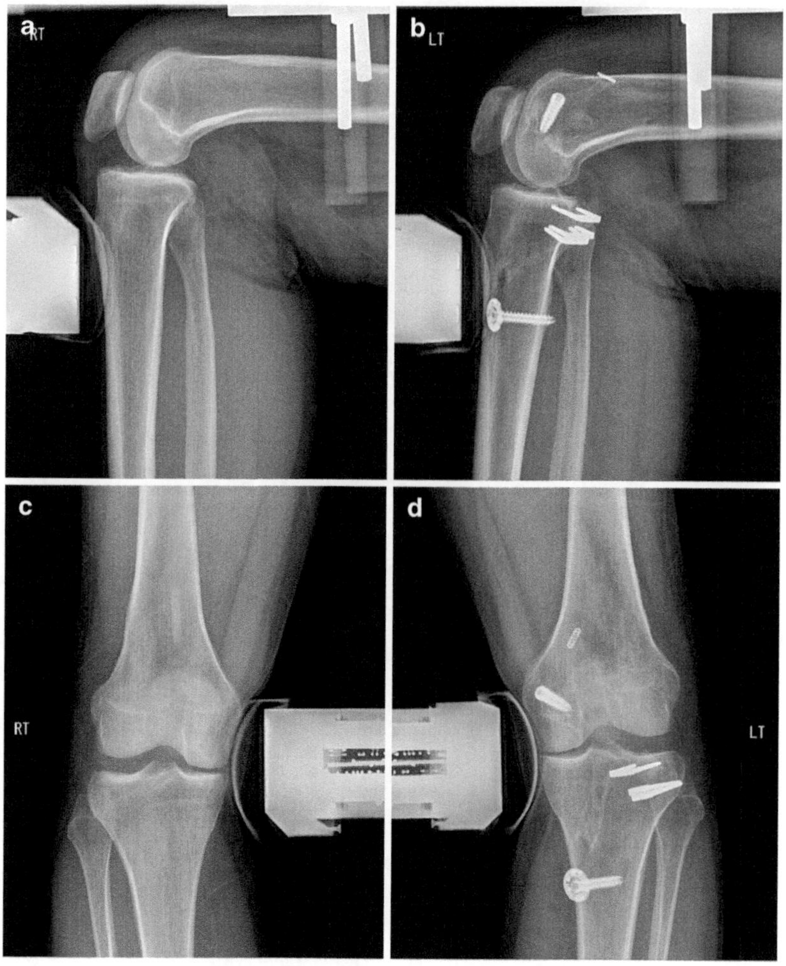

Fig. 12.9 After the surgery, postoperative 1 year, (**a**, **b**) There is no significant side-to-side difference on the pull stress view. (**c**, **d**) 0° varus stress view. (**e**, **f**) 30° flexion view; there is no significant side-to-side difference in the varus stress view

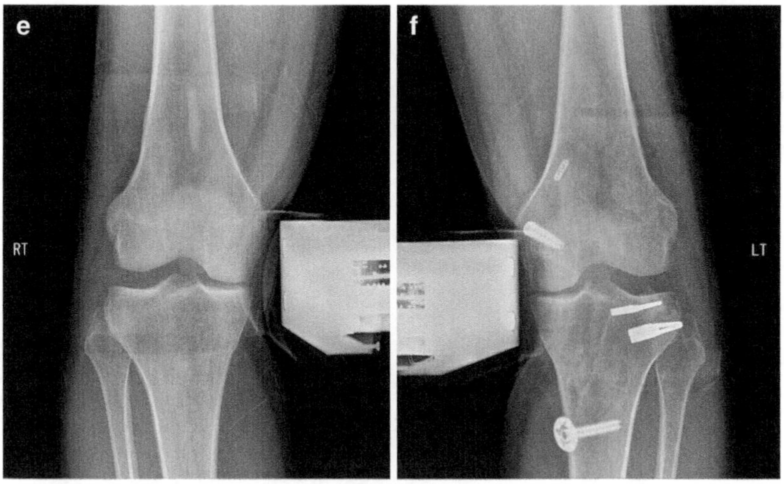

Fig. 12.9 (continued)

Fig. 12.10 (**a**, **b**) 14.2 mm side-to-side difference in push view. (**c**, **d**) Lateral joint space widening was observed in the varus stress view

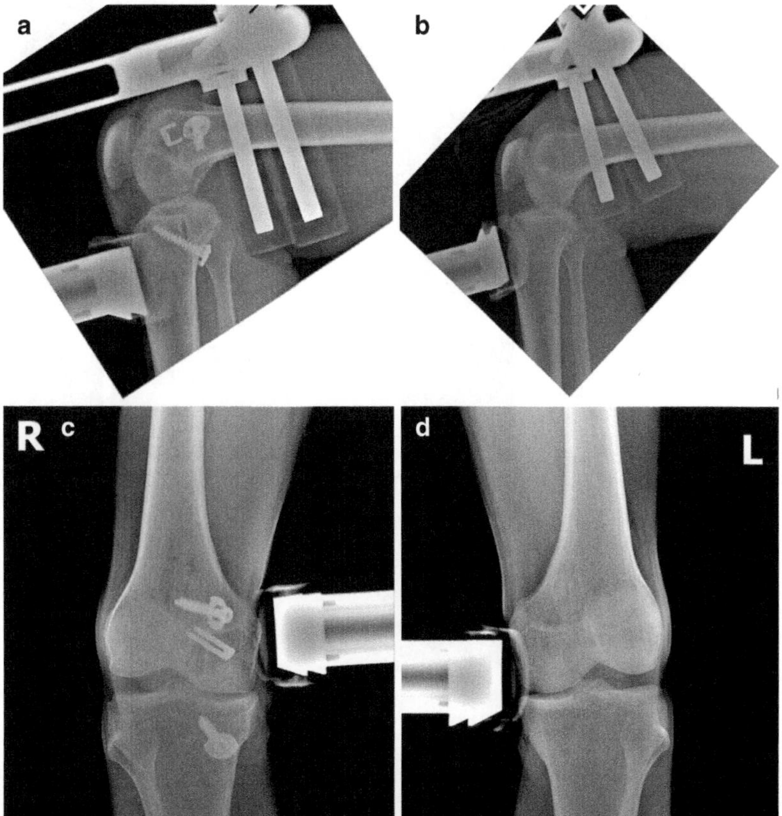

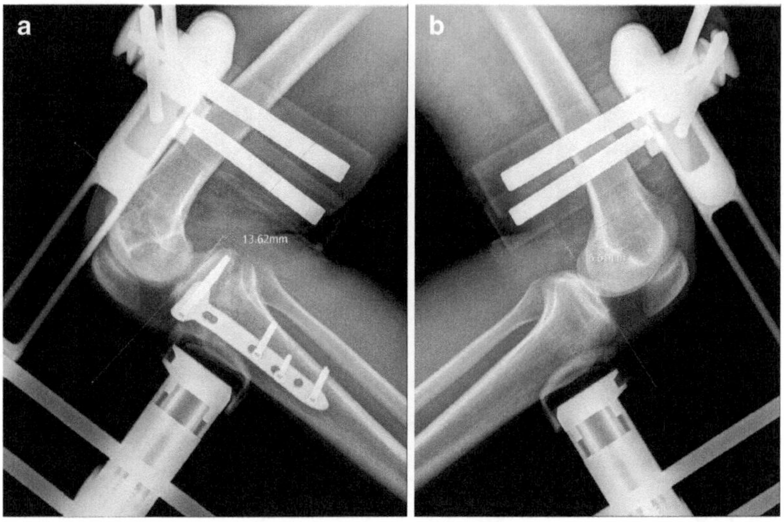

Fig. 12.11 (**a**, **b**) 12.4 mm side-to-side difference was checked compared to the unaffected side in the push stress view

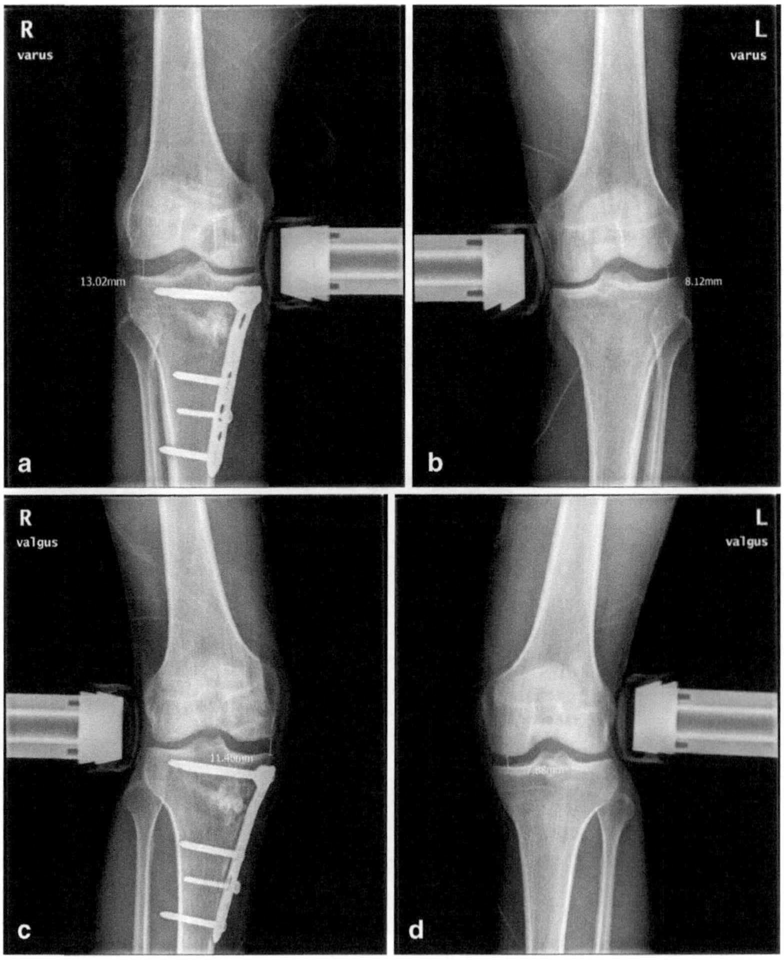

Fig. 12.12 (**a**, **b**) varus stress view (**c**, **d**) valgus stress view; Right knee medial and lateral joint space is wider than the left knee

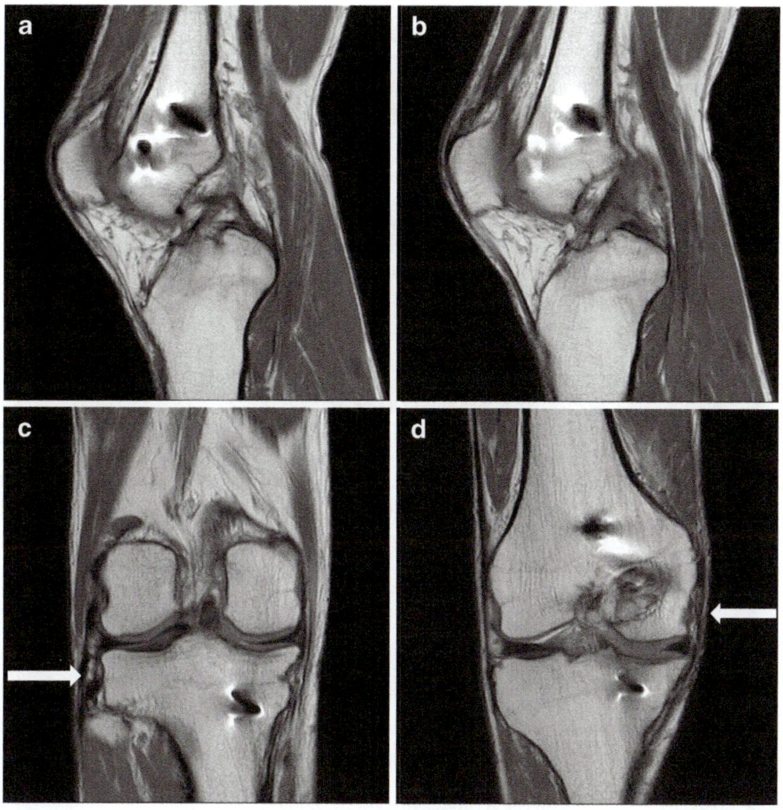

Fig. 12.13 (**a**, **b**) We found that the PCL graft is laxed and narrow, with medial collateral ligament and lateral collateral ligament injury on MRI. (**a**, **b**) Complete PCL rupture was found. (**c**) Suspicious LCL and posterolateral complex injury. (**d**) Chronic injury on the MCL, especially in the deep fiber, in the femoral attachment area

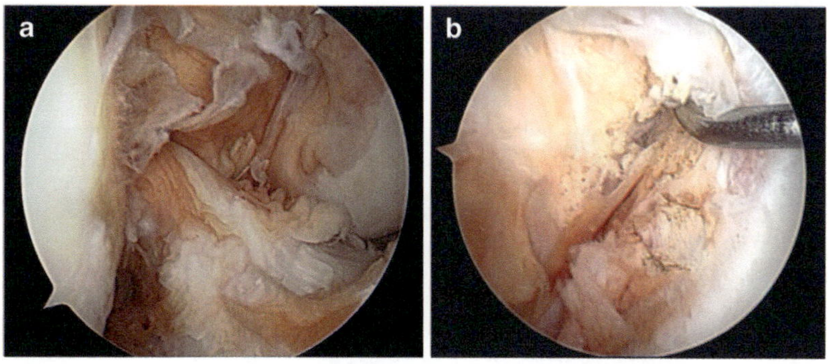

Fig. 12.14 (**a**, **b**) These are the intra-operative findings. Previous PCL graft could not be well seen

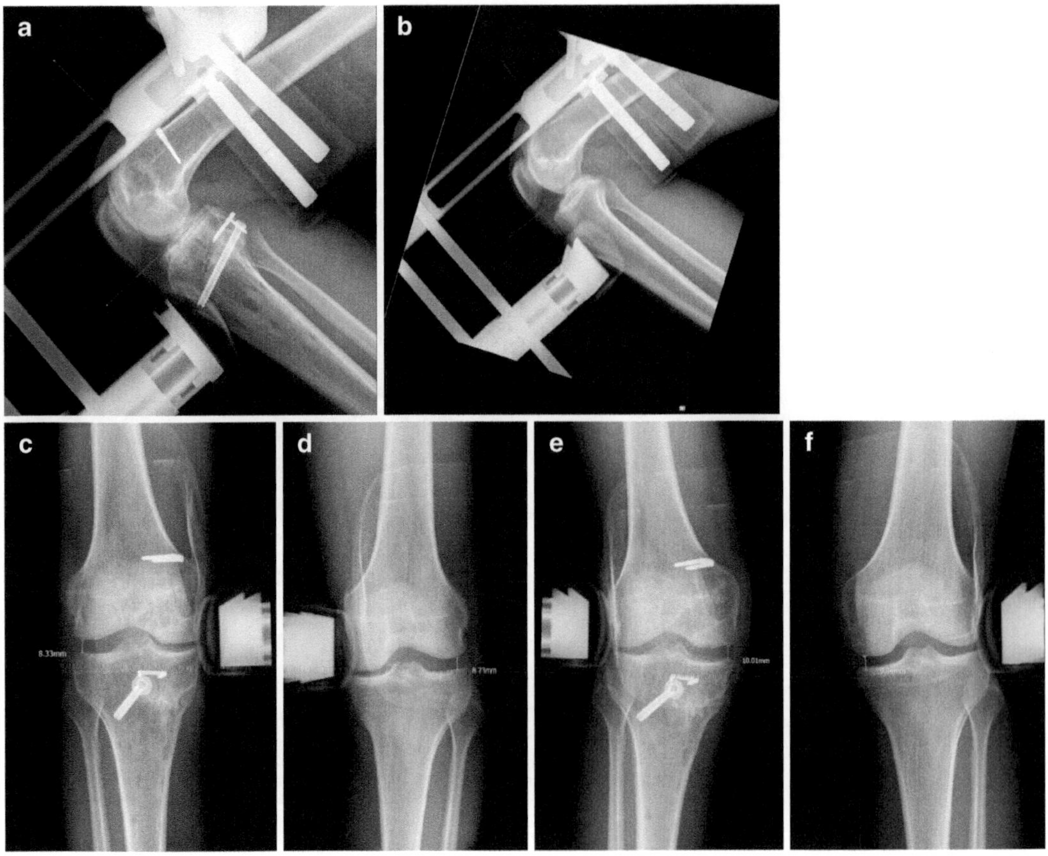

Fig. 12.15 Six months after PCL revision with PLCS, MCL reconstruction. (**a**, **b**) Posterior tibial sagging was significantly improved compared to preoperative (Fig. 12.12). (**c**, **d**) Varus and (**e**, **f**) valgus stress view of both knees. There is marked improvement in the varus and valgus stress views

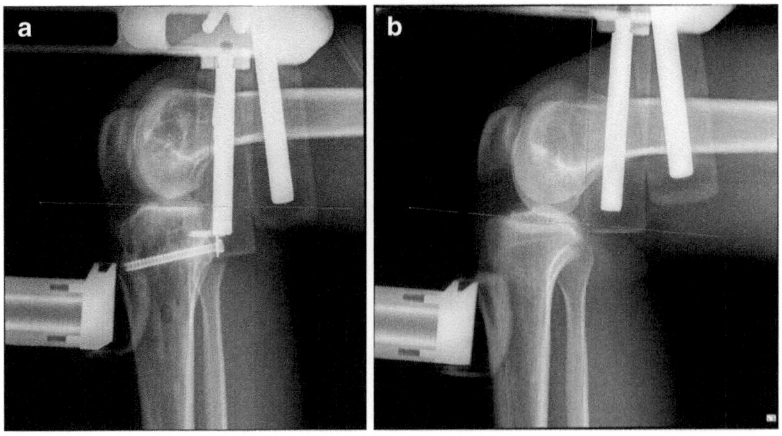

Fig. 12.16 19 months after PCL revision with PLCS, MCL reconstruction. (**a**, **b**) Push view; posterior sagging of the tibia was significantly improved compared to the preoperative view (Fig. 12.12). (**c**, **d**) Varus stress and (**e**, **f**) valgus stress views of both knees. There is marked improvement in the varus and valgus stress view. There is no instability in the varus stress view and pull view. However, the medial joint space of the right knee is slightly wider than that of the left knee

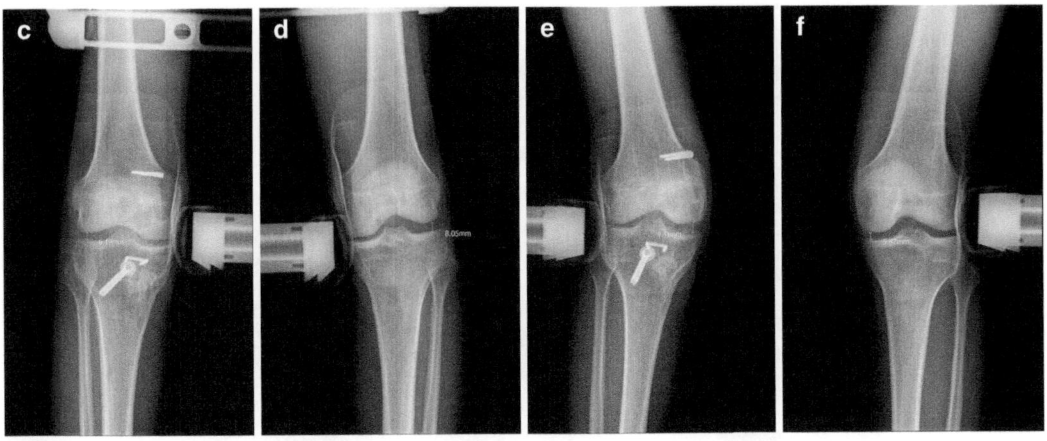

Fig. 12.16 (continued)

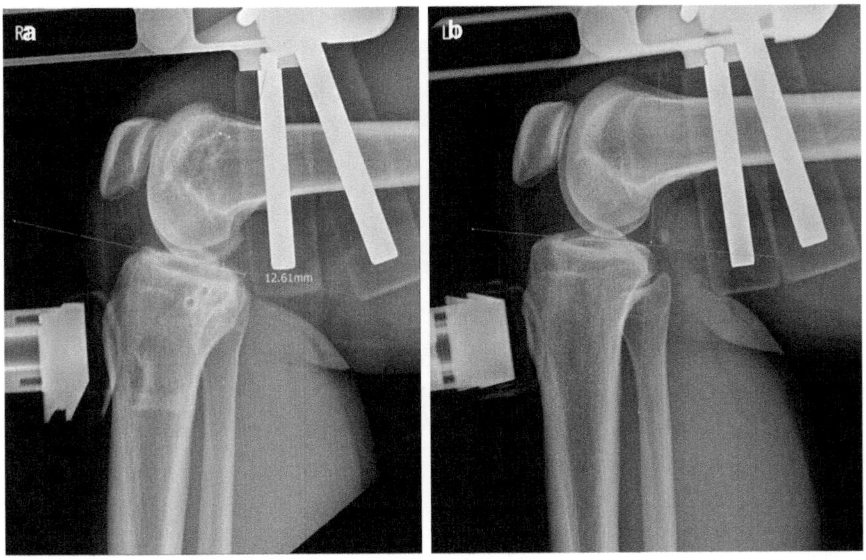

Fig. 12.17 (**a**, **b**) 12.6 mm side-to-side difference was checked compared to the unaffected side in the push stress test view

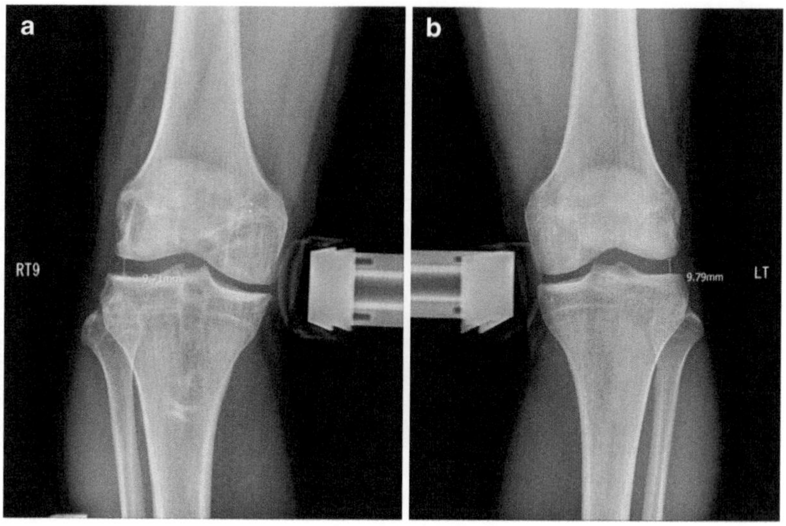

Fig. 12.18 (**a**, **b**) Varus stress view; no significant difference between both knees

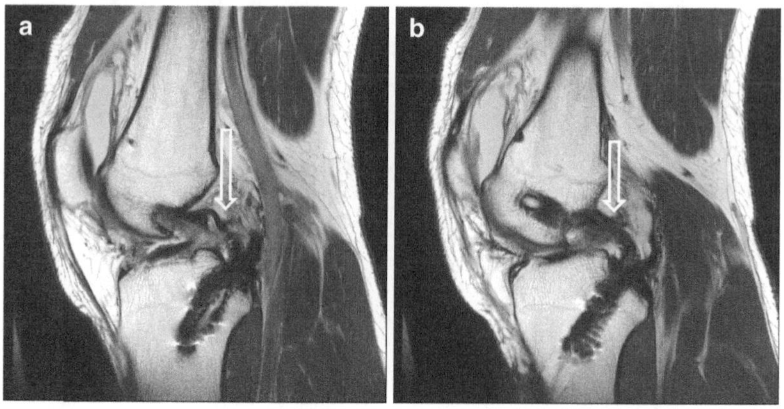

Fig. 12.19 (**a**, **b**) The placement of the tibial tunnel for the PCL was too anterior

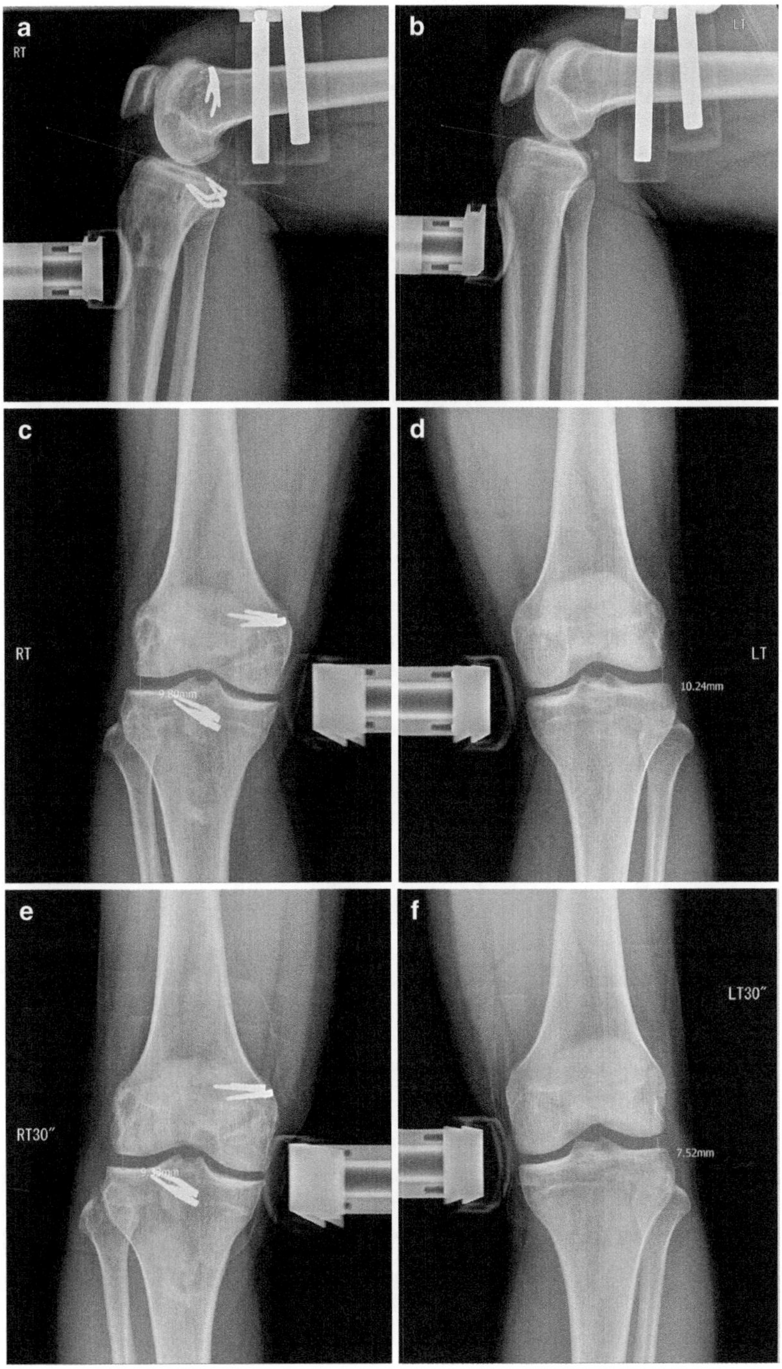

Fig. 12.20 16 months after PCL revision using the modified inlay technique. (**a**, **b**) Push view, improved posterior displacement of the tibia. (**c**, **d**) 0° varus stress view. (**e**, **f**) 30° flexion view, there is no instability in the varus stress views

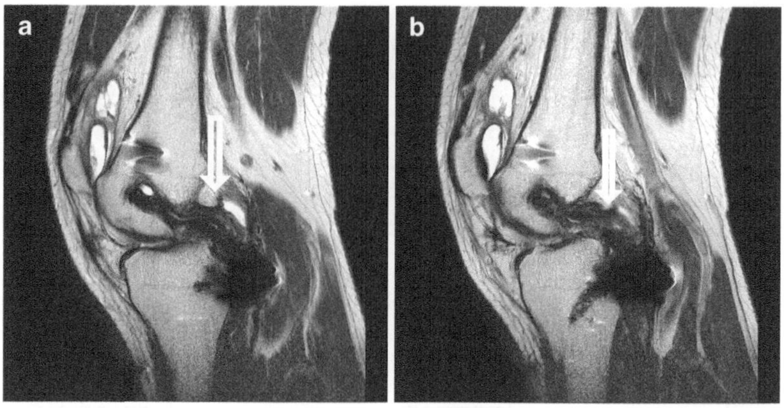

Fig. 12.21 (**a**, **b**) 16 months after PCL revision. Reconstructed PCL is well preserved on MRI

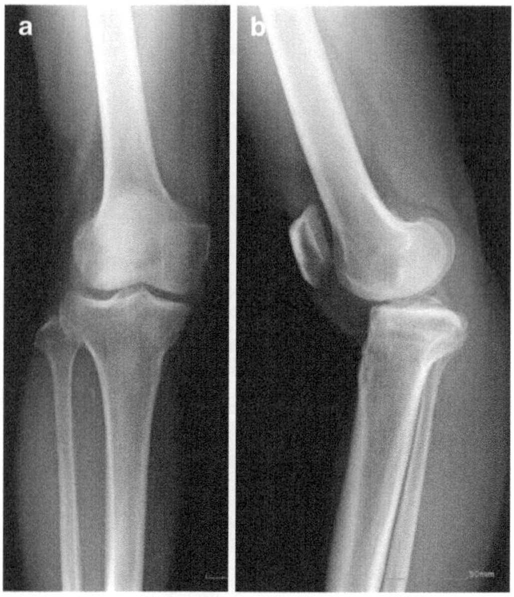

Fig. 12.22 (**a**, **b**) Genu recurvatum is seen on the plain radiograph. We can see that the posterior tibial slope of the patient is almost 0°

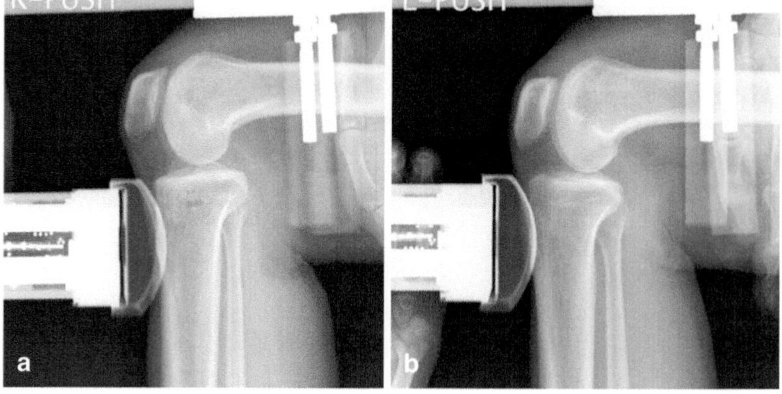

Fig. 12.23 (**a**, **b**) Grade 2 posterior instability was noted in the push view

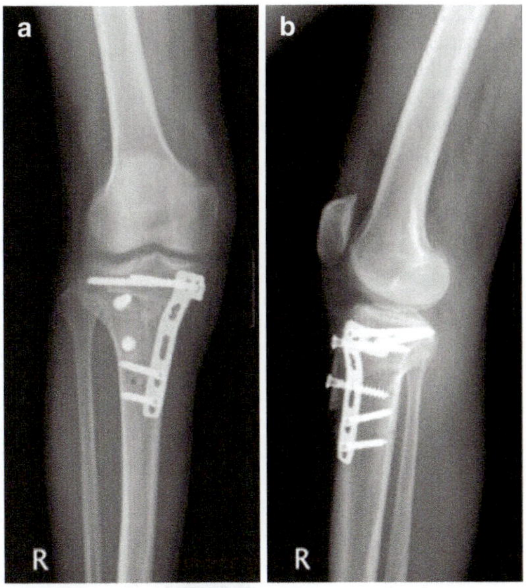

Fig. 12.24 (**a**, **b**) Two months after the osteotomy, these are postoperative radiographs.

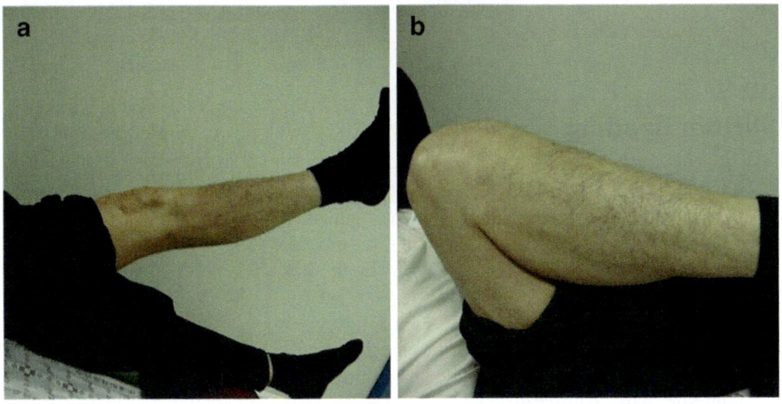

Fig. 12.25 (**a**, **b**) Two months after surgery, without PCL reconstruction, the genu recurvatum and posterior tibial sagging were completely resolved by tibial osteotomy alone (Video 11.1)

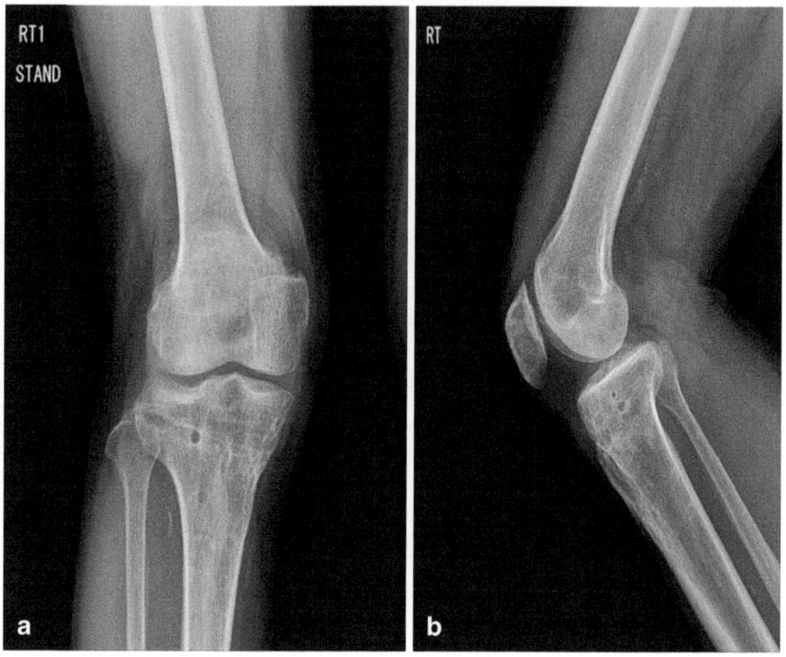

Fig. 12.26 (a, b) Six years after osteotomy. He is walking with a normal gait and no genu recurvatum

Further Reading

1. Jung YB, Jung HJ, Song KS, Kim JY, Lee HJ, Lee JS. Remnant posterior cruciate ligament-augmenting stent procedure for injuries in the acute or subacute stage. Arthroscopy. 2010;26(2):223–9. Epub 2009 Dec 21
2. Lee SH, Jung YB, Lee HJ, Jung HJ, Kim SH. Revision posterior cruciate ligament reconstruction using a modified tibial-inlay double-bundle technique. J Bone Joint Surg Am. 2012;94(6):516–22.
3. Gill GK, Gwathmey FW. Revision PCL reconstruction review/update. Curr Rev Musculoskelet Med. 2018;11(2):320–4.
4. Fanelli GC, Fanelli MG, Fanelli DG. Revision posterior cruciate ligament surgery. Sports Med Arthrosc Rev. 2017;25(1):30–5.
5. Winkler PW, Zsidai B, Wagala NN, Hughes JD, Horvath A, Senorski EH, Samuelsson K, Musahl V. Evolving evidence in the treatment of primary and recurrent posterior cruciate ligament injuries, part 2: surgical techniques, outcomes and rehabilitation. Knee Surg Sports Traumatol Arthrosc. 2021;29(3):682–93.
6. Winkler PW, Zsidai B, Wagala NN, Hughes JD, Horvath A, Senorski EH, Samuelsson K, Musahl V. Evolving evidence in the treatment of primary and recurrent posterior cruciate ligament injuries, part 1: anatomy, biomechanics and diagnostics. Knee Surg Sports Traumatol Arthrosc. 2021;29(3):672–81.
7. Johnson DH, Fanelli GC, Miller MD. PCL 2002: indications, double-bundle versus inlay technique and revision surgery. Arthroscopy. 2002;18(9 Suppl 2):40–52.
8. Lee SH, Jung YB, Rhee SM, Lee HJ, Jung HJ. Revision posterior cruciate ligament reconstruction with a modified tibial-inlay double-bundle technique. JBJS Essent Surg Tech. 2014;4(1):e1.

Part IV

Multiligament Injuries

13 ACL, PCL Injuries with PLRI or MCL Combined Injury

Abstract

In the acute stage of multi-ligament injuries, there should be a careful analysis of the neurovascular injury, and also as early as possible, as surgery will be better.

Early mobilization after the MLKI procedure results in less range of motion deficit. The order of fixation of the grafts id as follows: simultaneous tensioning of the ACL, PCL, and PLCS graft; cyclic loading about 10–15lbs tensioning; PCL first fixation at 90 flexion and then ACL graft fixation at 0–10 flexion of the knee; and, finally, PLCS fixation to the femoral tunnel at 70–90 flexion of the knee position. Usually I'd recommend 10lbs tension for the PLCS and check the lateral joint space in flexion and extension of the knee arthroscopically. Postoperative rehabilitation is almost same as PCL reconstruction with PLCS.

Keywords

Multi-ligament injury • ACL • PCL, PLRI, or MCL injury

In the acute stage of multi-ligament injury, we should carefully analyze the neurovascular injury, and also, as early as possible, surgery will be better. The best outcome in MLKI is achieved by operative treatment with acute or staged reconstruction.

An effective repair can only be performed within the first three weeks after the injury.

There is no difference between the repair and reconstruction of the medial collateral ligament and the posteromedial corner.

Reconstruction of the posterolateral corner has a lower rate of failure than repair.

Early mobilization after the MLKI procedure results in fewer deficits in the range of motion.

In this chapter, we'd like to deal with the chronic stage, especially ACL, PCL, with PLRI, or MCL injuries.

Treatment of posterolateral rotation instability with anterior and posterior cruciate ligament injuries. The surgical procedure for the anterior and posterior cruciate ligament and PLRI can be performed as described in the respective chapters, but the surgical sequence may vary, depending on the arthroscopic field of view (Fig. 13.10) in each case. However, in general, the ACL femoral tunnel, (accessary low anteromedial portal technique—in—out technique), PCL femoral tunnel (Fig. 13.10c), ACL femoral tunnel then PCL tibial tunnel (modified transseptal technique), ACL tibial tunnel, then PLCS through fibular head tunnel (modified Larson technique) - fibular head tunnel and femoral tunnel. The graft passing; PCL graft through AMP (anteromedial portal) to femoral tunnel and tibial tunnel respectively. Then ACL graft passing through tibial tunnel anterior to the femoral tunnel and then PLCS graft passing fibular head tunnel and then femoral

Y. B. Jung et al., *Treatment of the Cruciate Ligaments Injuries*,
https://doi.org/10.1007/978-981-95-9039-1_13

tunnel, lateral epicondyle area to the medial femoral side pulling. The order of fixation of the grafts, simultaneous tensioning of the ACL, PCL and PLCS graft, cyclic loading about 10–15lbs tensioning, PCL first fixation at 90 flexion and then ACL graft fixation at 0–10 flexion of the knee, finally PLCS fixation to the femoral tunnel at 70–90 flexion of the knee position usually I'd like recommend 10lbs tension for the PLCS and check the lateral joint space in flexion and extension of the knee arthroscopically. A long leg splint was applied in full knee extension to prevent posterior sagging of the knee for 2–3 weeks. A PCL brace was then applied with a spring to prevent posterior sagging of the proximal tibia. The QSE SLR exercise was taught to the patient preoperatively.

13.1 Cases of ACL, PCL Reconstruction Combined with PLCS

Case 1: ACL, PCL Reconstruction, MM Repair Combined with PLCS

A 40-year-old female patient with no history of knee problems presented to the outpatient clinic complaining of pain in his left knee. The pain started 2 months ago after slipping down while hiking. The Lachmann test (gr 2), posterior drawer test (gr 1), PLRI (gr 2), varus stress test, and pivot shift test were positive on physical examination (Figs. 13.1, 13.2, 13.3, 13.4, and 13.5).

Therefore, ACL and PLC reconstruction, MM repair, and PLCS were performed (Fig. 13.6).

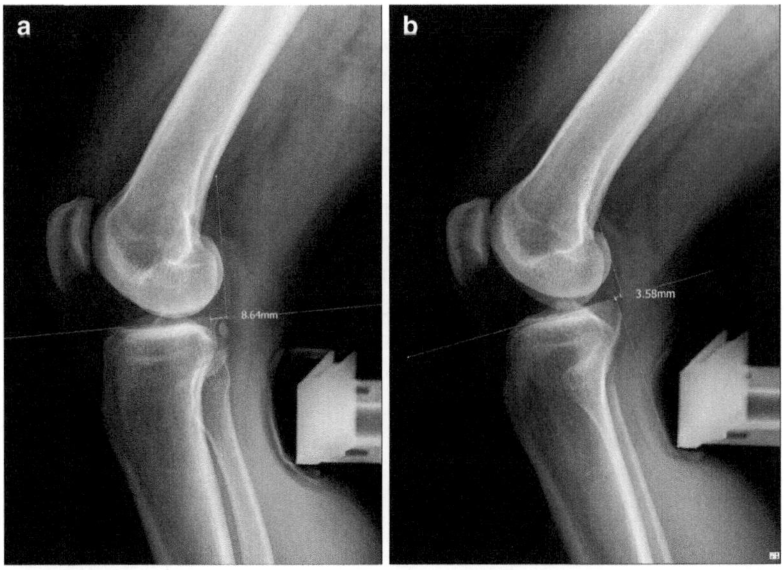

Fig. 13.1 (**a**, **b**) 5.1 mm side-to-side difference was checked compared to the unaffected side in the pull stress test imaging

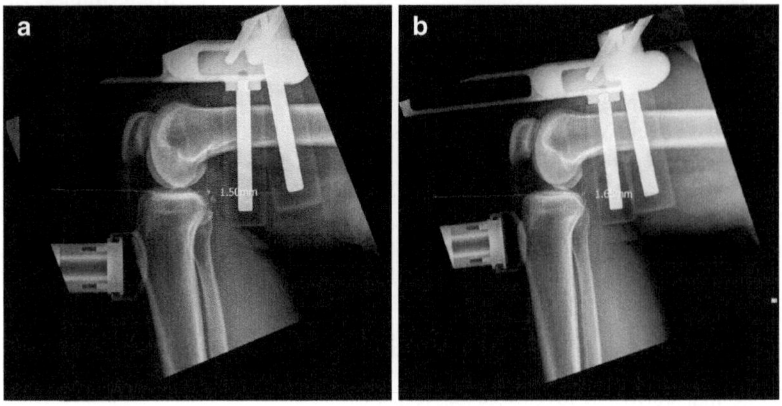

Fig. 13.2 (**a**, **b**) No significant difference was checked compared to the unaffected side in the push stress test imaging

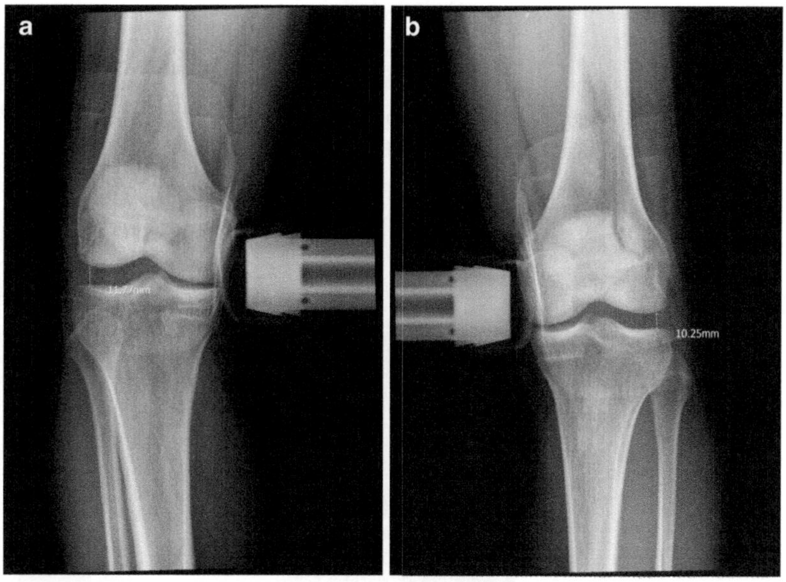

Fig. 13.3 (**a**, **b**) 30° flexion varus view; right knee lateral joint space is slightly wider than left knee

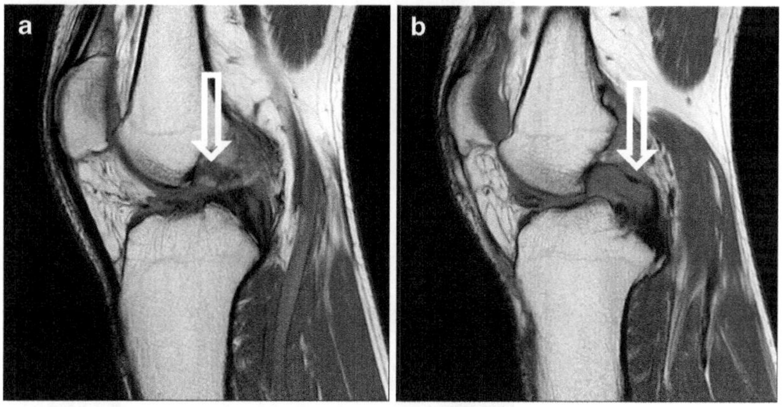

Fig. 13.4 (**a**, **b**) ACL complete rupture, PCL partial rupture can be seen

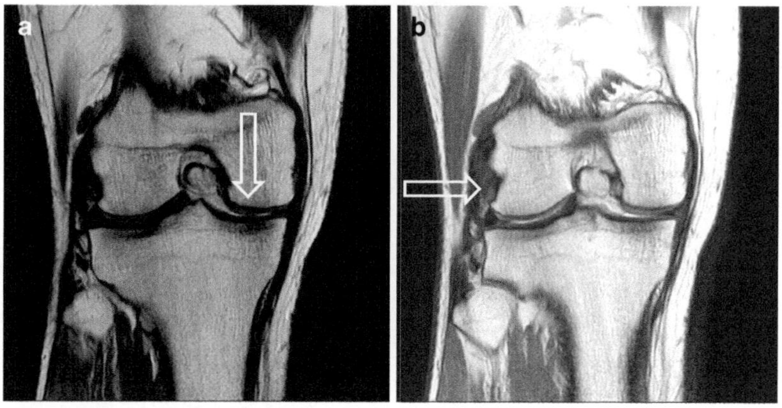

Fig. 13.5 (**a**, **b**) Medial meniscus complex tear, lateral collateral ligament injury can be seen

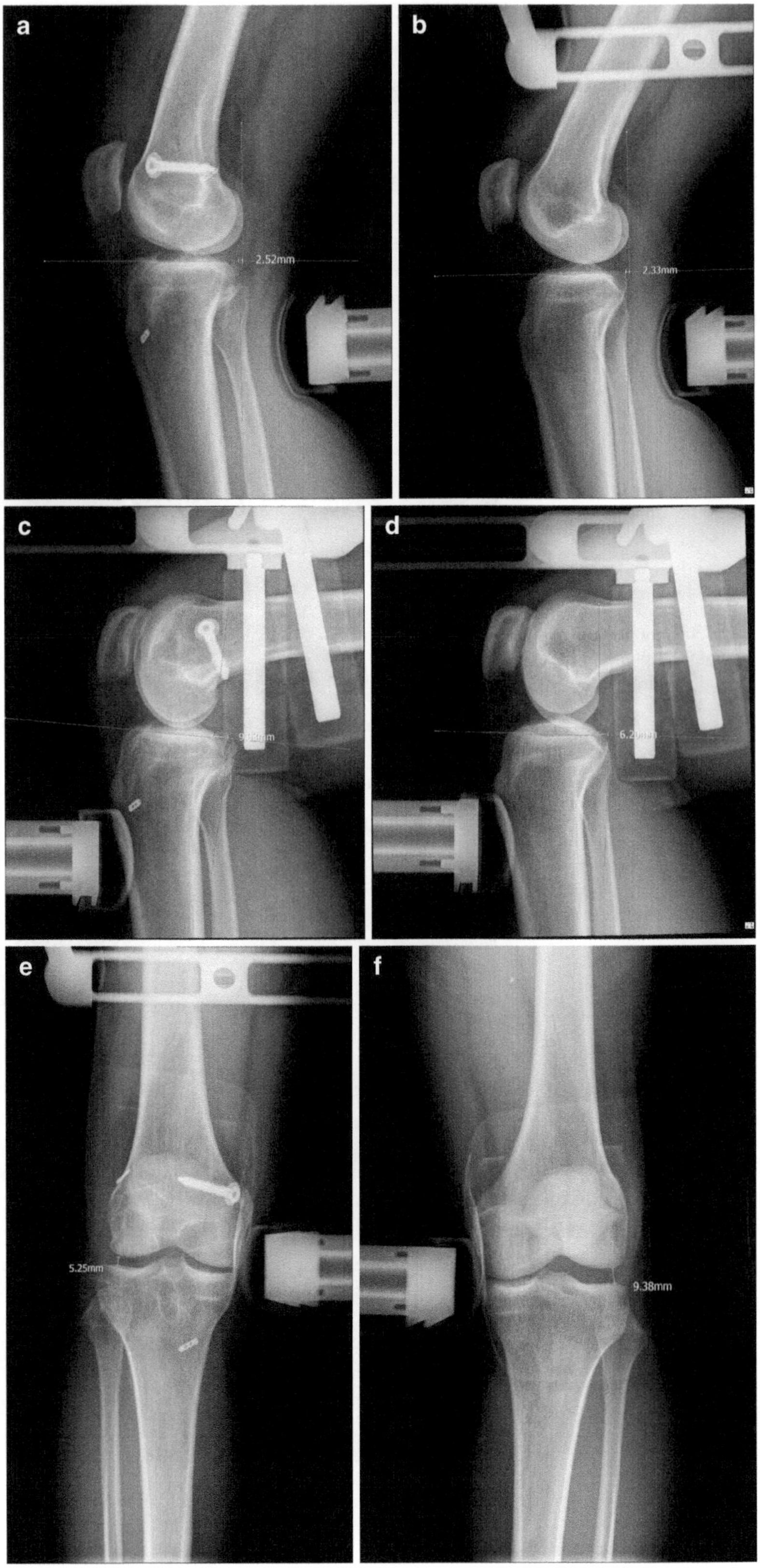

Fig. 13.6 (a–f) 8 months after ACL & PLC reconstruction, MM repair, and PLCS; There is no instability in the varus stress and pull, push views

Case 2: ACL, PCL Reconstruction, Combined with PLCS

A 41-year-old male patient with no history of knee problems presented to the outpatient clinic complaining of left knee pain. The pain started 5 months ago, right after a slip-down event. Lachmann test (gr 2), posterior drawer test (gr 3), varus stress test, and pivot shift test were positive on physical examination (Figs. 13.7, 13.8, 13.9, 13.10, 13.11, and 13.12).

The contralateral side (right knee) shows anterior instability. We recommended surgery, but the patient refused.

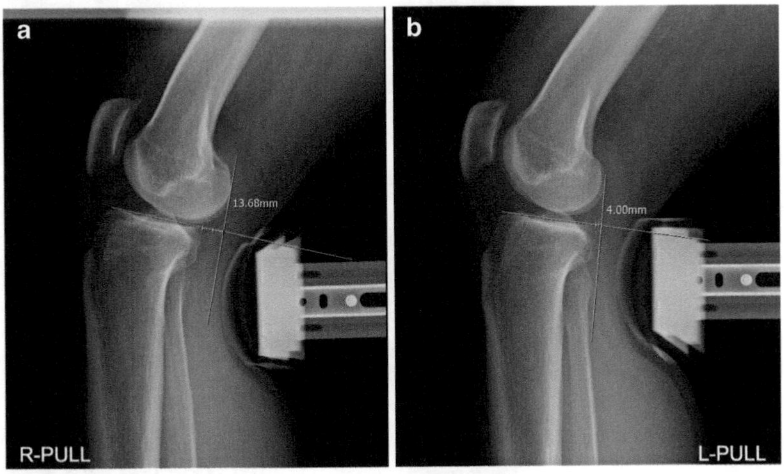

Fig. 13.7 (**a**, **b**) Unaffected side showed more side-to-side difference in the pull stress test

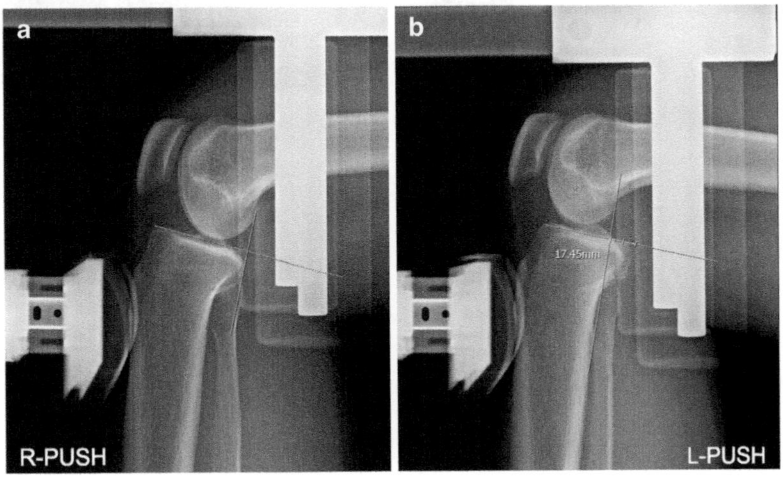

Fig. 13.8 (**a**, **b**) 17.4 mm side-to-side difference was checked compared to the unaffected side in the push stress test view

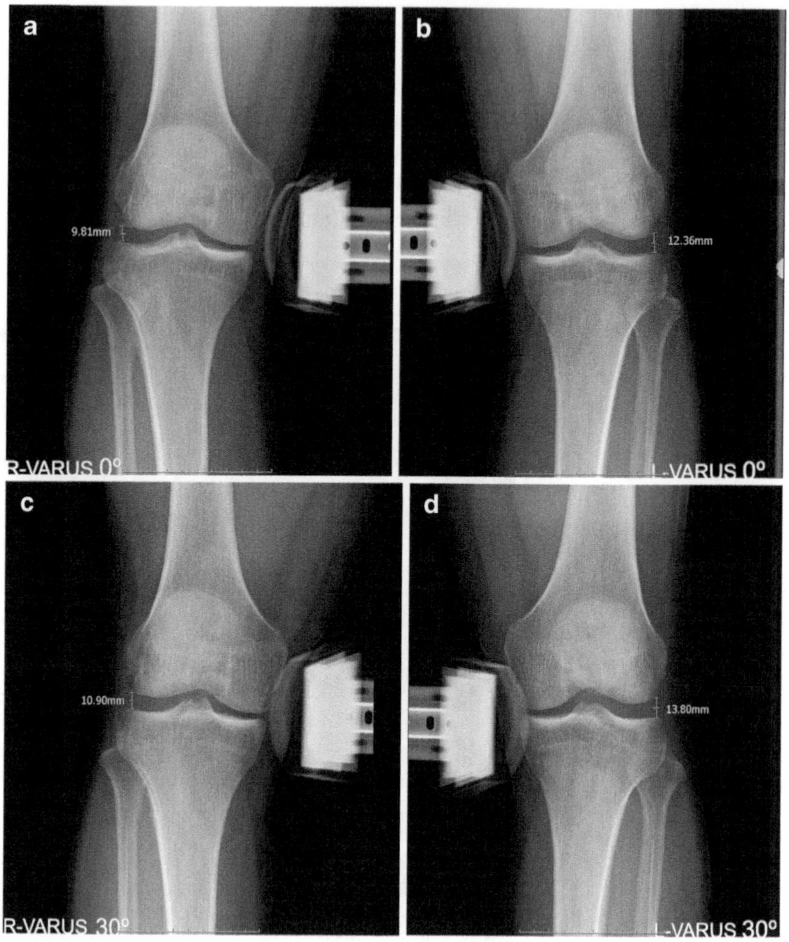

Fig. 13.9 (**a**, **b**) 0° varus stress view (**c**, **d**) 30° flexion varus stress view; lateral joint space of the left knee was wider than that of the right knee

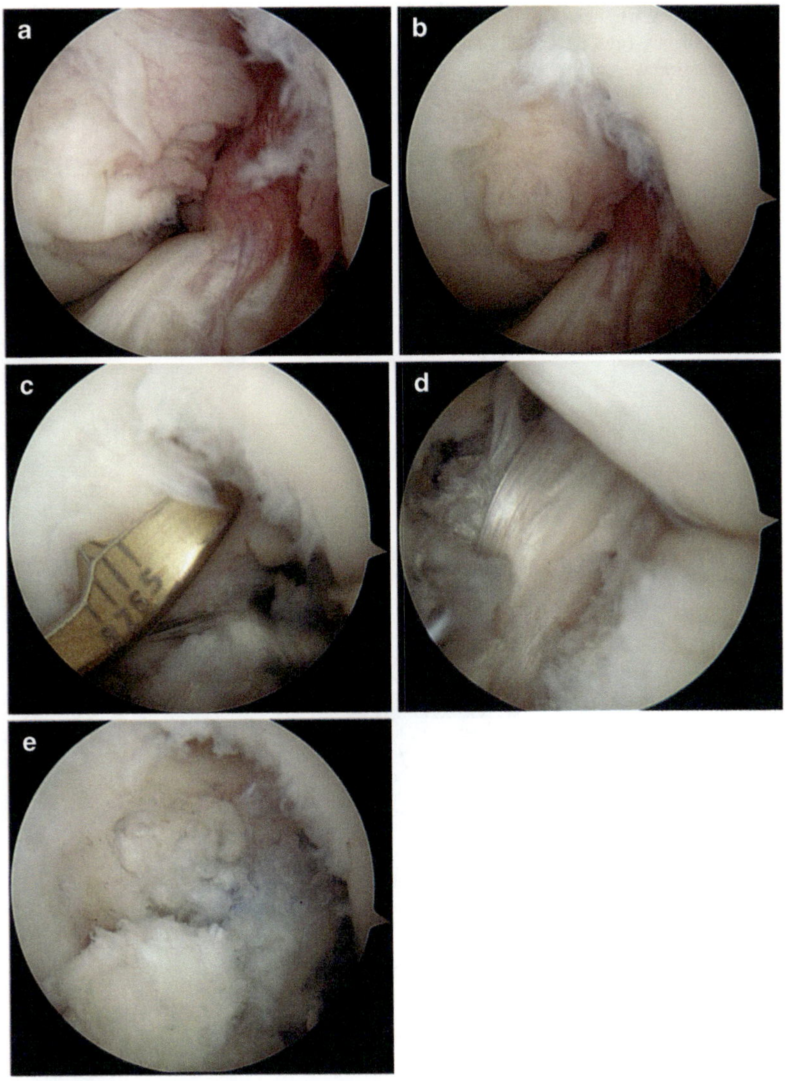

Fig. 13.10 (**a**, **b**) ACL insufficiency and laxity and PCL rupture were observed in the arthroscopic finding (**c**–**e**) ACL reconstruction with auto hamstring tendon and PCL reconstruction using Achilles tendon bone block were performed. Posterolateral corner reconstruction was also performed

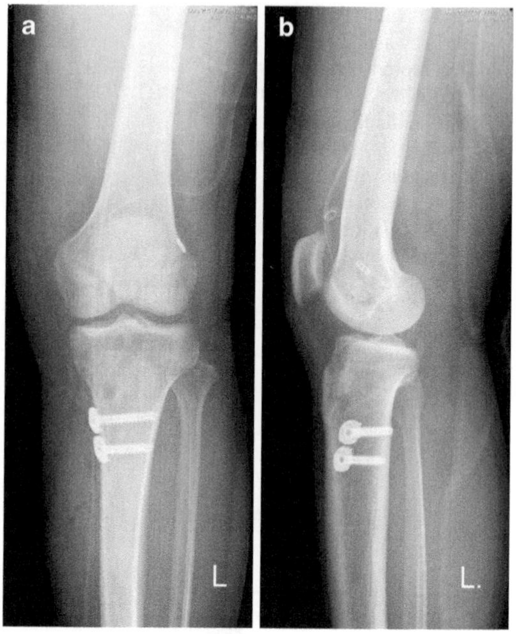

Fig. 13.11 (**a**, **b**) These are the postoperative X-rays. ACL, PCL, and PLC reconstruction were performed

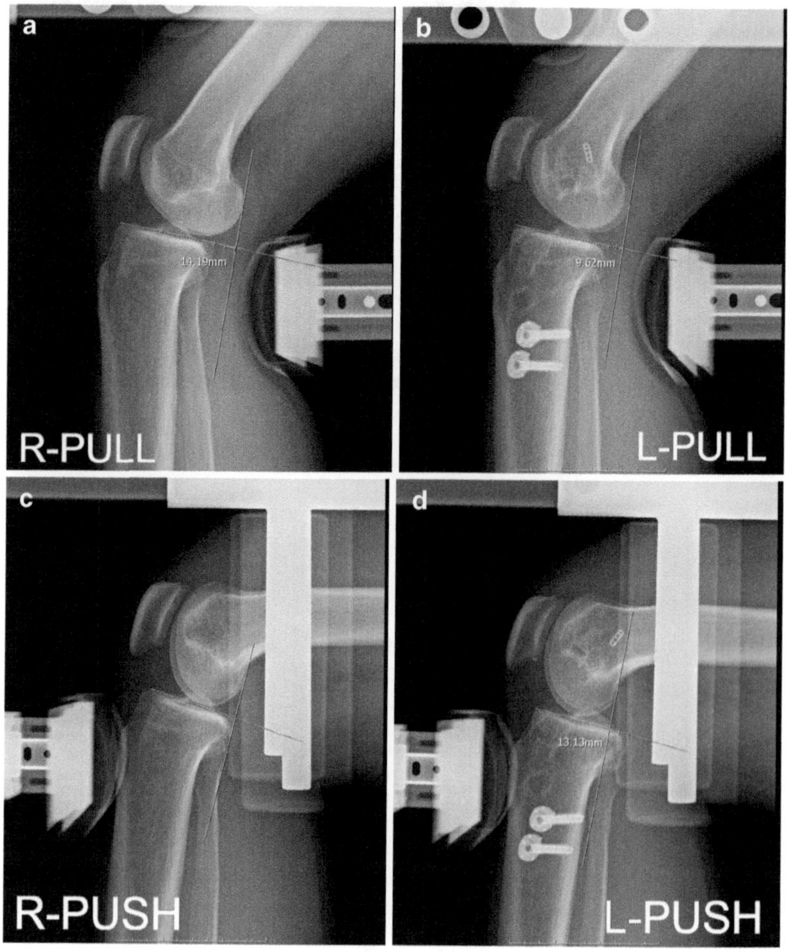

Fig. 13.12 Two years after surgery, (**a**, **b**) pull view (**c**, **d**) push stress view. Slight instability was noted

Further Reading

1. Ng JWG, Myint Y, Ali FM. Management of multiligament knee injuries. EFORT Open Rev. 2020;5(3):145–55.
2. Levy BA, Freychet B. Knee multiligament injury. Clin Sports Med. 2019;38(2):xv–xvi.
3. Neri T, Myat D, Beach A, Parker DA. Multiligament knee injury: injury patterns, outcomes, and gait analysis. Clin Sports Med. 2019;38(2):235–46.
4. Mook WR, Ligh CA, Moorman CT 3rd, Leversedge FJ. Nerve injury complicating multiligament knee injury: current concepts and treatment algorithm. J Am Acad Orthop Surg. 2013;21(6):343–54.
5. Perkins CA, Willimon SC. Multiligament knee injuries in young athletes. Clin Sports Med. 2022;41(4):611–25.
6. Patel NK, Lian J, Nickoli M, Vaswani R, Irrgang JJ, Lesniak BP, Musahl V. Risk factors associated with complications after operative treatment of multiligament knee injury. Orthop J Sports Med. 2021;9(3)
7. Braaten JA, Schreier FJ, Rodriguez AN, Monson J, LaPrade RF. Modern treatment principles for multiligament knee injuries. Arch Bone Jt Surg. 2022;10(11):937–50.